HAND REHABILITATION

A Quick Reference Guide and Review

HAND REHABILITATION
A Quick Reference Guide and Review

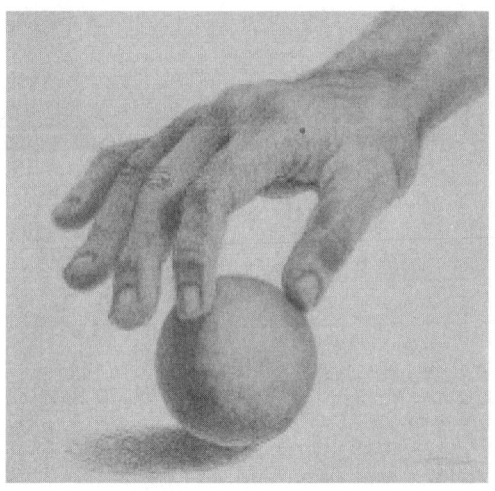

Nancy Falkenstein, OTR/L, CHT
Occupational Therapy Clinical Coordinator
Palms of Pasadena Hospital
St. Petersburg, Florida

Susan Weiss, OTR/L, CHT
Director of Hand Therapy
All Florida Orthopaedic Associates
St. Petersburg, Florida

with illustrations by Jan Cervone and Anita Smith
with 220 illustrations and photos

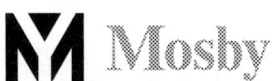

St. Louis   Baltimore   Boston   Carlsbad   Chicago   Minneapolis   New York   Philadelphia   Portland
London   Milan   Sydney   Tokyo   Toronto

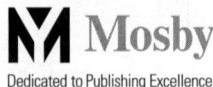

Copyright © 1999 by Mosby, Inc.

All rights reserved. No part of this publication may be reproduced, stored in a retrieval system, or transmitted, in any form or by any means, electronic, mechanical, photocopying, recording, or otherwise, without written permission of the publisher.

Permission to photocopy or reproduce solely for internal or personal use is permitted for libraries or other users registered with the Copyright Clearance Center, provided that the base fee of $4.00 per chapter plus $.10 per page is paid directly to the Copyright Clearance Center, 222 Rosewood Drive, Danvers, MA 01923. This consent does not extend to other kinds of copying, such as copying for general distribution, for advertising or promotional purposes, for creating new collected works, or for resale.

Mosby, Inc.
11830 Westline Industrial Drive
St. Louis, Missouri 63146

Library of Congress Cataloging-in-Publication Data

Falkenstein, Nancy.
    Hand rehabilitation : a quick reference guide and review / Nancy Falkenstein, Susan Weiss; with illustrations by Jan Cervone and Anita Smith.
      p.   cm.
    Includes bibliographical references and index.
    ISBN 0-323-00251-X
    1. Hand—Wounds and injuries—Patients—Rehabilitation—Examinations, questions, etc. 2. Hand—Wounds and injuries—Physical therapy. 3. Hand—Pathophysiology—Examinations, questions, etc. I. Weiss-Lessard, Susan. II. Title.
    [DNLM: 1. Hand Injuries—rehabilitation examination questions. 2. Hand—physiopathology examination questions. 3. Arm Injuries—rehabilitation examination questions. 4. Arthritis examination questions. WE 18.2 F192h 1999]
RD559.F34 1999
617.5′750446—dc21
DNLM/DLC   98-44802

99 00 01 / 9 8 7 6 5 4 3 2

DISCLAIMER

We are aware of the many techniques available to treat particular pathologies and realize this book may present debatable material. We have made every effort to verify the answers to the questions. References are provided to clarify controversial points. The material presents the technique, view, statement, or opinion of the authors and contributors, which is helpful and interesting to other practitioners. We have made every effort to ensure that the therapeutic modalities recommended are in accordance with accepted standards and the appendix material is current at the time of this publication. It is the practitioner's responsibility to evaluate the appropriateness of a particular opinion in clinical situations and to consider new developments.

One of the uses of this text is to help readers review for certification and/or exams related to the upper extremity. It does not, however, guarantee that you will pass any certification and/or exam, including the Hand Therapy Certification Exam or any other exam pertaining to or including the upper extremity. This book has not been endorsed by nor is affiliated with any organization that licenses or certifies in hand rehabilitation. The authors have not been assisted in the development or publication of this text by any licensing or certifying organization.

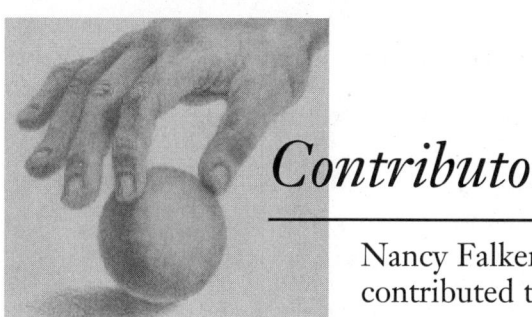

Contributors

Nancy Falkenstein and Susan Weiss developed and contributed to all chapters.

Patricia Anderson, OTR/L, BS
Coordinator, Harborside Hand/Burn Clinic
Tampa Regional Burn Center
Tampa General Healthcare
Tampa, Florida
Burns

Brett Bolhofner, MD
Chief, Orthopedic Surgery
Director, Orthopedic Trauma
Bay Front Medical Center
All Florida Orthopaedic Associates
Clinical Assistant Professor, University of South Florida
St. Petersburg, Florida
Fractures (Elbow and Forearm)

Dale Bramlet, MD
Chief, Orthopedic Surgery
St. Anthony's Medical Hospital
All Florida Orthopaedic Associates
St. Petersburg, Florida
Reconstructive Surgery (Arthritis), Fractures (Hand and Wrist)

Arlicia Brown
Medical Assistant
Drs. Smith, Nantais, Swiggett
St. Petersburg, Florida
OSHA

Phyllis J. Bruni, RN, BSN, CIC
Infection Control Manager
Palms of Pasadena Hospital
St. Petersburg, Florida
OSHA

Barbara A. Carmen, RN, BA, PhD
Research Consultant, Clearwater, Florida
Research and Statistics

Lisa Rementer Choe, OTR/L
Senior Staff Therapist
All Florida Orthopaedic Associates
St. Petersburg, Florida
Modalities (thermal)

Kate Cooper, PT
Formerly: Physical Therapy Coordinator
Palms of Pasadena Hospital
St. Petersburg, Florida
Modalities (electrical)

Gail P. Counts, PT
Senior Physical Therapist
Good Samaritan Hospital
Dayton, Ohio
Shoulder, Joint Mobilization

Lawrence Gnage, MD
Sports Medicine and Arthroscopy
All Florida Orthopaedic Associates
St. Petersburg, Florida
Shoulder

Daniel Greenwald, MD
Associate Professor, Biomedical Engineering
University of South Florida
Tampa, Florida
Biomechanics and Tendon Transfers

Barbara G. Henry, RPT, CHT
Senior Staff Therapist
Department of Physical Therapy
All Florida Orthopaedic Associates
St. Petersburg, Florida
Shoulder

Jeri Lynn Houck, PT, CHT
Independent Contractor
Physical Therapy and Hand Therapy
Palm Harbor, Florida
Shoulder, Joint Mobilization

Jennifer J. Jones King, OTR/L, CHT
Clinical Coordinator of Hand Therapy
Department of Occupational Therapy and Hand Therapy
Memorial Hospital of Tampa
Center for Comprehensive Rehabilitation
Tampa, Florida
Biomechanics and Tendon Transfers, Splinting

Contributed topics are italicized.

Jodi Jones Knauf, OTR, PAC
Occupational Therapist, Physician Assistant
All Florida Orthopaedic Associates
St. Petersburg, Florida
Drug Appendix

Amy Mills, OTR/L
Occupational Therapist
All Florida Orthopaedic Associates
St. Petersburg, Florida
Appendices on Vitamins, Websites, Equipment

John J. O'Brien Jr., MD
Private Practice
Plastic Reconstructive and Hand Surgery
St. Petersburg, Florida
Flaps and Grafts

Scott Raub, DO
Physical Medicine and Rehabilitation
All Florida Orthopaedic Associates
St. Petersburg, Florida
Reflex Sympathetic Dystrophy

John M. Rayhack, MD
Director
The Wrist and Hand Center
Tampa, Florida
Wrist

Lori Long Root, OTR, CHT
HealthSouth
Tampa, Florida
*Dupuytren's Disease and Tumors,
Evaluation, Wounds/Infection and Cumulative Trauma*

Douglas R. Shier, PhD
Professor, Department of Mathematical Sciences
Clemson University
Clemson, South Carolina
Research and Statistics

Sharon Root Spiegel, MS, OTR/L, CHT
Consultant, Hand Therapist
Cincinnati, Ohio
Prosthetics and Amputations

To my devoted children, David and Danielle, who have given me unconditional love and sacrificed their "mommy." To my loving mom, Joan Powers, for her guidance, strength, and devotion. To my dad, Christian G. Falkenstein, in loving memory. To my siblings, Judy, Gail, and Chris for being there for me. To my wonderful Aunt Trish and Uncle Ron Chiurazzi, for their wisdom and guidance.

Nancy

To Mom and Dad for inspiring me to achieve my goals and providing me with endless advice. To Jason for being a wonderful and supportive brother. To Aunt Joan and Uncle Doug for being excellent role models.

Susan

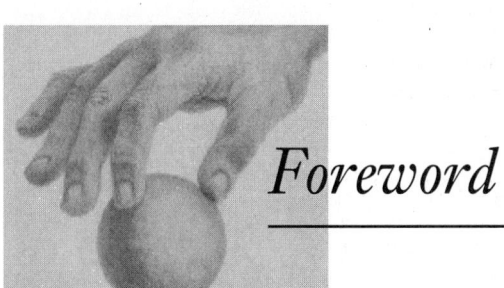

Foreword

No doubt Socrates is smiling. In *Hand Rehabilitation: A Quick Reference Guide and Review*, Nancy Falkenstein and Susan Weiss use a mostly Socratic method—question and answer format—to teach a wide range of topics on hand therapy. In so doing, the authors demonstrate their wealth of knowledge on hand therapy and their skills in *teaching* hand therapy. They also reveal their creativity and sense of fun.

In this long-awaited book, health professionals and students interested in hand therapy will finally have the opportunity to test and enhance their knowledge with a series of structured questions and comprehensive answers. While other disciplines have long enjoyed this format, hand rehabilitation has been without—until now. However, Falkenstein and Weiss go well beyond the basics of question and answer. Each answer includes a well-developed rationale with references in order to bring the reader to a higher level in his or her grasp of the information. With this approach, the authors bring the reader face to face with hand therapy's core literature.

Hand Rehabilitation: A Quick Reference Guide and Review offers a great deal of information and enjoyment for students and health professionals of all levels of expertise. Falkenstein and Weiss have walked the difficult path of incorporating the breadth of hand therapy wisdom—from the basic core concepts (that always seem to need review) to the most esoteric topics. I was thrilled to finally have a name for a sign that I commonly find in my patients but have never seen referenced—despite many years of reading. Who among us is familiar with Linburg's sign? This is the anatomic interconnection between the flexor pollicis longus and the index finger flexor digitorum profundus that causes the index distal interphalangeal joint to flex when the thumb interphalangeal joint flexes and *vice versa*. This is only one example of the answers to career-long questions that I found in this text.

The authors have carefully sifted through the huge range of hand therapy topics and selected strategic chapters, including: evaluation; flaps, grafts, and thermal conditions; wounds and infection; Dupuytren's disease and tumors; fractures; arthritis; reflex sympathetic dystrophy; tendons; splinting; congenital anomalies, amputations, prosthetics; modalities; cumulative trauma; joint mobilization and other treatment techniques; and several chapters on anatomy. This book covers all commonly seen pathologies, as well as some rarer hand pathologies. It also includes topics usually omitted from texts on hand therapy, notably: research and statistics, drugs commonly encountered in hand therapy, and a resource list of vendors offering hand therapy products. I commend Falkenstein and Weiss for including a nutritional quick reference—a topic so critical to excellent outcomes and so often ignored. In keeping with the up-to-date nature of this text, the authors have also included a list of hand therapy-related Internet websites. With such a wellspring of information, no therapist should ever want for references or resources.

I predict *Hand Rehabilitation: A Quick Reference Guide and Review* will be the number one publication sought by therapists studying for the Hand Certification exam. All health professionals and students interested in hand rehabilitation will find this to be a one-of-a-kind, quick reference text that provides a comprehensive overview. It is well thought out, creatively designed, and packed with the resources we all need as hand rehabilitation professionals. I cannot thank the authors enough for providing the hand therapy community with this book.

Karen Schultz-Johnson, MS, OTR, FAOTA, CHT
Director, Rocky Mountain Hand Therapy
President, U E TECH

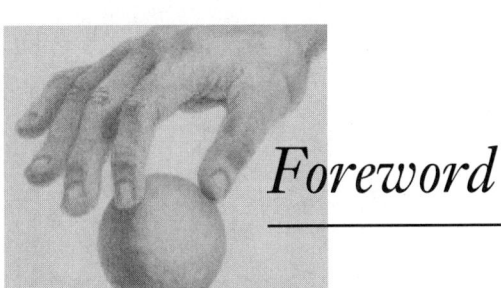

Foreword

Those in the upper extremity rehabilitation world know that it takes a Herculean effort to understand and keep up with massive amounts of information. We are now inundated with books, journals, and web pages. Continuing education and society meetings fill your calendar. So why would I agree to support yet another book on the hand and upper extremity? The reason is simple. This book amplifies and defines the areas of the upper extremity you need to bone up on and reviews the areas you are competent in. This aptitude assessment is easily evaluated with this book. As well, this book is another nice clinical resource that uses a creative and unique format (thank you Nancy Falkenstein and Susan Weiss) to present hand and upper extremity information.

At first glance this is a book of test questions and answers on the upper extremity. Although this conjures up images of hours spent reading preparatory books for standardized tests such as the SAT or GRE, **there is much more to this book.** "Clinical gems" permeate each chapter and provide easy-to-remember pearls of wisdom regarding various anatomic regions of the upper extremity, specific pathologic states, splinting, modalities, occupational considerations, and research. Answers to the questions are clearly and concisely stated and supplemented with informative illustrations. Quick referencing is made easy through a detailed index at the front of the book. The slide rule helps suppress the desire to check the correct answer before formulating it yourself.

Obviously, the structure of this book is designed to aid readers preparing for exams on the upper extremity. There is no other book on the upper extremity available that meets this need, and it serves that purpose extremely well. I hope, however, that readers use it for more than just preparing for "the test." The format of this book lends itself to self-assessment, which all too often stops once we leave the confines of professional schooling. The exercise of testing yourself is akin to looking at your professional image in the mirror. Is there substance to what you see or is it simply superficial and without state-of-the-art content? This book is the tool for such an assessment. Certainly when areas of weakness are identified, definitive books and specialized journals are essential for in-depth discussion.

I'll never forget how failing a test in school served as a well-defined signal that I had areas of study that needed significant attention. This type of critique should not be limited to your professional education. I encourage all upper extremity rehabilitation professionals to take advantage of this opportunity to assess your level of competence and better define your areas of need. After doing this, read, attend meetings, "surf the net," question mentors and colleagues, and encourage questions from students. Then combine these academic experiences with the art of treating patients. Good luck and fear not the "test" as it is the test that crystallizes and better defines opportunities for growth.

Paul LaStayo, MPT, CHT
**Northern Arizona University, Department of Biology and
DeRosa Physical Therapy, P.C.
Flagstaff, Arizona**

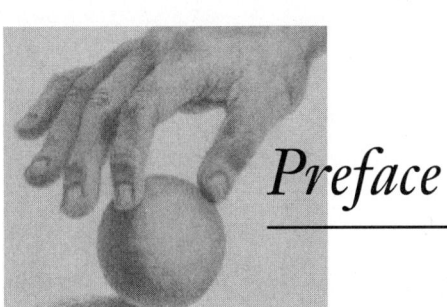

Preface

The art and science of asking questions is the source of all knowledge.
--Adolf Berle

The question and answer format of *Hand Rehabilitation: A Quick Reference Guide and Review* provides readers with the unique opportunity to answer questions and the inspiration to ask more. We have written this book to challenge readers to learn and develop a better understanding of the exciting art of hand rehabilitation. We hope that this book will become a premiere resource for many individuals in the health sciences, including hand specialists, certified hand therapists, occupational and physical therapists and students, occupational therapy and physical therapist assistants in hand rehabilitation settings, medical and nursing students, physicians, physician assistants, operating room technicians, and orthopedic technicians. This book can be used in a classroom setting or by practitioners who work with or would like to work with patients who have hand or upper extremity disorders. In addition, of course, it is an excellent resource and study guide for professionals preparing for specialty examinations such as the Certified Hand Therapy exam, the Board Certified Hand Surgery exam, and the Certified Orthopaedic Specialty exam. Students preparing for general registration exams will also greatly benefit from the self-study method presented.

This book provides a comprehensive overview of hand rehabilitation through a detailed question and answer format that consists of multiple choice, true and false, matching, and fill-in-the-blank questions. Following the questions and answer choices, we have provided detailed explanations of the correct answer. The references, including page numbers, are cited with each question to provide the reader with a simple avenue for further study on a particular subject. In addition, many illustrations have been included to aid in the ease of learning and understanding the topics presented. This book is designed with a thorough Quick Reference Guide, found at the beginning of the book, to assist the reader in quickly finding information on any topic. A wealth of special features are provided in this book, including clinical gems, case studies, advanced question icons, bulleted lists of topics covered in each chapter, a slide rule to aid in self testing, a list of drugs commonly encountered in hand rehabilitation, nutrition resources, vendors, website resources, and practice questions.

There are several different ways to use this text: (1) Readers can review questions and answer explanations as a method of learning the material. (2) The book can be used as a quick reference to access information on a particular topic or clinical problem. (3) Readers can perform self assessments using the slide rule method, covering up the answer portion with the slide rule provided in the back of the book. (This is part of the back cover and perforated for easy removal.) To use the text in this way, readers should place the slide rule at the top of a page and slowly slide it down the page until they come to the marbled line below the answer choices. This line indicates the end of the choices and marks the beginning of the correct answer explanation. Readers can take their time to come up with the correct answer and then move the slide rule down to reveal the answer. Readers may want to write their answers on a separate sheet of paper so they can test themselves more than once. (4) Of course, any combination of these uses is possible.

Each chapter begins with a bulleted list of topics that will be discussed. Chapters are generally organized in a building block fashion—beginning with anatomy and progressing to clinical application. We selected a chapter sequence that we feel provides an understandable progression for the reader. Chapter 1, Anatomy Extravaganza, is a collection of fundamental information and obscure anatomy facts and concepts. We have not gone into great detail in this chapter as we reserved specific, detailed anatomic knowledge for designated chapters. Chapter 2, Intrinsic Mechanism, has been included as its own chapter because of the complexity of the intrinsic system. Chapter 3, Evaluation, is an overview of common hand and upper extremity evaluation methods. Chapter 4, Neuroanatomy and Sensory Re-education, is an excellent synopsis of the nervous system in relation to hand and upper extremity rehabilitation.

Chapter 5, Wrist, and Chapter 6, Shoulder, include anatomy, diagnostic testing, surgical intervention, and rehabilitation. We decided not to isolate the elbow and digits in separate chapters and instead dispersed this information throughout several chapters. Chapter 7, Flaps/Grafts/Thermal Conditions, is a thorough review of surgical and therapeutic techniques for these topics. Chapter 8, Wounds/Infection, is a comprehensive outlook on basic wound and infection management. Chapters 9 through 13 help the readers evaluate and expand their knowledge of specific pathologies, including Dupuytren's disease, tumors, fractures, arthritis, reflex sympathetic dystrophy, and tendon disorders.

Chapter 14, Biomechanics and Tendon Transfers, and Chapter 15, Splinting, help readers improve their clinical approach to restoring function and motion in hand and upper extremity patients. Chapter 16, Congenital Anomalies/ Amputations/ Prosthetics, is designed for the reader to obtain a fundamental understanding of these complex topics. Chapter 17, Modalities, Chapter 18, Cumulative Trauma, and Chapter 19, Joint Mobilization/Other Treatment Techniques enhance the reader's knowledge of treatment techniques.

Chapter 20, Occupational Safety and Health Administration (OSHA), covers issues of state and federal inspections and worker safety. Guidelines vary from state to state. Consumer and provider concerns relating to blood-borne pathogens are an issue in our society and this chapter identifies state and federal laws addressing protection in the workplace.

Chapter 21, Research and Statistics, aids readers in understanding commonly used terms and concepts. Research is vital to the survival of hand rehabilitation. We hope readers will become less intimidated with research and will incorporate it into their clinical practices.

There are five appendices at the end of the book to use as a quick reference on various subjects. Appendix 1, Drugs Commonly Encountered in Hand Therapy, introduces the reader to some of the most commonly prescribed drugs used in hand rehabilitation. Appendix 2, Nutrition, is a reference for healthcare professionals to use when discussing optimal nutrition with their patients. Appendix 3, Resource List of Vendors, is a superior resource for therapists when ordering durable medical equipment. It is an alphabetical list with specific categories provided such as splinting, exercise equipment, wound care, and ergonomic equipment. Appendix 4, Internet Websites, is a list of sites, descriptions, and addresses for healthcare professionals. Appendix 5, Practice Questions, includes 100 questions that the reader can use to practice test-taking skills and as a self-review of information throughout the book. Explanations to the correct answers are discussed throughout the text. This Appendix is perforated and can be removed from the book and used repeatedly.

We have included more than 100 clinical gems compiled by therapists, physicians, and educators. Clinical gems range from splinting tips to mnemonics for remembering hand surgery and rehabilitation facts. The clinical gems provide invaluable clinical information.

Advanced questions are denoted with an icon placed after the explanation. Answering advanced questions correctly shoud be rewarding for readers because we feel that these will be the most difficult to anwer. If these questions are answered incorrectly, readers will have an indication of difficult or complicated topic areas that require further self-study. The advanced questions are randomly dispersed throughout chapters. Some questions overlap or are presented in various formats to reinforce difficult concepts. Case studies have been used throughout the book to show the reader how content applies to clinical practice.

This book has been developed through years of experience, preparation for specialty certification, and the desire to learn the art of hand rehabilitation. We have devoted countless hours to preparing and writing this book. Our goal is to provide a quick reference resource that will fill a void in hand rehabilitation literature. We developed all of the chapters with the assistance of our contributors who have diverse professional backgrounds. We express our deep appreciation to the contributors for sharing their knowledge.

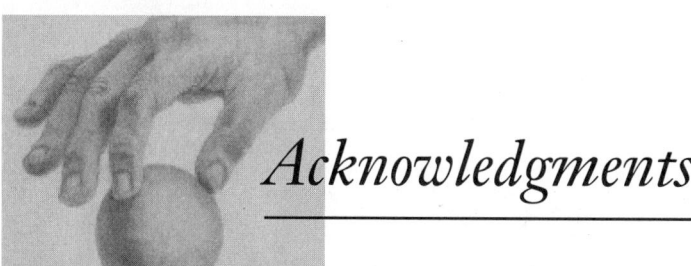

Acknowledgments

We appreciate everyone who made contributions to this book, especially the following:

- Allyson Burnett for keeping us in line and typing the manuscript over and over again.

- Lori Long Root for helping with the groundwork and envisioning the book's conception. Our warm thanks to Lori for offering her priceless wisdom.

- Amy Mills for her persistence in pursuing all the information needed for her contribution.

- A. Lee Dellon, MD for taking the time to review the Neuroanatomy and Sensory Re-education chapter. We appreciate his valuable input.

- Anita Smith, COTA and Jan Cervone, PTA for their beautiful talents in designing the artwork in this book.

- Our gratitude to Jonathan Rogers for his creative cover illustrations that depict function and therapeutic touch.

- Sincere appreciation to all of the contributors who helped make this book possible.

- Thank you to Beth Reigart, MPH, OTR/L, CHT and Sally E. Poole, MA, OTR, CHT for carefully reading and reviewing the entire manuscript.

- Thank you to Amy Christopher and Martha Sasser at Mosby for their guidance, time, and direction. We are indebted to them.

- Jim Fielding for allowing this book to happen.

- Laura Chamberlain and Sean O'Neal for their support on this project.

- Dr. Jorge Rodriquez for his wisdom and the use of his books.

- Dr. Thomas Greene for his input.

- The Founders of the Hand Society for inspiring us.

- Thank you to the following people for reviewing and commenting on various chapters:
  - Gina Angelastro
  - Nancy Buckley, OTR/L, CHT
  - Jennifer Coutre
  - Roxanne Crespo-Bottom, OTR/L, CHT
  - Dr. A. Lee Dellon
  - Marc Droste, PT

- Ed Durfer, PT
- Amy Eriksson, OTR/L
- Lisa Ferguson, PT
- Debi Harriott, PTA
- Barbara Henry, PT, CHT
- Jeri-Lynn Houck, PT, CHT
- Joy Langworthy
- Lori Long-Root, OTR/L, CHT
- Cindy Modesitt
- Amy Parker, PT
- Dr. Scott Raub
- Lisa Rementer-Choe, OTR/L
- Dominiek Schelfaut Senior, PT
- Doug Shier, PhD
- Drexey Smith, PT
- Dan Teaney, ATC
- Rosemary Thompson, PTA
- Matt Webb, PT

Nancy specially recognizes:

- Debbie Murray for her unconditional support and friendship.
- Bess Powers, my Gram, for listening.
- Nancy Brome and Nan MacDonald for their infinite love.
- Glenn Hunt for her inspiration.
- Gloria Vinciguerra for her support.
- Madlyn Weir for her prayers.
- My co-author Susan Weiss for her dedication, knowledge, connections, and perseverance. Her drive, commitment, and friendship have made this book possible.
- My special buddy Nancy Brome for the computer and her friendship.

Susan expressly thanks:

- Dr. Dale Bramlet for his inspiration and for being my mentor.
- Ali Goldenfarb and Angie Clark for their friendship and support.
- Naomi Zimmerman for listening.
- Rachel, Bob, Maureen, and Ernie for always allowing me to miss family events.
- Tigger (my dog) for staying up late and keeping us company while writing the book.
- My co-author Nancy Falkenstein for everything. Now I know it can be done: maintaining a friendship and writing a book simultaneously. My gratitude is limitless. Thanks!

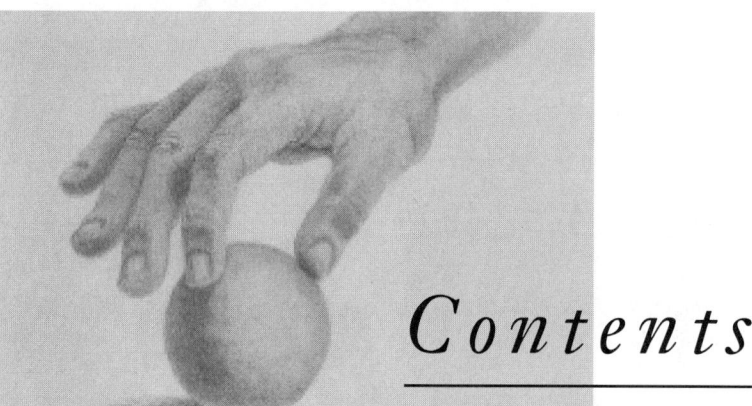

Contents

1 Anatomy Extravaganza *1*

2 Intrinsic Mechanism *15*

3 Evaluation *25*

4 Neuroanatomy and Sensory Re-education *35*

5 Wrist *53*

6 Shoulder *69*

7 Flaps/Grafts/Thermal Conditions *83*

8 Wounds/Infection *97*

9 Dupuytren's Disease and Tumors *107*

10 Fractures *113*

11 Arthritis *131*

12 Reflex Sympathetic Dystrophy *143*

13 Tendons *153*

14 Biomechanics and Tendon Transfers *167*

15 Splinting *177*

16 Congenital Anomalies/Amputations/Prosthetics *193*

17 Modalities *205*

18 Cumulative Trauma *219*

19 Joint Mobilization/Other Treatment Techniques *233*

20 Occupational Safety and Health Administration (OSHA) *241*

21 Research and Statistics *245*

Appendix 1 Drugs Commonly Encountered in Hand Therapy *251*

Appendix 2 Nutrition *259*

Appendix 3 Resource List of Vendors *263*

Appendix 4 Internet Websites *271*

Appendix 5 Practice Questions *275*

Quick Reference Guide

A

A-β fibers, 35
   constant-touch pressure, 36
A-α motor fibers, 37
Abduction wedge, thoracic outlet syndrome and, 51
Abductor pollicis brevis, 4, 41
   description of, 4
   innervation of, 6
   interphalangeal joint of thumb after extensor pollicis longus rupture, 157-158
   median nerve and, 40
Abductor pollicis longus, 2, 41
   de Quervain's disease and, 220
   posterior interosseous nerve and, 42
Acetaminophen, osteoarthritis management, 134
ACL: *see* Collateral ligaments, accessory
Acromioclavicular injury, 76
   shoulder limitations after, 76-77
   types of, 76
Acromion
   coracoacromial arch and, 71
   shape of, 72-73
Acromioplasty, supraspinatus tendon tear and acromiohumeral impingement, 77
Acrosyndactyly, 193
Activities of daily living

Activities of daily living—cont'd
   adaptive products for, resource list of vendors, 265-268
   Jebsen hand function test, 28
   with only one hand, 199
Adalat, 253
Adaptic dressing, crush injury and, 102
Adaptive equipment
   meal preparation and, 238-239
   resource list of vendors, 265-268
   rheumatoid arthritis and, 239
Adductor digiti minimi, 41
Adductor pollicis, 41
   description of, 4
   innervation of, 6
Adhesions
   prevention after tendon repair, 155-156
   tendon healing and, 154
Adson maneuver, 80
Advil, 252
AIN: *see* Anterior interosseous nerve
Alcohol
   implications in therapy, 254
   side effects of, 254
Aldomet, 253
Aleve, 252
Alfalfa, 262
Algodystrophy, 150-151
Allen's test, 26-27
Allograft, 90

Aloe vera, 262
American Burn Association, 85
Amitriptyline, 253
Amoxicillin/clavulanate, 252
Ampicillin/sulbactam, 252
Amplitude, 213
Amputation, 193-203
   above-elbow
      mechanical elbow in prosthesis, 200
      terminal device opening, 201
   below-elbow, Krukenberg procedure, 199
   fingertips, treatment objectives in, 90
   high-pressure injection injuries and, 100-101
   one-handed activities of daily living, 199
   phantom limb sensation, 197-198
   phantom pain, 198
   prosthetic management after, 198
   replantation and, 104-105
   residual limb desensitization and, 197
   shoulder level, upper extremity impairment, 197
   transradial, terminal device for, 203
Anacin, 254
Analgesics, narcotic, 251
Anaprox, 252

Q-1

Anastomosis, Riche Cannieu, ulnar nerve palsy and, 175
Anatomic interconnections, Linburg's sign, 2
Anatomic snuffbox
  arterial anatomy of, 7
  scaphoid fracture and, 7
  tenderness during palpation, 62
Ancef, 252
Anconeus, 41
  nerve innervation, 42
  radial nerve and, 42
Andre-Thomas sign, 44
Aneurysm, 8
Angulation, metacarpal shaft fracture and, 118
Animal bites, 101
Ansaid, 252
Antebrachial cutaneous nerve, lateral, 37
Anteposition, abductor pollicis brevis and, 4
Anterior interosseous nerve
  flexor digitorum profundus and, 42
  flexor pollicis longus and, 42
  injury to, 42
  median nerve and, 42
  pronator quadratus, 42
  volar wrist capsule and, 42
Anterior interosseous nerve syndrome, 228-229
Anthropometry, 229
Antiadrenergic agents, 253
Antibiotics, 252
  open wounds and, 98
  side effects of, 252
Anticoagulant therapy, 252-253
  bleeding in, 253
Antiinflammatory agents
  barley grass and, 262
  corticosteroids as, 252
  nonsteroidal: see Nonsteroidal antiinflammatory drugs
Antimicrobial therapy, 252
  infection and, 101
  side effects of, 252

Antiseptics, honey and, 262
Antithrombotic therapy, 252-253
Anxiety, function testing and, 29
APB: see Abductor pollicis brevis
APL: see Abductor pollicis longus
Aponeurosis, bicipital, 9
Apprehension test, 72
Arcuate ligament, 219
Ardeparin, 253
Aristocort, 252
Arterial blood supply
  to forearm, 4
  to hand, 4, 6
Arterial flux, Allen's test and, 27
Arterial insufficiency
  intermittent compression pumps and, 209
  replant failure and, 102
  signs of, 14
Arterial occlusion, anticoagulants and, 252
Arterial reconstruction, venous grafts in, 10
Arteries: see also specific artery
  brachial, 4
  median, 6
  radial
    Allen's test and, 26-27
    evaluation in hand, 26-27
  ulnar
    Allen's test and, 26-27
    blood supply to hand and, 6
    evaluation in hand, 26-27
Arterio-occlusive disorders, Raynaud's phenomenon and, 84
Arthritis, 131-142
  basal joint
    ligament reconstruction tendon interposition arthroplasty and, 140
    splinting of, 189
  dexamethasone and, 215
  flaxseed and, 262

Arthritis—cont'd
  food supplements for, 262
  NSAIDs and, 251
  osteoarthritis: see Osteoarthritis
  pantrapezial, treatment of, 140
  posttraumatic, postoperative therapy, 138
  psoriatic, 135
  rheumatoid: see Rheumatoid arthritis
  sea cucumber and, 262
  sea mussel and, 262
  shark cartilage and, 262
  triscaphe, triscaphe joint fusion and, 63
Arthrodesis
  elbow, positioning of, 128
  first metacarpophalangeal joint, 140
  proximal interphalangeal joint fracture-dislocation and, 126-127
  total wrist, rheumatoid arthritis and, 141
Arthrography
  ligament injuries in wrist and, 65
  shoulder evaluation, 77
  SLAP lesion detection, 74-75
Arthrogryposis, 195
Arthroplasty
  carpometacarpal joint implant, rehabilitation of thumb after, 140-141
  elbow, complication rates of, 142
  joint mobilization and, 234
  ligament reconstruction tendon interposition
    basal joint arthritis and, 140
    pantrapezial arthritis and, 140
    rehabilitation after, 141
  metacarpophalangeal joint, 21

Arthroplasty—cont'd
  metacarpophalangeal joint—cont'd
    flexion outrigger and, 139
    lateral pinch after, 139
    pronation/supination deformities after, 139
    range-of-motion goals after, 139
    swan-neck deformity and, 138
  proximal interphalangeal joint, treatment of, 138
  Silastic
    indications in metacarpophalangeal joint, 137
    metacarpophalangeal joint, 138
    postoperative treatment, 142
  volar plate, 126
  wrist, rehabilitation after, 142
Arthroscopy
  rotator cuff repair and, 80
  SLAP lesion detection, 74-75
  subacromial decompression, range of motion exercises after surgery, 74
  supraspinatus tendon tear and acromiohumeral impingement, 77
Articular cartilage
  joint pain in osteoarthritis and, 133
  osteoarthritis and, 133
Ascorbic acid, 260
Aspirin, 252, 254
Assessment/evaluation, 25-34
  Adson maneuver, 80
  Allen's test, 26-27
  apprehension test, 72
  axon regeneration, 33
  biceps head stability, 32-33
  caput ulnae syndrome, 136
  clunk test, 73

Assessment/evaluation—cont'd
  coefficient of variation and, 28-29
  crank test, 72
  Crawford small parts dexterity test, 28
  de Quervain's disease, 221
  Dellon test, 31
  dorsal interossei, 27
  drop-arm test, 72
  dynamic splinting of joints, 179-180
  edema, volumeter and, 30
  Froment's sign, 175
  goniometry, 27-28
  grind test of thumb, 28
  Halstead maneuver, 80
  Hawkins-Kennedy impingement test, 72
  hitchhiker's test, 221
  Jamar dynamometer, 29
  Jebsen hand function test, 28
  labral tear, 73
  ligament injuries in wrist, 65
  Lippman test, 72
  lunotriquetral ligament, ballottement test, 60
  malrotation, 118
  manual muscle testing, 26
  Minnesota rate of manipulation test, 28
  Moberg pick-up test, 29-30, 31
  moving two-point discrimination, 31
  nerve supply integrity, 25
  neural tension test, 31
  ninhydrin test, 31
  osteoarthritis, 28
  pain perception, 31
  Purdue pegboard, 28
  radial tunnel syndrome, 226
  reflex sympathetic dystrophy, 144
  reflex testing, 25
  Rosenbusch test of finger dexterity, 28
  Semmes-Weinstein monofilaments, 26, 30, 31
  shoulder, 72

Assessment/evaluation—cont'd
  shoulder—cont'd
    after brachial plexus injury, 47-48
  static two-point discrimination, 31
  sudomotor function testing, 31
  tactile gnosis, 31
  thoracic outlet syndrome, 80
  threshold testing, 31
  Tinel's sign, 33
  total active range of motion, 32
  triangular fibrocartilage complex, 64
  ulnar nerve palsy, 175
  ulnar nerve status, 27
  visual analog scale, 33
  Watson's test for S-L ligament assessment, 61
  Weber test, 31
  Weber two-point discrimination test, 32
  Yergason test, 32-33
Astroglia in central nervous system, 38
Atrophy
  muscle, "fracture disease" and, 57
  skin, reflex sympathetic dystrophy and, 143
  soft tissue, sympathetic nervous system mediation of, 45-46
  Sudeck's, 150-151
Augmentin, 252
Autograft, 90
Avascular necrosis, scaphoid and, 7
Avulsion fracture, mallet finger injury and, treatment of, 125-126
Axillary nerve
  deltoid and, 45
  injury, 70
  shoulder abduction and, 72
Axillary vein formation, 10
Axis, 167

Axonal continuity, neuropraxic injury and, 43
Axonotmesis, 43
Axons
  myelin sheath around, 38
  regeneration, 33
    neuromas and, 44
      Tinel's sign and, 46
  sensory neuron, 37
  Wallerian degeneration and, 43
Azithromycin, 252

B

Bacterial contamination level, 99-100
Balloon edema testing, 30
Ballottement test, 60
Baltimore Therapeutic Equipment tools, 238
Bankart lesion, 75
  external rotation after repair, 75
Barley grass, 262
Barton's fracture, 56
  dislocation on radiograph and, 56
Basal joint pain, 238-239
Base fractures, 116
Basilic vein
  axillary vein and, 10
  in forearm, 8
Bell curve, 247
Bennett's fracture, 122
  reverse, 122-123
Betamethasone, 252
Biaxin, 252
Biceps brachii, supination and, 173-174
Biceps head
  stability in bicipital groove, 32
  Yergason test for stability of, 32-33
Biceps tenodesis, range-of-motion exercises after, 79
Bicipital aponeurosis, 9

Bicipital aponeurosis—cont'd
  pronator syndrome and, 231-232
Bicipital groove
  biceps head stability in, 32
  pectoralis major and, 11
Bicipital tendinitis, 72
Biofeedback
  thermal
    Raynaud's phenomena and, 84
    vasodilation in reflex sympathetic dystrophy and, 146
    thoracic outlet syndrome and, 80-81
Bioflavonoids, 260
Biomechanical load, lunate and, 60
Biomechanics, 167-176
  axis and, 167
  creep and, 169-170
  drag and, 169
  of flexor tendons, 14
  hysteresis and, 169
  levers and, 169
  mechanical advantage, 167
  shear stress and, 167
  shoulder, 71
  stress and, 167
  stress relaxation and, 169
  terminology in, 167
  work and, 169
Biomedical waste
  body excretions and, 242
  cleaning with EPA-approved disinfectant, 242-243
  contaminated dressings as, 242
  precautions for, 242
  protective equipment for disposal in sink, 242
Black wounds, 99
Bleeding, anticoagulant therapy and, 253
Blix curve, muscle tension and, 172
Blood exposure reporting, 243-244

Blood vessels, after surgical repair, 5
Blood-borne disease transmission, 243
Body fluids/excretions, 242
  Universal Precautions and, 242
Bone avulsion, mallet finger and, 20
Bone growth stimulator, fracture healing and, 127
Bone healing, manual muscle testing and, 26
Bone mass, osteoporosis and, 117
Bone ossification, heterotopic, after elbow fracture, 129
Bone scan, reflex sympathetic dystrophy assessment, 144
Bones
  capitate fracture, 54
  cylindrical shaft of, 114
  diaphysis of, 114
  epiphysis of, 114
  fracture frequency
    distal phalanx, 115
    hand, 115
  hamate fracture, 54
  lunate fracture, 54
  metaphysis of, 114
  pisiform
    fracture of, 54
    as sesamoid bone, 55
  scaphoid fracture, 54
  sesamoid, 55
  trapezium fracture, 54
  trapezoid fracture, 54
  triquetrum fracture, 54
Boron, 261
Bouchard's nodes, 134
Boutonnière deformity
  causes of, 16
  disabling elements of, 16
  exercise for, 16
  oblique retinacular ligament and, 12
  presenting signs of, 16
  rheumatoid thumb and, 131

Boutonnière deformity—cont'd
   terminal tendon tenotomy for, 18
   triangular ligament and, 22
Bovine cartilage, 262
Bowen disease, 108
Bower's hemiresection, 63
Bowler thumb, 108
Boxer's fracture, 113
   location of, 116
   metacarpophalangeal neck and, 116
   treatment and splinting for, 117
Braces
   Galveston, metacarpal shaft fracture and, 182
   Sarmiento fracture, for humeral shaft fracture, 187
Brachial artery, 4
Brachial plexus
   anatomy of, 48
   compression in thoracic inlet, 39
   injury
      C5 and C6 damage after, 47
      contracture prevention after, 48
      limb protection after, 48
      muscle paralysis after, 47
      muscle return after, 42
      psychological distress after, 48
      sensory recovery after, 48
      shoulder joint assessment after, 47-48
      therapy goals, 48
   Klumpke palsy and, 48
   median nerve and, 40
   suprascapular nerve and, 45
   traction lesion of, 44
   ulnar nerve in, 42-43
Brachial vein, axillary vein and, 10
Brachialis muscle insertion, 11
Brachioradialis, 41
   radial nerve and, 42
   wad of Henry and, 11

Brachioradialis reflex, C6 assessment, 25
Brachydactyly, 193
Bracing: see Splinting
Bruit, 8
Budding strapping splint, 190-191
Bunnell tendon transfer, 173
Bupivacaine, corticosteroids and, 252
Burns
   aloe vera and, 262
   classification of, 85, 86
   continuous passive motion and, 213
   dorsum of hand, split-thickness skin graft for, 89
   edema and, 87
   exercise program after, 87
   first-degree: see Burns, superficial
   food supplements for, 262
   full-thickness, 86
   honey and, 262
   hypertrophic scarring and, 86
      predictors of, 87
   joint mobilization after, 88
   keloid scarring and, 86
   partial-thickness, 86
      excision and grafting of, 93-94
   pressure therapy after, 91
   products for, resource list of vendors, 265-268
   "rule of nines" and, 85
   second-degree: see Burns, partial-thickness
   skin graft for, sensory loss after, 90
   superficial, 86
   superficial heat in treatment of, 87
   tendon adhesion release, 88
   third-degree: see Burns, full-thickness
Bursitis
   dexamethasone and, 215
   glucosamine and, 262
Butalbital, 254

Butorphanol, 251

C

C5
   brachial plexus injury and, 47
   dermatome covering deltoid muscle and, 45
C6, brachial plexus injury and, 47
C8, dermatome for, 50
C8 nerve root damage, sensation loss and, 50
CAD: see Calcium alginate dressings
Cafergot, 254
Caffeine, 254
Calcium, 261
Calcium alginate dressings, 103
   infected wounds and, 103-104
Calcium channel blockers, 253
Calcium soft-tissue deposition, indomethacin and, 62
Callus formation, fracture stability and, 114
Camitz tendon transfer, 173
   opposition in median nerve palsy, 176
Camper's chiasm, 156
Camptodactyly, 196
Cancer, intermittent compression pumps and, 209
Capillary refill, 14
Capitate
   fracture frequency, 54
   location of, 28
   measuring ulnar/radial deviation of wrist, 27-28
Capitulum, 11
Capsaicin, 253
   osteoarthritis management, 134
Capsulectomy
   metacarpophalangeal joint contractures and, splinting after, 184

Capsulectomy—cont'd
  volar metacarpophalangeal joint, indications for, 118-119
Capsulitis
  adhesive, ultrasound treatment of, 76
  primary adhesive, 75
Capsulotomy, continuous passive motion and, 213
Caput ulnae syndrome, 135-136
Cardiac dysfunction, intermittent compression pumps and, 209
Cardiovascular disease, calcium channel blockers and, 253
Carpal bones
  carpal instability dissociative, 58
  pisiform as sesamoid bone, 55
  proximal transverse arch and, 177
  scaphoid fracture, 54
Carpal canal, transverse carpal ligament and, 3
Carpal instability, triscaphe joint fusion and, 63
Carpal instability dissociative, 58
Carpal instability nondissociative, 58
Carpal row, in ulnar deviation of wrist, 65
Carpal tunnel
  anatomy of, 1
  Linburg's syndrome and, 2
  structures through, 1
Carpal tunnel release, pillar pain after, 231
Carpal tunnel syndrome
  nocturnal pain in, 221
  rehabilitation for, 225
  splinting position, 224
Carpi radialis brevis, 41
Carpi radialis longus, 41
Carpometacarpal boss, 108-109
Carpometacarpal joint

Carpometacarpal joint—cont'd
  carpometacarpal boss of, 108
  osteoarthritis assessment, 28
Carpus, ulnar translation of, Preiser's disease and, 66
Cartilage thickness in osteoarthritis, 133
Casting
  air, lateral epicondylitis and, 224
  preconditioning before, 186
  serial
    fixed proximal interphalangeal joint contracture and, 185-186
    materials for, 186
Cathode, 214
Causalgia, 150-151
Cayenne, 262
Ceclor, 252
Cefaclor, 252
Cefadroxil, 252
Cefazolin, 252
Cefotan, 252
Cefotaxime, 252
Cefotetan, 252
Cefprozil, 252
Ceftin, 252
Ceftriaxone, 252
Cefuroxime, 252
Cefzil, 252
Celestone, 252
Cell body
  of motor neuron, 37
  of sensory neuron, 37
Cell excitability, 40
Cell membrane, 40
Cells, content of, 40
Cellulitis, 100
Central nervous system
  astroglia in, 38
  oligodendrocytes in, 38
Central slip, 16
  rupture of, 16
Central tendency, 246
Cephalexin, 252
Cephalic vein, in forearm, 8

Cerebrovascular accident, reflex sympathetic dystrophy and, 144
Cervical nerves, subclavius muscle and, 71
Chauffeur fracture, 65
Check rein ligaments, 2
Chemotaxis, 98
Chilblains, 84
Children
  cubitus varus after supracondylar fracture, 127
  functional level of sensibility testing, 29-30
  hemangiomas and, 112
  Moberg pick-up test and, 29-30
  reflex sympathetic dystrophy in, 150
  soft-tissue tumors, 112
Chlorhexidine gluconate, 102
Chlorine, splint cleaning and, 179
CIND: *see* Carpal instability nondissociative
Cipro, 252
Ciprofloxacin, 252
Claforan, 252
Clarithromycin, 252
Clavicle
  coracoclavicular ligament and, 70
  medial epiphysis of, 115
Claw deformity
  hand burn and, 88
  treatments for, 175-176
Clawing, Riche Cannieu anastomosis and, 175
Cleland's ligament, function of, 5
Cleocin, 252
Clindamycin, 252
Clinoril, 252
Closed-chain exercise, 239
Clunk test, 73
Coalition, lunotriquetral, 53-54
Coban wrap/dressing, 103
  edema and, 83
Codeine, 251

Codman's exercises, 75
 use of, 78
Coefficient of variation, 28-29
Cold exposure, Hunting reaction and, 84
Cold flashes, during nerve regeneration, 34
Cold injury
 frostbite
  management of, 85
  rewarming after, 84-85
 Neoprene glove for, 84
 Raynaud's phenomenon and, 84
 types of, 84
Cold sensitivity, immersion injuries and, 84
Cold therapy, 206
 lateral epicondylitis and, 213
 skin redness after, 206-207
Collagen, 98
Collagen synthesis, wound healing and, 98-99
Collapse deformity, rheumatoid thumb, 131
Collar button infection, 100
Collateral ligaments
 accessory, 22
  joint capsule and, 22
  volar plate and, 22
 medial, elbow dislocation and, 117
 proper, 22
  volar plate and, 22
  splinting of, 22
 ulnar
  gamekeeper's thumb and, 121
  splinting of injuries to, 188
Colles' fracture, 17, 56
 reflex sympathetic dystrophy after, 150
 volar flexion and, 56-57
Comminuted fracture, of proximal phalanx, treatment for, 126
Compartment syndrome, 103
 crush injury and, 119
 symptoms of, 120

Compartment syndrome—cont'd
 treatment for, 119
Complex regional pain syndrome, 150-151
Compression, 233-234
 median nerve, 33
Compression device, pneumatic, edema treatment and, 83
Compression neuropathy, 193
Compression pump
 intermittent, 206
  intermittent compression pumps, 209
 Jobst, contraindications for, 210
Compression stress, 169
Computed tomography, ligament injuries in wrist and, 65
Computer use, ergonomics and, 231
Conduction, 205
Conduction block, neuropraxic injury and, 43
Congenital anomalies/deformities, 193-203
 arthrogryposis, 195
 camptodactyly, 196
 congenital constriction band syndrome, 193
 duplication, 193
 ectrodactyly, 195
 failure of differentiation, 193
 failure of formation, 193
 hypoplastic thumb, 197
 Kirner's deformity, 194
 lunotriquetral coalition, 53-54
 Madelung's deformity, 194
 Maffucci's syndrome, 196
 overgrowth, 193
 phocomelia, 195
 polydactyly, 195
 pterygium cubital, 195
 skeletal, 193
 undergrowth, 193
 webbed fingers, 193-194
 windblown hand, 195

Connective tissue, 38
 regenerating nerves and, 44
Connective tissue disorders, Raynaud's phenomenon and, 84
Constant-touch pressure, 36
 Merkel cells and, 36
 Ruffini end organs and, 36
Constriction band syndrome, congenital, 193
Contractile tension, Blix curve and, 172
Contraction
 concentric, isotonic exercise and, 238
 metacarpophalangeal joint, in Dupuytren's disease, 110
 muscle, 26
  resting length in, 167-168
Contractures
 after skin graft, 90
 Dupuytren's, 2, 107
  volar metacarpophalangeal joint capsulectomy for, 118-119
 first web space, splinting for, 186
 fixed proximal interphalangeal joint, serial casting for, 185-186
 intrinsic muscle, volar metacarpophalangeal joint capsulectomy for, 118-119
 metacarpophalangeal joint
  Dupuytren's disease and, 108
  splinting after capsulectomy for, 184
  splinting of, 183
 preventing after brachial plexus injury, 48
 in proximal interphalangeal joint, 2
 proximal interphalangeal joint flexion, dynamic splinting of, 181

Contractures—cont'd
  soft-tissue, static splinting and, 179
Contrast baths, 211
Convection, fluidotherapy and, 205
Convex-concave rule, 233
Coordination
  fine-motor: see Fine-motor coordination
  gross-motor: see Gross-motor coordination
Copper, 261
Coracoacromial arch, 71
Coracoacromial ligament, coracoacromial arch and, 71
Coracobrachialis
  action of, 14
  innervation of, 71
  insertion of, 11
Coracoclavicular ligament, 70
Coracoid process, coracoacromial arch and, 71
Coronal abduction, after brachial plexus injury, 47-48
Coronal plane, 11-12
Coronoid fossa, 11
Corpuscles: see also specific corpuscles
  Meissner's, 35-36
  Pacinian, 35
  Ruffini, 35
Correlation coefficient, 248
Corticosteroid cream, hypergranulation tissue and, 210
Corticosteroids, 252
  osteoarthritis management, 134
  side effects of, 252
Cortisone, 252
Coulomb friction, 168
Coumadin, 253
COV: see Coefficient of variation
Co-wraps, 91
Crank test, 72

Crawford small parts dexterity test, 28
Creep
  definition of, 169
  heat before stretching and, 169-170
  serial splinting for joint contractures and, 178
Crepitation, 79
CREST syndrome, 132-133
Crossed-intrinsic transfer, 137
Crush injury
  compartment syndrome and, 119
  distal phalanx fracture and, 115
  dressing for, 102
  open, 98
  tuft fractures and, 116
  volar advancement flap for, 93
CT: see Computed tomography
Cubital tunnel
  anatomy of, 219
  nerve compression at, 227
Cubital tunnel syndrome
  conservative treatment for, 228
  splinting for, 228
  therapy after release, 228
Cubitus valgus, after lateral epicondyle fracture, 127
Cubitus varus, after supracondylar fracture, in child, 127
Cumulative trauma disorders, 221
  anthropometry and, 229
  ergonomic tool design and, 230
  job-site analysis, 229
  force measurement during, 230
  temperature and, 229-230
Cushingoid features, corticosteroids and, 252
Cutaneous nerve, lateral antebrachial, 37
Cyanocobalamin, 260

Cyanosis, 14
  after nerve injury, 45-46
  Raynaud's phenomena and, 84
Cyriax's description of end-feel, 236
Cyriax's technique, 235
Cyst
  inclusion, 111
  synovial, 108

D

Daily living tasks, grip strength and, 134-135
Danaparoid, 253
Darrach procedure, 63
Darvocet-N, 251
Darvon, 251
Daypro, 252
de Quervain's disease, 220
  Finkelstein test and, 220-221
  splinting for, 222
  symptoms of, 240
Decadron, 252
Decompression, compartment syndrome and, 103
Deformity prevention, static splinting and, 179
Deftazidime, 252
Degeneration, Wallerian, 43
Degenerative joint disease, 62
Dehiscence, 98
Dellon two-point discrimination test, 31
Deltasone, 252
Deltoid
  action of, 14
  dermatome covering, 45
  humeral elevation and, 71
  paralysis after brachial nerve injury, 47
  paralysis after brachial plexus injury, 47
  shoulder extension and, 70
Demerol, 251
Depo-Medrol, 252
Depression, amitriptyline and, 253
Dermatome

Dermatome—cont'd
    for C8, 50
    of deltoid muscle, 45
Dermis, papillary ridges in, 12
Dermofasciectomy, strengthening after, 110
Desensitization
    contact mediums for, 48
    neuromas and, 44
    residual limb, 197
    vibration texture after, 48
Deviation
    radial: see Radial deviation
    ulnar: see Ulnar deviation
Dexamethasone, 252
    iontophoresis and, 215
    phonophoresis and, 206
Dexterity, Rosenbusch test of finger dexterity, 28
Diabetes
    corticosteroids and, 252
    reflex sympathetic dystrophy and, 144
Diaphysis, 114
Dibenzyline, 253
Diclofenac, 252
Diffusion barrier, perineurium as, 38-39
Diffusion through cell membrane, 40
Diflunisal, 252
Digital nerve repair, sensation return after, 46
Digits
    boutonniere deformity of, 16
    bowler thumb, 108
    boxer's fracture and, 113
    clawing of, Riche Cannieu anastomosis and, 175
    cold injury to, Neoprene glove for, 84
    cross-finger flaps and, 92
    Dupuytren's disease and, 109
    extension, Klumpke palsy and, 48
    extensor mechanism injury and, 16
    flexion
        distal transverse arch and, 177

Digits—cont'd
    flexion—cont'd
        Klumpke palsy and, 48
        median nerve palsy and, tendon transfer in, 172
    giant cell tumors of, 56
    immobilization after trauma, 182
    index
        flexor digitorum profundus in, 1
        sensory loss after brachial plexus injury, 47
    intrinsic function, Klumpke palsy and, 48
    Jersey finger, 163
    little
        adduction of, 44
        C8 nerve-root damage and, 50
        clawing of, 44
        Dupuytren's disease and, 109
        extensor tendon rupture in rheumatoid arthritis and, 135
        Kirner's deformity and, 194
        numbness of, 39
        sensation loss, 50
    mallet finger injury with avulsion fracture, treatment of, 125-126
    middle, radial/ulnar abduction of, 44
    missing, 195
    reverse Bennett's fracture of, 122-123
    ring
        C8 nerve-root damage, 50
        clawing of, 44
        Dupuytren's disease and, 109
        flexion contracture of, 9
        flexor digitorum profundus tendon graft, 21
        management after tip amputation, 88-89

Digits—cont'd
    ring—cont'd
        sensation loss, 50
        Rosenbusch test of finger dexterity and, 28
    syndactyly of, 193-194
    thumb
        basal joint arthritis, 189
        basal joint reconstruction, 140
        Bennett's fracture of, 122
        boutonnière deformity of, 131
        collapse deformity in rheumatoid arthritis, 131
        crush injury to, 93
        hypoplastic, 197
        pulleys in, 154
        retroposition, 62
        sensory loss of, 47
        vibratory trauma to, Raynaud's phenomenon and, 84
Dilaudid, 251
Dipyridamole, 253
Discoloration, reflex sympathetic dystrophy and, 145
Discrimination testing
    Dellon two-point, 31
    moving two-point, 31
        Meissner's corpuscles and, 36
    static two-point, 31
        constant-touch pressure and, 36
    Weber two-point, 32
Discriminative sensory re-education, 26
DISI: see Dorsal intercalated segment instability
Disinfectant
    EPA-approved, biomedical waste cleaning and, 242-243
    tuberculocidal, vomit cleanup and, 243
Dislocation
    Barton's fracture and, 56

Dislocation—cont'd
  distal radioulnar joint, radial head fracture and, 58
  lunate, 66
  perilunate, 66
  shoulder, Bankart lesion and, 75
Distal interphalangeal joint
  active extension of, 20
  bony enlargement of, 134
  boutonnière deformity and, 16
  flexion
    limitations in, 16
    longitudinal arch and, 177
    terminal tendon tenotomy and, 18
  functional flexion of, 116
  Heberden's nodes and, 134
  hyperextension of, 16
  isolated flexion of, 16
  loss of flexion in, 16
  paradoxical extension of, 21
Distal phalanx, 13, 17, 21
  base fractures of, 116
  fracture frequency, 115
Distal radius fracture: see Radius fracture, distal
Distraction, 233-234
Distribution
  gaussian, 247
  normal, 247
Dog bites, 101
Dolobid, 252
Dolophine, 251
Doppler echocardiography, 8
Dorsal hood, 15
Dorsal intercalated segment instability, scapholunate dissociation and, 57
Dorsal interossei
  actions of, 27
  first
    description of, 4
    ulnar nerve status testing and, 27
Dorsal root ganglion, sensory neuron and, 37

Dorsal scapular nerve, levator scapulae muscles and, 71
Dorsal subscapular nerve, rhomboid major/minor muscles and, 70
Dorsal wrist compartments, tendons in, 2
Dorsal wrist ganglion, 56
Dorsiflexion in hypomobile wrist, 236
Doxycycline, 252
Drag, 169
Dressings
  Adaptic, 102
  calcium alginate, 103
    infected wounds and, 103-104
  Coban, 102, 103
  contaminated, 242
  crush injury, 102
  dry sterile, 102, 103
  elastic wrap, 103
  infected wounds, 103-104
  Kaltostat, 103
  Kerlix, 103
  pouch, 103
  semipermeable film, 103
  Tegaderm, 103
  wet-to-dry, 102
Drop-arm test, 72, 77
Drugs of abuse, 253-254
Duchenne sign, 44
Dupuytren's contracture, 2, 107
  splinting after surgical release, 108-109
  volar metacarpophalangeal joint capsulectomy for, 118-119
Dupuytren's disease, 107-112
  adhesions and, 112
  complications of, 112
  fingers affected by, 109
  flexion problems and, 112
  Grayson's ligament and, 5
  hand trauma and, 110
  initial manifestation of, 107
  joint stiffness and, 112
  McCash open-palm technique for, 111

Dupuytren's disease—cont'd
  metacarpophalangeal joint contraction in, 110
  proximal interphalangeal joint flexion contractures and, 112
  reflex sympathetic dystrophy and, 112
  surgical intervention for, 108
  wound dehiscence and, 112
Duran protocol, 158
  flexor tendon passive motion and, 158-159
Duricef, 252
Dynamometer, Jamar, handle position on, 29
Dystrophy
  posttraumatic, 150-151
  reflex sympathetic: see Reflex sympathetic dystrophy
  shoulder-hand, 148

E

Echocardiography, Doppler, 8
ECRB: see Extensor carpi radialis brevis
ECRL: see Extensor carpi radialis longus
Ectrodactyly, 195
ECU: see Extensor carpi ulnaris
ED: see Extensor digitorum
EDC: see Extensor digitorum communis
Edema
  balloon, 30
  brawny, reflex sympathetic dystrophy and, 143
  burn injuries and, 87
  contrast baths and, 211
  corticosteroids and, 252
  elevation and, 83
  flaxseed and, 262
  fracture disease and, 57
  pitting, reflex sympathetic dystrophy and, 143
  prevention in reflex sympathetic dystrophy, 147
  prevention/reduction of, 83

Edema—cont'd
  tendon repair and, 162
  treatment of, 83
  trigger finger and, 220
  volumeter assessment, 30
EDM: see Extensor digiti minimi
E.E.S., 252
Egawa sign, 44
EIP: see Extensor indicis proprius
Elastic stretch, Blix curve and, 172
Elastic wrap dressing, 103
Elasticity, 170
Elavil, 253
Elbow
  arthrodesis, positioning of, 128
  arthroplasty, complication rates of, 142
  fracture, heterotopic bone ossification and, 129
  golfer's, 223
    splinting for, 186
  lateral antebrachial cutaneous nerve in, 37
  position, during Jamar dynamometry, 29
  tennis
    splinting for, 184-185
    testing for, 227
  webbing, 195
Electrical stimulation
  amplitude of, 213
  cathode and, 214
  current for muscle tissue denervation, 215
  frequency, 213
  interferential, frozen shoulder and, 76
  neuromuscular, reflex sympathetic dystrophy and, 146
  pain reduction and, 216
  parameters of, 213
  polarity, 214
  pulse duration, 213
  rheobase and, 214-215
  rise time in, 213

Electrical stimulation—cont'd
  strength-duration testing, 214-215
  on time/off time, 213
  wave forms, 214
Electrodiagnostics, reflex sympathetic dystrophy and, 144
Electromyogram feedback, tremor control in multiple sclerosis, 217
Electromyography, thoracic outlet syndrome and, 39
Electrotherapy, products for, resource list of vendors, 265-268
E-mycin, 252
Enchondroma, 108, 111
  Maffucci's syndrome and, 110
End organ protection, ulnar nerve repair and, 45
Endocrine problems, frozen shoulder and, 75
Endoneural tubes, perineurium and, 38-39
Endoneurium, 38
Enophthalmos, 44
Enoxaparin, 253
Environmental Protection Agency, biomedical waste cleanup, 242-243
EPA: see Environmental Protection Agency
EPB: see Extensor pollicis brevis
Epicondyle fracture, cubitus valgus after, 127
Epicondylitis
  acute lateral, wrist immobilization splint for, 223
  lateral
    air casts for, 224
    cold therapy for, 213
    splinting of, 184-185
    tendon injury in, 223

Epicondylitis—cont'd
  lateral—cont'd
    testing for, 227
  medial, 223
    management of, 223
    splinting for, 186
Epineurium, 38
  external, 38
  internal, 38
    gliding and, 38
Epiphysis, 114
  medial, of clavicle, 115
Epitenon suture in tendon repair, 162
EPL: see Extensor pollicis longus
Eponychium, 12
Erb's palsy, C5/C6 nerve roots and, 51
Ergonomics
  computer use, 231
  products for, resource list of vendors, 265-268
  program management guidelines, 230
  tool design, 230
Ergotamine, 254
Erythema, Raynaud's phenomena and, 84
Erythematous, 9
Erythematous skin rash, psoriatic arthritis and, 135
Erythromycin, 252
Esgic, 254
Essex-Lopresti fracture-dislocation, 58
Etodolac, 252
Evaluation: see Assessment/evaluation
Excedrin, 254
Excision, partial-thickness burns and, 93-94
Exercise program
  after burn injury, 87
  home
    after shoulder surgery, 78
    edema treatment and, 83
  osteoporosis and, 117

Exercises
- closed-chain, 239
- flexion, distal interphalangeal joint, 16
- isokinetic, 239
- isotonic, concentric contraction and, 238
- products for, resource list of vendors, 265-268
- thoracic outlet syndrome, 39

Extension
- active, of proximal interphalangeal joint, 16
- deficits, summation of, 32
- paradoxical, 21
- passive, of proximal interphalangeal joint, 16
- of proximal interphalangeal joint, 16

Extension moment arm, 3
Extensor carpi radialis brevis, 2
- description of, 4
- nerve innervation, 42
- origination of, 3
- paralysis after brachial plexus injury, 47
- radial nerve and, 42
- strength of, 171
- wad of Henry and, 11

Extensor carpi radialis brevis tendon, tendon transfer for radial nerve palsy and, 174

Extensor carpi radialis longus, 2
- paralysis after brachial plexus injury, 47
- radial nerve and, 42
- sustained work and, 171
- wad of Henry and, 11

Extensor carpi ulnaris, 2, 41
- description of, 4
- posterior interosseous nerve and, 42
- subluxation of, 224

Extensor digiti minimi, 2, 41
- posterior interosseous nerve and, 42

Extensor digiti minimi tendon, 165

Extensor digitorum, 2
Extensor digitorum communis, 41
- posterior interosseous nerve and, 42
- return after brachial plexus injury, 42
- tendon transfer for radial nerve palsy and, 174

Extensor digitorum communis tendon, lumbrical muscles and, 22

Extensor indicis muscle, innervation of, 6

Extensor indicis proprius, 41
- posterior interosseous nerve and, 42
- radial nerve innervation, 27

Extensor indicis proprius tendon, 165

Extensor pollicis brevis, 2, 41
- posterior interosseous nerve and, 42

Extensor pollicis brevis tendon, de Quervain's disease and, 220

Extensor pollicis longus, 2, 41
- description of, 4
- Lister's tubercle and, 10-11
- posterior interosseous nerve and, 42
- rupture of, after distal radius fracture, 62
- tendon transfer for radial nerve palsy and, 174

Extensor tendon zones, 153
Extensor tendons
- mallet finger and, 20
- nutritional pathway in, 155
- repair, treatment protocol for, 164-165
- stabilization in metacarpophalangeal joint, 20
- subluxation, central tendon involvement, 162-163
- synovial diffusion in, 155
- wrist ganglion and, 109

Extensors, tightness of, 17

External fixation, 124
- device, pin care and, 104
- pilon fractures and, 127

Exudate, 98
Eyeglasses, protective side shields, 241

F

Fascia, definition of, 9
Fascicles
- endoneurium in, 38
- perineurium and, 38-39
- perineurium in, 38

Fasciotomy, compartment syndrome and, 119
Feldene, 252
Felon, 100
Fenoprofen, 252
Fibroblasts, wound healing and, 98-99
Fibromatosis, palmar, 107
- reflex sympathetic dystrophy and, 145

Fibrosis
- lacertus, pronator syndrome and, 231-232
- perineural, posterior interosseous nerve injury and, 60

Fine-motor coordination, Crawford small parts dexterity test and, 28
Finger cuff, torque range of motion and, 32
Fingernails
- anatomy of, 27
- cellulitis of, 100
- changes in
    - psoriatic arthritis and, 135
    - sympathetic nervous system mediation of, 45-46
- growth of, 39
    - reflex sympathetic dystrophy and, 143
- nerve supply to, 13
- staphylococcus and, 100

Fingerprint, 12
Fingers: *see* Digits

Fingertips
  amputations, treatment objectives in, 90
  nerve regeneration after repair, 47
  protective sensation of, 26
  reconstruction, cross-finger flaps and, 92
  ring, management after tip amputation, 88-89
Finkelstein test
  de Quervain's disease and, 220-221
  performing, 221
Fioricet, 254
Fiorinal, 254
Fish oil, 262
Fist, hook, 42-43
Fixation/stabilization
  disadvantages of, 124
  external fixation, 124
  intramedullary device for, 124
  Kirschner pins for, 124
  Kirschner wires and, 123
  oblique fracture of proximal phalanx, 125
  open reduction internal: *see* Open reduction internal fixation
  percutaneous pin, 126
  plate and screws for, 124
  summation of, 32
Flagyl, 252
Flaps, 83-95
  cross-finger, 92
  groin, 95
  index cross-finger, 93
  pedicles of, 89
  radial forearm, dorsal tissue loss of hand and, 94
  random pattern, 92-93
  temporoparietal fascia free, 94
  thenar, 94
  thoracoabdominal, 92-93
  volar advancement, 93
Flashes during nerve regeneration, 34
Flaxseed oil, 262

Flexion
  distal interphalangeal joint, 16
    terminal tendon tenotomy and, 18
  functional, 116
  limitations in, distal interphalangeal joint and, 16
Flexion contracture
  in proximal interphalangeal joint, 2
  of ring finger, 9
Flexion exercises, distal interphalangeal joint, 16
Flexion outrigger, after metacarpophalangeal arthroplasty, 139
Flexor carpi radialis, 41
  medial epicondyle and, 10
  median nerve and, 40
  in palmar oblique ligament reconstruction, 140
Flexor carpi ulnaris, 41
  medial epicondyle and, 10
  strength of, 171
  ulnar nerve and, 42-43
  ulnar nerve in forearm and, 48
Flexor carpi ulnaris tendon
  tendinitis, 231
  tendon transfer for radial nerve palsy and, 174
Flexor digiti minimi, 41
Flexor digitorum profundus, 1, 41
  anterior interosseous nerve and, 42
  median nerve and, 40
  shortness after laceration, pullout suture and, 158
  ulnar nerve and, 42-43
Flexor digitorum profundus tendon
  full-fist exercise for, 159
  graft to ring finger, 21
  lumbrical muscles and, 22
Flexor digitorum superficialis, 1, 41

Flexor digitorum superficialis—cont'd
  boutonniere deformity and, 16
  dynamic traction of fingers and, 164
  medial epicondyle and, 10
  median nerve and, 40
Flexor muscles
  proximal transverse arch and, 177
  tightness of, 17
Flexor pollicis brevis, 41
  median nerve and, 40
Flexor pollicis longus, 1, 41
  after median nerve injury, tendon transfer for, 173
  anterior interosseous nerve and, 42
  index finger flexor digitorum profundus and, 1
  median nerve and, 40
  tendon rupture, in rheumatoid arthritis, 135
Flexor tendon zones, 154
  "no man's land," 155
Flexor tendons, 13
  adhesion prevention after repair, 155-156
  blood supply to, 155
  Duran protocol for passive motion, 158-159
  pulleys in, 14
  repair
    immobilization splinting after, 161
    rupture risks after, 165-166
    tenolysis after, 165
  vincula and, 155
Floxin, 252
Fluidotherapy
  disadvantages of, 207
  temperature of, 209
Fluori-methane spray, 205, 209-210
Flurbiprofen, 252
Folic acid, 260
Food supplements, natural, 262

Force
  description of, 168
  in dynamic splinting, 179
  in joint mobilization, 180-181
Forearm
  arterial supply to, 4
  both bone fractures of
    internal fixation of, 125
    synostosis after ORIF, 125
  crush injury, compartment syndrome and, 119
  functional rotation of, 129
  lateral antebrachial cutaneous nerve in, 37
  length of trough in splint, 178-179
  median nerve in, 40, 48
  median nerve innervation in, 40
  position, during Jamar dynamometry, 29
  radial nerve in, 42
  radial tunnel syndrome and, 226
  venous anatomy of, 8
Fortaz, 252
Fracture disease, immobilization and, 57
Fracture-dislocation, Barton's fracture and, 56
Fractures, 113-128: see also specific site or type
  base, 116
  boxer's, 113, 116
  continuous passive motion and, 213
  fixation of: see Fixation/stabilization
  healing of, 114
    bone growth stimulator and, 127
  immobilized, healing in, 115
  internal fixation of, 114
  primary healing in, 115
  range of motion after fixation, 121
  reflex sympathetic dystrophy and, 144
  secondary healing in, 115

Fractures—cont'd
  shaft, 116
  stability of, callus formation and, 114
  stable, continuous passive motion and, 213
  tuft, 116
Friction
  coulomb, description of, 168
  description of, 168
  static, description of, 168
Froment's sign, 44
  ulnar nerve palsy and, 175
Frontal plane, 11-12
Frostbite, 84
  management of, 85
  rewarming after, 84-85
Frozen shoulder, 75
  shoulder taping and, 236-237
  therapy for, 76
Function testing
  coefficient of variation in, 28-29
  Crawford small parts dexterity test, 28
  inconsistent effort during, 28-29
  Jebsen hand function test, 28
  Minnesota rate of manipulation test, 28
  Moberg pick-up test, 29-30, 31
  patient performance on, 29
  Purdue pegboard, 28
  Rosenbusch test of finger dexterity, 28
  sudomotor, 31
  for tactile gnosis, 29-30, 31
  threshold, 31
Fusion
  lunotriquetral, flexion loss after, 67
  triscaphe joint, 63
Futuro wrist splint, 62

G

Gabapentin, 253
Galeazzi fracture, 117

Galvanic stimulation, high-voltage, 217
Galveston brace, metacarpal shaft fractures and, 182
Gamekeeper's thumb, 121
  tip pinch after surgery for, 122
  treatment of, 121
Ganglion, 108
  dorsal wrist, 56
  of wrist, 109
  wrist, range of motion after removal, 109
Gantzer's muscle, 221
Garlic, 262
Gate-control theory, 210
Gaussian distribution, 247
Genetic factors/conditions
  osteoarthritis and, 133
  reflex sympathetic dystrophy and, 144
Germanium, 261
Giant cell tumors, 56
Gigantism, 193
Glabrous skin, sensory receptors in, 35
Glenohumeral joint
  osteoarthritis of, 79
  shoulder abduction and, 71
  stability of, 6
Glenohumeral ligament, anterior inferior, 75
Glenoid labrum, 6
Glenoid process, shoulder stability and, 6
Gliding, 233-234
  internal epineurium and, 38
Gloves
  sensory receptors while wearing, 36
  skin tears and, 243
Glucosamine, 262
Gnosis, tactile, 30, 31
Golfer's elbow, 223
  management of, 223
  splinting for, 186
Goniometry
  radial deviation of wrist, 27-28

Goniometry—cont'd
   torque range of motion and, 32
   ulnar deviation of wrist, 27-28
Gooseflesh, 39, 51
Gout
   radiographic evaluation of, 62
   uric acid level and, 107-108
Grafts, 83-95
   allograft, 90
   autograft, 90
   full-thickness groin, 93
   heterograft, 90
   isograft, 90
   partial-thickness burns and, 93-94
   skin: *see* Skin graft
   split-thickness hypothenar skin, 93
   xenograft, 90
Granuloma, pyogenic, 108
Grasp
   Cleland's ligament and, 5
   Grayson's ligament and, 5
   lumbrical muscles and, 22
   psoriatic arthritis and, 135
Grayson's ligament, function of, 5
Greater tubercle, supraspinatus and, 11
Grind test
   osteoarthritis assessment, 28
   of thumb, 28
Grip
   loss after ulnar nerve palsy, 176
   ulnar nerve palsy and, 176
Grip strength, 134-135
   lateral epicondylitis and, 227
   muscles crossing wrist, 171
Gross-motor coordination, Minnesota rate of manipulation test and, 28
Ground substance, 98
Growth factors
   nerve, 38
   tissue repair and, 99

Guanethidine, 253

H

Habitrol, 254
Hair growth, 39
   reflex sympathetic dystrophy and, 143
   sympathetic nervous system mediation of, 45-46
Halstead maneuver, 80
Hamate, hook of: *see* Hook of the hamate
Hamate fracture, 123
   frequency of, 54
Hand
   Allen's test of radial/ulnar arteries, 26-27
   arterial supply to, 4
   balloon edema in, 30
   blood supply to, 6
   burns
      classification of, 85
      claw deformity and, 88
      "rule of nines" and, 85
      splinting of, 88
      superficial heat in treatment of, 87
   distal palmar crease, splinting and, 177-178
   distal transverse arch of, 177
   dorsal tissue loss of, radial forearm flap and, 94
   intrinsic minus deformity, treatments for, 175-176
   Jebsen hand function test, 28
   longitudinal arch of, 177
   Maffucci's syndrome and, 110
   malignant tumors of, 56
   Mycobacterium marinum infection of, 101
   neural tension test of, 31
   Ollier disease and, 110
   palmar wounds, full-thickness skin graft for, 92
   proximal interphalangeal joint stiffness and, 114

Hand—cont'd
   proximal transverse arch of, 177
   psoriatic arthritis and, 135
   radial artery evaluation in, 26-27
   reconstruction of, skin graft for, 89
   Rosenbusch test of finger dexterity, 28
   sarcomas of, 56
   trauma, Dupuytren's disease and, 110
   ulnar artery evaluation in, 26-27
   volumeter testing of, 30
Hand function, Moberg pick-up test and, 29-30
Hand therapy
   medications used in, 251-258
   pin care in external fixation device, 104
Handlebar palsy, 227
Hansen's disease, 45
   nerves and, 45
Hawkins-Kennedy impingement test, 72
Hazards, personal protective equipment and, 241
Head injury, reflex sympathetic dystrophy and, 144
Healing, rate of, sympathetic nervous system mediation of, 45-46
Heat
   frozen shoulder and, 76
   infection and, 101
Heberden's nodes, 134
Hemangiomas
   in children, 112
   definition of, 8
   Maffucci's syndrome and, 110
Hematoma, skin graft failure and, 89
Hemiresection, Bower's, 63
Heparin, 253
Hepatitis B, 243
   vaccine, blood donation and, 243

Hepatitis C, 243
Herbert-Whipple screw, proximal interphalangeal joint fracture-dislocation, 126-127
Herpetic whitlow, 111
30-Hertz movement/vibration
   Meissner's corpuscles and, 35-36
   moving two-point discrimination and, 36
   sensory re-education and, 46
   sensory return after nerve injury, 37
256-Hertz movement/vibration
   after median nerve injury, 36
   Pacinian corpuscles and, 36
   sensory re-education and, 46
   sensory return after nerve injury, 37
Heterograft, 90
Hibiclens, 102
   pin care in external fixation device, 104
High-voltage galvanic stimulation, 217
Hip necrosis, corticosteroids and, 252
Histogram, 246
Hitchhiker's test, 221
Home exercise program, edema treatment and, 83
Honey, 262
Hook fist, ulnar nerve injury and, 42-43
Hook of the hamate, 1
   transverse carpal ligament and, 3
Horner's syndrome, 44
Hosmer-Dorrance voluntary opening hook, 202
Hot flashes, during nerve regeneration, 34
Hot packs, in hydrocollator, temperature of, 209
Huber tendon transfer, 173
   opposition in median nerve palsy, 176
Human immunodeficiency virus, 243

Humeral head depression, 72
Humeral shaft fracture, splinting of, 187
Humeral ulnar aponeurotic arcade, 219
Humerus
   elevation of, 71
   fracture bracing of, 187
   head of, shoulder stability and, 6
   muscle anatomy of, 10
   quadrangular space and, 7
   radial nerve and, 42
   shaft of, coracobrachialis and, 11
   supracondylar fracture, cubitus varus and, in child, 127
Humerus fracture
   distal, ulnar nerve and, 127
   proximal, treatment for, 78
Hunting reaction, cold exposure and, 84
Hydrocodone, 251
Hydrocortisone, phonophoresis and, 206
Hydrogen peroxide, 102
   pin care in external fixation device, 104
Hydromorphone, 251
Hyperglycemia, corticosteroids and, 252
Hypergranulation tissue, treatment of, 210
Hyperhidrosis, immersion injuries and, 84
Hypersensitivity
   contact mediums for desensitization program, 48
   vibration texture for desensitization program, 48
Hypertension, calcium channel blockers and, 253
Hypertrophic scar
   capillary pressure for reduction of, 91
   etiology of, 86-87
   predictors of, 87
Hyponychium, 12, 13

Hypoplasia, 193
Hypothesis
   experimental, 249
   null, 249
Hysteresis
   definition of, 169
   serial splinting for joint contractures and, 178

I

Ibuprofen, 252
Idiopathic conditions, reflex sympathetic dystrophy and, 144
Immersion injuries, 84
Immobilization
   acute lateral epicondylitis and, 223
   after flexor tendon repair, 161
   after radial nerve tendon transfer, 174
   after ulnar nerve repair, 44-45
   cast
      after Silastic implant arthroplasty of wrist, 142
      of thumb after carpometacarpal joint implant arthroplasty, 140-141
   of digits after trauma, 182
   distal radius fracture, 56
   extensor tendon closed injury management, 159
   fracture disease and, 57
   infection and, 101
   mallet finger with bone avulsion, 20
   metacarpal fracture, 120-121
   prolonged, volar metacarpophalangeal joint capsulectomy for, 118-119
   proximal humeral fracture, 78

Immobilization—cont'd
   reflex sympathetic dystrophy and, 144
   SLAP lesion repair and, 74-75
   static splinting and, 179
Immune system
   garlic and, 262
   shark cartilage and, 262
Immunologic disorders, frozen shoulder and, 75
Impingement
   acromiohumeral, 77
   Bower's hemiresection and, 63
   rotator cuff tendon, management of, 74
   shoulder, rehabilitation of, 74
   shoulder taping and, 236-237
Impingement syndrome, at shoulder, 73-74
Impulses, neurons and, 37
Inclusion cyst, 111
Index finger, sensory loss after brachial plexus injury, 47
Indocin, 252
Indomethacin, 252
   calcium soft-tissue deposition and, 62
Infection
   antimicrobial therapy and, 101
   cellulitis, 100
   chlorhexidine gluconate, 102
   collar button, 100
   dog bites and, 101
   felon, 100
   food supplements for, 262
   hand, *Mycobacterium marinum* and, 101
   heat and, 101
   Hibiclens, 102
   hydrogen peroxide and, 102
   immobilization and, 101
   intermittent compression pumps and, 209
   joint mobilization and, 234

Infection—cont'd
   lymphangitis, 100
   management of, 102
   povidone-iodine and, 102
   pus and, 100
   retrograde massage and, 101
   saline and, 102
   wound, 97-105
      bacterial contamination level and, 99-100
Infectious disease, Hansen's disease, 45
Inflammation
   bovine cartilage and, 262
   corticosteroids and, 252
   flaxseed and, 262
   frozen shoulder and, 75
Infraspinatus muscle
   in rotator cuff, 71
   suprascapular nerve innervation in, 45
Injection injuries, high-pressure, 100-101
Innervation
   density, 32
   median nerve, 40
   proprioceptive, posterior interosseous nerve and, 60
   radial nerve, 42
      order of, 42
   suprascapular nerve and, 45
   ulnar nerve, 42-43, 43
Insomnia, corticosteroids and, 252
Instability
   carpal, triscaphe joint fusion and, 63
   carpal instability dissociative, 58
   dorsal intercalated segment, scapholunate dissociation and, 57
   dorsiflexion, 57
   multidirectional, shoulder taping and, 236-237
   palmarflexion, 57
   shoulder, nonoperative treatment of, 79

Interferential electrical stimulation, frozen shoulder and, 76
Interossei, 41
   actions of, 27
   dorsal: *see* Dorsal interossei
   palmar: *see* Palmar interossei
Interosseous muscle, location of, 15
Interosseous nerves: *see* Anterior interosseous nerve; Posterior interosseous nerve
Interosseous wiring, proximal interphalangeal joint fracture-dislocation, 126-127
Interphalangeal joints, 13
   distal: *see* Distal interphalangeal joint
   extension of, lumbrical muscles and, 22
   paradoxical extension of, 21
   proximal: *see* Proximal interphalangeal joint
   thumb
      flexion of, 44
      Froment sign and, 44
   volar plate and, 22
Interposition grafts
   arteries in, 10
   veins in, 10
Intersection syndrome, 222
   symptoms of, 240
Interval scale of measurement, 245
Intraarticular fracture, proximal interphalangeal joint, 126
Intrafascicular environment, perineurium and, 38-39
Intramedullary device, 124
Intrinsic mechanisms, 15-23
Intrinsic minus hand deformity, treatments for, 175-176
Intrinsic muscles
   cross transfers, 21
   ulnar

Intrinsic muscles—cont'd
    ulnar—cont'd
        paralyzed, 175-176
        rheumatoid arthritis and, 21
    wasting of, 39
Iodine test, 33
Iontophoresis, 215
    neuromas and, 44
    setting up treatment, 215-216
Ipsilateral Horner's syndrome, 44
Iron, 261
Irritability, corticosteroids and, 252
Ismelin, 253
Isograft, 90
Isokinetic exercise, 239
Isotoner gloves, 91
Isotonic exercise
    concentric contraction and, 238
    constant loading and, 238
    eccentric contraction and, 238
    plyometric loading, 238
    variable loading, 238

J

Jamar dynamometer, handle position on, 29
Jeanne sign, 44
Jebsen hand function test, 28
Jersey finger, 163
Job safety
    eyeglasses and, 241
    personal protective equipment and, 241
Job-site analysis
    cumulative trauma disorder and, 229
    force measurement during, 230
Jobst compression pump, contraindications for, 210
Jobst pressure garment, edema and, 83

Joint capsule
    accessory collateral ligament and, 22
    tightness of, 17
Joint contractures, serial splinting for, stress relaxation and, 178
Joint disease, degenerative: see Degenerative joint disease
Joint dislocation, distal radioulnar, radial head fracture and, 58
Joint injury, proximal interphalangeal, volar plate damage and, 120
Joint mobilization, 233-240
    accessory movements in, 233-234
    after burn injury, 88
    benefits of, 234
    constant force in, 180-181
    contraindications for, 234
    convex-concave rule, 233
    crepitation during, 79
    distraction prior to, 235
    dorsal glide in, 235
    physiological movements in, 233-234
    positioning during, 234
    precautions for, 234
    shoulder external rotation and, 235
    volar glide, 236
Joint protection
    muscle strength and, 132
    pain and, 132
    principles of, 132
    range of motion maintenance and, 132
    rheumatoid arthritis and, 239
Joint replacement, complication rates of, 142
Joints: see also specific joint
    acromioclavicular
        injury to, 76
        shoulder limitations after injury, 76-77
    carpometacarpal

Joints—cont'd
    carpometacarpal—cont'd
        carpometacarpal boss of, 108
        osteoarthritis assessment, 28
    distal interphalangeal
        active extension of, 20
        functional flexion of, 116
        hyperextension of, 16
        isolated flexion of, 16
        longitudinal arch and, 177
    distal radioulnar, triangular fibrocartilage complex and, 53
    dynamic splinting of, 179-180
    glenohumeral
        osteoarthritis of, 79
        shoulder abduction and, 71
        stability of, 6
    immobilization of, static splinting, 179
    internal derangement of, 236
    interphalangeal, 13
        paradoxical extension of, 21
    metacarpophalangeal, 13
        contraction of, in Dupuytren's disease, 110
        flexion during scleroderma treatment, 133
        functional flexion of, 116
        longitudinal arch and, 177
        proximal interphalangeal joint flexion and, 19
        rotation of, 44
        splinting of, 183
        splinting of contractures, 183
    motor function loss, dynamic splinting and, 179-180
    proximal interphalangeal
        camptodactyly and, 196
        central tendon rupture and, 16

Joints—cont'd
    proximal interphalangeal—cont'd
        extension of, 16
        flexion of, 16
        fracture-dislocation of, 126-127
        functional flexion of, 116
        intrinsic tightness in, 19
        longitudinal arch and, 177
        palmar plate stability and, 19-20
        splinting for dorsal dislocation of, 183
        stiffness of, 114
    scaphoid, trapezium, trapezoid, fusion of, 63
    static splinting of, 179
    subluxation of, 134
    triscaphe, fusion of, 63
Juncturae tendinum, 160

K

Kaltenborn's technique, 235
Kaltostat dressing, 103
Kanavel, cardinal signs of, 101
Keflex, 252
Kefzol, 252
Keloid scar, 86, 99
Kelp, 262
Kenalog, 252
Kerlix dressing, 103
Ketoprofen, 252
Ketorolac, 252
Key pinch, ulnar nerve palsy and, 176
Kidney dysfunction, intermittent compression pumps and, 209
Kienböck's disease, 58
    etiology of, 59
    signs of, 59
    treatment options for, 60
    triscaphe joint fusion and, 63
Kirner's deformity, 193, 194
Kirschner pins, disadvantages of, 124
Kirschner wires, 123

Kirschner wires—cont'd
    proximal interphalangeal joint fracture-dislocation, 126-127
Kleinert protocol, 158
    dynamic traction and, 164
Klumpke palsy, brachial plexus and, 48
Krukenberg procedure, 199
K-wires: *see* Kirschner wires

L

Labral tear, clunk test and, 73
Labrum
    shoulder stability and, 6
    superior, biceps tendon and, 74-75
Lacertus fibrosus: *see* Bicipital aponeurosis
Lactated Ringer's solution, 102
Lactobacillus bifidus, 262
Landsmeer's ligament, 12
Lasso technique, clawing in ulnar nerve palsy and, 176
Lateral antebrachial cutaneous nerve, 37
Lateral bands, 16
    location of, 15
    subluxation in swan-neck deformity, 18
    subluxation of, 16
Lateral epicondylitis
    air casts for, 224
    tendon injury in, 223
    testing for, 227
    wrist immobilization splint for, 223
Lateral pinch, ulnar nerve palsy and, 176
Latissimus dorsi
    action of, 14
    innervation of, 71
    paralysis after brachial plexus injury, 47
    shoulder extension and, 70
Leeches, 253
Leprosy: *see* Hansen's disease

Lesions
    supraganglionic, ipsilateral Horner's syndrome and, 44
    traction, of brachial plexus, 44
Lesser tubercle, subscapularis and, 11
Levator scapulae
    innervation of, 71
    strengthening, thoracic outlet syndrome and, 80-81
    strengthening of, 39
Levers in human body, 169
Lidocaine
    corticosteroids and, 252
    phonophoresis and, 206
Ligaments: *see also* specific ligament
    accessory collateral, 22
    acromioclavicular
        injury to, 76
        shoulder limitations after injury, 76-77
    anterior inferior glenohumeral, 75
    arcuate, 219
    check rein, 2
    Cleland's, 5
    collateral, splinting of, 22
    coracoacromial, coracoacromial arch and, 71
    coracoclavicular, 70
    Grayson's, 5
    injuries in wrist
        arthrography and, 65
        diagnosing, 65
    Landsmeer's, 12
    lunotriquetral
        ballottement test and, 60
        carpal instability dissociative and, 58
    medial collateral, elbow dislocation and, 117
    oblique retinacular, 12
        tightness of, 16-17
    Osborne's, 219

Ligaments—cont'd
  palmar oblique, flexor carpi radialis tendon in reconstruction of, 140
  proper collateral, 22
  radioscapholunate, 55
  role of, 12
  scapholunate
    carpal instability dissociative and, 58
    Watson's test and, 61
    wrist ganglion and, 109
  scapholunate interosseous, dorsal wrist ganglion and, 56
  of Struthers, pronator syndrome and, 231-232
  tension stress in, 169
  of Testut, 55
  transverse retinacular, rupture of, 22
  triangular, 219
    boutonniere deformity and, 16, 22
    location of, 15
    rupture of, 22
  ulnar collateral, gamekeeper's thumb and, 121
Light touch, Semmes-Weinstein monofilament classification and, 30
Limb
  protection, after brachial plexus injury, 48
  residual, desensitization of, 197
  seal, 195
Linburg's sign, 2
  assessment for, 2
Linburg's syndrome, 2
Lipomas, 108
  of wrist, 56
Lipoproteins, myelin, 38
Lippman test, 72
Lister's tubercle, 10-11
Lodine, 252
Long extensor tendon, 15
Lorcet, 251
Lortab, 251

Lovenox, 253
LT: see Lunotriquetral
Lumbrical muscles, 21, 41
  interphalangeal joint extension and, 22
  location of, 15
  median nerve and, 40
  metacarpophalangeal joint flexion and, 22
  role of in hand, 22
  tendon and, 22
Lunate
  compression of, 59
  Kienböck's disease and, 58, 60
  shear stress of, 59
Lunate dislocation, 66
Lunate fracture, frequency of, 54
Lunotriquetral coalition, 53-54
Lunotriquetral fusion, flexion loss after, 67
Lunotriquetral ligament
  ballottement test and, 60
  carpal instability dissociative and, 58
Lunula, 12
Lymphangitis, 100
Lymphatic channel obstruction, intermittent compression pumps and, 209
Lymphedema, intermittent compression pumps and, 209

M

Maceration, 104
Macrodactyly, 193
Macrophages, growth factors in tissue repair and, 99
Madelung's deformity, 193, 194
  ulnar impaction syndrome and, 64
Maffucci's syndrome, 110, 193, 196
Magnesium, 261
Magnetic resonance imaging

Magnetic resonance imaging—cont'd
  ligament injuries in wrist and
  shoulder evaluation, 77
  SLAP lesion detection, 74-75
Maitland's technique, 234, 235
Malignancy, joint mobilization and, 234
Malignant tissue, ultrasound and, 207
Mallet finger
  bone avulsion and, 20
  extensor tendon and, 20
  swan-neck deformity and, 19-20
  terminal tendon and, 20
  treatment of, 125-126
Malrotation
  assessment of, 118
  metacarpal shaft fracture and, 118
Manganese, 261
Manipulation
  frozen shoulder and, 76
  Purdue pegboard for assessment, 28
Manual muscle testing
  after tendon transfer, 171
  contraindications to, 26
  muscle contraction and, 26
  Scott's grading system for, 26
  triceps muscle, 26
  Trombly's grading system for, 26
Marcaine, corticosteroids and, 252
Martin-Gruber anastomosis, prevalence of, 3
Massage
  frozen shoulder and, 76
  ice
    indications for, 213
    lateral epicondylitis and, 213
  retrograde
    edema and, 83
    infection and, 101

Massage—cont'd
  ulnar nerve repair and, 45
Masse sign, 44
McCarron-Dial vocational rehabilitation system, 238
McCash open-palm technique, Dupuytren's disease and, 111
McGill pain assessment questionnaire, 33
Meal preparation, basal joint pain and, 238-239
Mechanical advantage, 167
Medial collateral ligament, elbow dislocation and, 117
Medial epicondyle, muscle anatomy of, 10
Medial epicondylitis, 223
  management of, 223
  splinting for, 186
Median artery, 6
Median cubital vein, 8
Median nerve, 1, 4
  abductor pollicis brevis and, 40
  abductor pollicis brevis innervation by, 27
  anatomy of, 40
  anterior interosseous nerve and, 42
  brachial plexus and, 40
  compression, Phalen's sign and, 33
  flexor carpi radialis and, 40
  flexor digitorum profundus and, 40
  flexor digitorum superficialis and, 40
  flexor pollicis brevis and, 40
  flexor pollicis longus and, 40
  in forearm, 48
  injury
    256-Hertz vibration and, 36
    late-phase re-education after, 36
    sensory return sequence after, 37

Median nerve—cont'd
  injury—cont'd
    tactile gnosis after, 30
    tendon transfer for, 173
    Weber two-point discrimination test and, 32
  innervation, 40
  laceration, muscle return after, 40
  lumbricals and, 40
  Martin-Gruber anastomosis and, 3
  opponens pollicis and, 40
  palmaris longus and, 40
  palmaris longus innervation by, 27
  palsy
    Camitz technique for opposition in, 176
    finger flexion in, tendon transfer in, 172
    Huber technique for opposition in, 176
    Royle-Thompson technique for opposition in, 176
  pronator quadratus and, 40
  pronator teres and, 40
  terminal branches of, 41
  testing status of, 27
  in wrist, 40
Medications, in hand therapy, 251-258, 255-258
Medicine administration, phonophoresis and, 206
Medrol, 252
Meissner's corpuscles, 35
  moving two-point discrimination and, 36
  tuning fork and, 36
Mennel's technique, 235
Meperidine, 251
Merkel cells, 35-36, 36
  constant touch perception, 36
Mesocapsule, ligament of Testut, 55
Metacarpal arch, 44

Metacarpal fracture, immobilization and, 120-121
Metacarpal heads, distal transverse arch and, 177
Metacarpal shaft fracture
  angulation and, 118
  Galveston brace for, 182
  malrotation and, 118
Metacarpals, boxer's fracture and, 113
Metacarpophalangeal joints, 13
  arthroplasty, 21
    flexion outrigger and, 139
    lateral pinch after, 139
    postoperative therapy, 138
    range-of-motion goals for, 139
  extensor tendon stabilization in, 20
  first, arthrodesis of, for basal joint arthritis, 140
  flexion
    longitudinal arch and, 177
    lumbrical muscles and, 22
    scleroderma treatment and, 133
  functional flexion of, 116
  neck of, boxer's fracture and, 116
  proximal interphalangeal joint flexion and, 19
  reconstruction, cross-intrinsic transfer for, 137
  rotation of, 44
  Silastic arthroplasty indications, 137
  splinting, 183
    in rheumatoid arthritis, 137
  volar plate of, 20
Metaphysis, 114
Methadone, 251
Methyldopa, 253
Methylprednisolone, 252
Metronidazole, 252
Microvascular surgery
  Nifedipine and, 253
  replantation and, 104-105
Middle phalanx, 17
  fracture of, 16-17

Minerals, 261
Minipress, 253
Minnesota rate of manipulation test, 28
MMT: see Manual muscle testing
Moberg pick-up test, 29-30, 31
Mobile wad of Henry, 11
Mobilization
　joint: see Joint mobilization
　passive, tendon therapy and, 159
　soft-tissue, 237
Modalities: see Treatment modalities
Monofilament testing, protective sensation and, 26
Monteggia lesion, 118
Morphine, 251
Motion, immediate active, after tendon repair, 161
Motor neurons, 37
　ventral horn of spinal cord and, 37
Motor re-education, Moberg pick-up test and, 29-30
Motrin, 252
Mottling, after nerve injury, 45-46
Moving two-point discrimination, Meissner's corpuscles and, 36
MRI: see Magnetic resonance imaging
MS Contin, 251
Muenster socket, below-elbow amputee and, 200
Multiple sclerosis, tremor control in, 217
Muscle atrophy, "fracture disease" and, 57
Muscle contraction
　manual muscle testing and, 26
　resting length in, 167-168
Muscle fibers
　extensor carpi radialis longus and, 3
　sarcomere and, 168

Muscle movement, neuromas and, 44
Muscle tension, 170
　Blix curve and, 172
Muscle tissue
　potassium content, 40
　sarcomere and, 168
Muscle tissues, viscoelasticity of, 170
Muscle wasting
　immersion injuries and, 84
　reflex sympathetic dystrophy and, 143
Muscles: see also specific muscle
　abductor pollicis brevis
　　innervation of, 6
　　median nerve and, 40
　　median nerve testing and, 27
　abductor pollicis longus, posterior interosseous nerve and, 42
　adductor pollicis, innervation of, 6
　anconeus, radial nerve and, 42
　brachialis, insertion of, 11
　brachioradialis
　　radial nerve and, 42
　　wad of Henry and, 11
　coracobrachialis
　　action of, 14
　　innervation of, 71
　　insertion of, 11
　crossing wrist, grip strength and, 171
　definition of, 9
　deltoid
　　action of, 14
　　axillary nerve and, 45
　　dermatome covering, 45
　　paralysis after brachial nerve injury, 47
　　paralysis after brachial plexus injury, 47
　　shoulder extension and, 70
　denervation of, electrical stimulation current, 215

Muscles—cont'd
　extensor carpi radialis brevis
　　paralysis after brachial plexus injury, 47
　　radial nerve and, 42
　　strength of, 171
　　wad of Henry and, 11
　extensor carpi radialis longus
　　paralysis after brachial plexus injury, 47
　　radial nerve and, 42
　　sustained work and, 171
　　wad of Henry and, 11
　extensor carpi ulnaris, posterior interosseous nerve and, 42
　extensor digiti minimi, posterior interosseous nerve and, 42
　extensor digitorum communis
　　posterior interosseous nerve and, 42
　　return after brachial plexus injury, 42
　extensor indicis muscle, innervation of, 6
　extensor indicis proprius
　　posterior interosseous nerve and, 42
　　radial nerve testing and, 27
　extensor pollicis brevis, posterior interosseous nerve and, 42
　extensor pollicis longus
　　posterior interosseous nerve and, 42
　　rupture after distal radius fracture, 62
　flexor carpi radialis, median nerve and, 40
　flexor carpi ulnaris, 171
　　strength of, 171
　　ulnar nerve and, 42-43
　　ulnar nerve in forearm and, 48
　flexor digitorum profundus
　　anterior interosseous nerve and, 42

Muscles—cont'd
  flexor digitorum profundus—cont'd
    median nerve and, 40
    return after median nerve injury, 40
    ulnar nerve and, 42-43
  flexor digitorum superficialis, median nerve and, 40
  flexor pollicis brevis, median nerve and, 40
  flexor pollicis longus
    anterior interosseous nerve and, 42
    median nerve and, 40
  healing, manual muscle testing and, 26
  infraspinatus
    in rotator cuff, 71
    suprascapular nerve innervation in, 45
  interosseous, location of, 15
  intrinsic, wasting of, 39
  latissimus dorsi
    action of, 14
    innervation of, 71
    paralysis after brachial plexus injury, 47
    shoulder extensors and, 70
  levator scapulae
    innervation of, 71
    strengthening of, 39
  lumbrical, 22
    location of, 15
  lumbricals, median nerve and, 40
  manual testing of: *see* Manual muscle testing
  opponens pollicis, median nerve and, 40
  palmaris brevis, innervation of, 6
  palmaris longus
    median nerve and, 40
    median nerve testing and, 27
  pectoralis major, insertion of, 11

Muscles—cont'd
  pectoralis minor, action of, 14
  pronator quadratus
    anterior interosseous nerve and, 42
    innervation of, 6
    median nerve and, 40
  pronator teres, median nerve in forearm and, 48
  return after brachial plexus injury, 42
  rhomboid major, dorsal subscapular nerve and, 70
  rhomboid minor, dorsal subscapular nerve and, 70
  of rotator cuff, 71
  scalene, stretching of, 39
  serratus anterior
    scapular winging and, 69
    strengthening of, 39
  shoulder girdle, 39
  subclavius, innervation of, 71
  subscapularis
    innervation of, 71
    insertion of, 11
    in rotator cuff, 71
  supinator
    radial nerve and, 42
    radial nerve in forearm and, 48
  supraspinatus
    insertion of, 11
    in rotator cuff, 71
    suprascapular nerve innervation in, 45
  teres major, shoulder extension and, 70
  teres minor
    in rotator cuff, 71
    shoulder extension and, 70
  trapezius, action of, 14
  triceps
    radial nerve and, 42
    shoulder extension and, 70
    in wad of Henry, 11

Musculocutaneous nerve, coracobrachialis muscle and, 71
Musculoskeletal disorders, NSAIDs and, 251
Musculoskeletal pathology, musicians and, 39
Musculoskeletal tissue, healing of, continuous passive motion and, 212-213
Musicians, musculoskeletal pathology and, 39
Mycobacterium marinum, hand infection and, 101
Myelin, 38
Myofascial therapy, stretch and spray technique in, 237
Myositis ossificans, 110
Myotester, muscle group strength and, 203

N

Nabumetone, 252
Nafcillin, 252
Nail: *see* Fingernail
Nail bed, 13
Nail plate, 13
Nalbuphine, 251
Nalfon, 252
Naprosyn, 252
Naproxen, 252
Naproxen sodium, 252
Narcotic analgesics, 251
Neoprene glove, cold injury and, 84
Neosporin, pin care in external fixation device, 104
Nerve block, stellate ganglion, 149-150
Nerve compression
  at cubital tunnel, 227
  median, 33
Nerve conduction, neuropraxic injury and, 43
Nerve entrapment, radial sensory, 226
Nerve fibers, 38

Nerve fibers—cont'd
　　Pacinian corpuscle and, 35
Nerve growth factor, Schwann cells and, 38
Nerve injury
　　axonotmesis, 43
　　brachial, C5/C6 damage after, 47
　　median, late-phase re-education after, 36
　　neuropraxia, 43
　　neurotmesis, 43
　　peripheral
　　　　axonotmesis, 43
　　　　neuropraxia, 43
　　　　neurotmesis, 43
　　posterior interosseous, 60
　　Seddon classification of, 43
　　sensory return sequence after, 37
　　sympathetic dysfunction after, 45-46
　　sympathetic nervous system and, 45-46
　　ulnar
　　　　functional outcome after repair, 45
　　　　modalities after repair, 45
　　　　protective techniques after repair, 45
　　　　range of motion after repair, 45
　　　　splinting after repair, 45
　　　　splinting for, 176
　　Wallerian degeneration and, 43
Nerve regeneration
　　after digital nerve repair, 46
　　connective tissue and, 44
　　to fingertips, after repair at wrist, 47
　　neuroma and, 44
　　sensations during, 34
　　Tinel's sign and, 33
　　ulnar, after injury, 42-43
Nerve repair
　　regeneration to fingertips after, 47
　　Tinel's sign as indicator, 33

Nerve root injury, Klumpke palsy and, 48
Nerve roots
　　C5/C6, Erb's palsy and, 51
　　C5/C6 damage after brachial nerve injury, 47
Nerve supply, reflex testing and, 25
Nerve tissue, potassium content, 40
Nerves: see also specific nerve
　　anterior interosseous
　　　　distal radial shaft fracture fixation and, 125
　　　　flexor digitorum profundus, 42
　　　　flexor pollicis longus, 42
　　　　injury to, 42
　　　　pronator quadratus and, 42
　　　　volar wrist capsule and, 42
　　axillary
　　　　injury to, 70
　　　　shoulder abduction and, 72
　　cervical, subclavius muscle and, 71
　　digital, sensory return after injury, 46
　　dorsal scapular, levator scapulae muscles and, 71
　　dorsal subscapular, rhomboid major/minor muscles and, 70
　　epineurium and, 38
　　fascicles and, 38
　　to fingernail, 13
　　Hansen's disease and, 45
　　injury to: see Nerve injury
　　innervation of: see Innervation
　　lateral antebrachial cutaneous, 37
　　median, 1, 4
　　　　abductor pollicis brevis and, 40
　　　　abductor pollicis brevis innervation by, 27
　　　　anatomy of, 40

Nerves—cont'd
　　median—cont'd
　　　　anterior interosseous nerve and, 42
　　　　brachial plexus and, 40
　　　　compression of, 33
　　　　flexor carpi radialis and, 40
　　　　flexor digitorum profundus and, 40
　　　　flexor digitorum superficialis and, 40
　　　　flexor pollicis brevis and, 40
　　　　flexor pollicis longus and, 40
　　　　in forearm, 40, 48
　　　　lumbricals and, 40
　　　　Martin-Gruber anastomosis and, 3
　　　　muscle return after injury to, 40
　　　　opponens pollicis and, 40
　　　　palmaris longus and, 40
　　　　palmaris longus innervation by, 27
　　　　pronator quadratus and, 40
　　　　pronator teres and, 40
　　　　tactile gnosis after injury to, 30
　　　　terminal branches of, 41
　　　　testing status of, 27
　　musculocutaneous, coracobrachialis muscle and, 71
　　neuroma-in-continuity and, 44
　　peripheral
　　　　in forearm, 48
　　　　Hansen's disease and, 45
　　　　Seddon classification of injury, 43
　　　　Sunderland's injury classification, 38
　　posterior interosseous
　　　　abductor pollicis longus and, 42
　　　　extensor carpi ulnaris and, 42

Nerves—cont'd
  posterior interosseous—cont'd
    extensor digiti minimi and, 42
    extensor digitorum communis and, 42
    extensor indicis proprius and, 42
    extensor pollicis brevis and, 42
    extensor pollicis longus and, 42
    injury of, 60
    innervation and, 60
    radial nerve and, 42
    symptoms of injury, 222
  radial
    anatomy of, 42
    anconeus and, 42
    assessing function of, 25
    brachial plexus injury and, 42
    brachioradialis and, 42
    extensor carpi radialis brevis and, 42
    extensor carpi radialis longus and, 42
    extensor indicis proprius and, 27
    in forearm, 48, 225
    forearm and, 42
    humerus and, 42
    innervation of, 42
    motor and sensory branches of, 42
    posterior interosseous nerve and, 42
    supinator and, 42
    terminal branches of, 41
    testing status of, 27
    triceps and, 42
    wrist drop and, 173
  subscapular, subscapularis muscle and, 71
  suprascapular
    in brachial plexus, 45
    shoulder abduction and, 72
    shoulder capsule and, 45

Nerves—cont'd
  sympathetic, changes after injury, 45-46
  thoracodorsal, latissimus dorsi and, 71
  ulnar
    anatomy of, 42-43
    brachial plexus and, 42-43
    clawing in, 176
    distal humerus fracture and, 127
    in forearm, 48
    functional outcome after repair, 45
    handlebar palsy and, 227
    immobilization after repair, 44-45
    innervation, 43
    Martin-Gruber anastomosis and, 3
    paralysis of, 44
    regeneration after injury, 42-43
    reinnervation after injury, 44-45
    sensory re-education after repair of, 44-45
    terminal branches of, 41
    testing status of, 27
Nervous system
  central
    astroglia in, 38
    oligodendrocytes in, 38
  peripheral, Schwann cells in, 38
  sensory neurons in, 37
  sympathetic, functions mediated from, 45-46
Neural gliding, thoracic outlet syndrome and, 50-51
Neural pathways, reflexes and, 26
Neural tension test, 31
Neuralgia, amitriptyline and, 253
Neuroanatomy, 35-50
Neuroma-in-continuity, 44
Neuromas
  muscle movement and, 44
  regenerating axons and, 44

Neuromas—cont'd
  regenerating nerves and, 44
  scar tissue and, 44
  tendon movement and, 44
  treatment of, 44
Neuromuscular electrical stimulation, reflex sympathetic dystrophy and, 146
Neurons
  motor, 37
    ventral horn of spinal cord and, 37
  sensory, 37
    axon of, 37
    cell body of, 37
Neurontin, 253
Neuropathy, compression, 193
Neuropraxic injury, 43
  axonal continuity and, 43
  conduction block and, 43
  nerve conduction and, 43
  prognosis of, 43
Neuroreceptive afferents, 36
Neurotmesis, 43
Neurovascular bundle, 5
  Cleland's ligament and, 6
Niacin, 260
Nicoderm CQ, 254
Nicorette gum, 254
Nicotine, 253-254
Nicotrol, 254
Nifedipine, 253
Ninhydrin test, 31
NMES: *see* Neuromuscular electrical stimulation
No man's land, 155
Nodule, Dupuytren's disease and, 107
Nominal scale of measurement, 245
Nonsteroidal antiinflammatory drugs, 251-252
  frozen shoulder and, 76
  osteoarthritis management, 134
  side effects of, 252
Norgesic, 254
Normiflo, 253

NSAIDs: *see* Nonsteroidal anti-inflammatory drugs
Nubain, 251
Null hypothesis, 249
Numbness
  of little finger, 39
    during nerve regeneration, 34
  neural tension test and, 31
Nuprin, 252
Nutcracker effect, 59
Nutrition, 259-262
  food supplements, 262
  minerals required, 261
  vitamins required, 260

O

Obesity, osteoarthritis and, 133
Object recognition, after median nerve injury, 36
Oblique retinacular ligament, 12
  joint blocking exercises, 17
  reconstruction of, 19-20
  stretching exercises for, 17
  tightness of, 16-17
  treating, 17
Obstetric palsy, C5/C6 nerve roots and, 51
Occupational Safety and Health Administration, 241-244
  biomedical waste precautions and, 242
  blood exposure reporting, 243-244
  hazard exposure and, 241
  personal protective equipment and, 241
  sharps disposal precautions and, 242
Occupational therapy, frozen shoulder, 76
Oedema: *see* Edema
Ofloxacin, 252
Olecranon fossa, 25
Olecranon fracture, wound after casting, 103

Oligodendrocytes, in central nervous system, 38
Ollier disease, 110
Open reduction internal fixation
  both bone forearm shaft fractures, synostosis and, 125
  pilon fractures and, 127
Opponens digiti minimi, 41
Opponens pollicis, 41
  median nerve and, 40
Opposition, 4
  abductor pollicis brevis and, 4
Opposition transfer, methods of, 172-173
Ordinal scale of measurement, 245
Orgaran, 253
ORIF: *see* Open reduction internal fixation
ORL: *see* Oblique retinacular ligament
Orphenadrine, 254
Orudis, 252
Osborne's band, 219
OSHA: *see* Occupational Safety and Health Administration
Osseous demineralization, reflex sympathetic dystrophy and, 145
Ossification, heterotopic bone, after elbow fracture, 129
Ossification center, 114
Osteoarthritis
  basal joint pain and, 238-239
  cartilage thickness in, 133
  of glenohumeral joint, 79
  grind test for assessment, 28
  joint pain in, 133
  NSAIDs and, 252
  pharmacologic management of, 134
  risk factors in, 133
  short opponens splint for, 189

Osteophytes
  degenerative joint disease and, 62
  radiographic evaluation of, 62
Osteoporosis
  bone mass loss and, 117
  corticosteroids and, 252
  detection in reflex sympathetic dystrophy, 145
  "fracture disease" and, 57
  reflex sympathetic dystrophy and, 143
Otoform, 240
Oxaprozin, 252
Oxycodone, 251

P

P1: *see* Proximal phalanx
P2: *see* Middle phalanx
P3: *see* Distal phalanx
Pacinian corpuscles, 35-36
  median nerve injury and, 36
  tuning fork and, 36
Padding
  closed-cell, 178
  open-cell, absorbency of, 178
Pain
  assessment of
    McGill questionnaire for, 33
    Schultz questionnaire for, 33
    visual analog scale and, 33
  flaxseed and, 262
  "fracture disease" and, 57
  free endings and, 35
  gate-control theory and, 210
  during nerve regeneration, 34
  nocturnal, carpal tunnel syndrome and, 221
  perception, assessment of, 31
  pillar, 231
  posterior interosseous nerve injury and, 60
  receptors, location of, 37

Pain—cont'd
  reflex sympathetic dystrophy and, 143, 145
  sensory return after nerve injury, 37
  tolerance, in rheumatoid arthritis, 132
Pallor, 14
  Raynaud's phenomena and, 84
Palmar crease, distal, splinting and, 177-178
Palmar fibromatosis, 107
  reflex sympathetic dystrophy and, 145
Palmar interossei, actions of, 27
Palmar oblique ligament, flexor carpi radialis tendon in reconstruction of, 140
Palmar plate stability, 19-20
Palmar tilt, in wrist, 55
Palmaris brevis, 41
  innervation of, 6
Palmaris longus, 1, 13, 41
  carpal tunnel in, 1
  median nerve and, 40
  tendon transfer for radial nerve palsy and, 174
Palsy
  Erb's, C5/C6 nerve roots and, 51
  handlebar, 227
  median nerve
    Camitz technique for opposition in, 176
    Huber technique for opposition in, 176
    Royle-Thompson technique for opposition in, 176
  radial nerve
    splint for, 190-191
    standard tendon transfers for, 174
    supination in, 173-174
    wrist extension restoration after, 173, 174
  ulnar nerve

Palsy—cont'd
  ulnar nerve—cont'd
    Froment's sign and, 175
    function loss after, 176
    key pinch loss after, 176
    lasso technique for clawing in, 176
    lateral pinch loss after, 176
    proficient grip loss after, 176
    Riche Cannieu anastomosis and, 175
    tip pinch loss after, 176
Pantothenic acid, 260
Papillary ridges, fingerprints and, 12
Paradoxical extension, 21
Paraffin wax, temperature of, 209
Paralysis
  muscular, brachial plexus injury and, 47
  ulnar nerve, 44
Parameters, statistics and, 248-249
Paronychia, 12, 100
Patella, 55
PCL: see Collateral ligaments, proper
Pectoralis major
  insertion of, 11
  strengthening, thoracic outlet syndrome and, 80-81
Pectoralis minor
  action of, 14
  strengthening, thoracic outlet syndrome and, 80-81
  stretching of, 39
Pectoralis muscle, strengthening of, 74
Pedicle, 89
Penetrating injury, inclusion cyst and, 111
Penicillin V, 252
Pentazocine, 251
Pen-Vee K, 252
Percocet, 251

Percodan, 251
Percussion, Tinel's sign and, 33
Perilunate dislocation, 66
Perineural fibrosis, posterior interosseous nerve injury and, 60
Perineurium, 38
  function of, 38-39
Peripheral nerve diseases, Hansen's disease, 45
Peripheral nerves
  brachial nerve injury and, 47
  in forearm, 48
  Hansen's disease and, 45
  injury
    classification, 43
      Seddon's, 43
      Sunderland's, 43
    Seddon classification of, 43
    Sunderland's classification of, 38
Peripheral nervous system, Schwann cells in, 38
Persantine, 253
Personal protective equipment, 241
  biomedical fluid disposal, 242
  eyeglass safety, 241
  skin tears and, 243
  vomit cleanup, 243
Phalanx
  distal: see Distal phalanx
  middle: see Middle phalanx
  proximal: see Proximal phalanx
Phalen/Miller tendon transfer, 173
Phalen's sign, median nerve compression and, 33
Phantom limb sensation, 197-198
Phantom pain, treatment of, 198
Phenoxybenzamine, 253
Phentolamine, 253
Phocomelia, 193, 195
Phonophoresis, 206
Phosphorus, 261

Physical therapy, frozen shoulder, 76
Physiology, of cell excitability, 40
Piano-key sign, 136
Pillar pain, 231
Pillow, thoracic outlet syndrome and, 51
Pilomotor activity, reflex sympathetic dystrophy and, 145
Pilomotor function, 39, 51
   sympathetic nervous system mediation of, 45-46
Pilon fractures, dynamic traction and, 127
PIN: see Posterior interosseous nerve
Pin care, in external fixation device, 104
Pinch
   key, loss after ulnar nerve palsy, 176
   lateral
      after metacarpophalangeal arthroplasty, 139
      loss after ulnar nerve palsy, 176
   tip, loss after ulnar nerve palsy, 176
Piroxicam, 252
Pisiform, 1
   fracture of, frequency of, 54
   as sesamoid bone, 55
   transverse carpal ligament and, 3
Pitting edema, reflex sympathetic dystrophy and, 143
PL: see Palmaris longus
Plaster of Paris, 186
Plastofit, 186
Platelets, growth factors in tissue repair and, 99
Pneumatic compression device, edema treatment and, 83
Poirier, space of, 8
Polydactyly, 193, 195
   incidence of, 193-194

Posterior interosseous nerve
   abductor pollicis longus and, 42
   extensor carpi ulnaris and, 42
   extensor digiti minimi and, 42
   extensor digitorum communis and, 42
   extensor indicis proprius and, 42
   extensor pollicis brevis and, 42
   extensor pollicis longus and, 42
   injury, 60, 222
   supinator and, 42
Postinfarctional sclerodactyly, 150-151
Posttraumatic dystrophy, 150-151
Postural correction exercise, rotator cuff impingement and, 74
Potassium, 261
   level in cells, 40
   in muscles, 40
   in nerves, 40
Pourfour del petit syndrome, 150-151
Povidone-iodine, 102
Prazosin, 253
Prednisone, 252
Pregnancy, ultrasound and, 207
Prehension
   below-elbow amputee and, 200
   loss of, 16
Preiser's disease, ulnar translation of carpus and, 66
Pressure, constant-touch, 36
Pressure garments, 91
Primary adhesive capsulitis, 75
Priscoline, 253
Probability, 249
Procardia, 253
Profundus, 21
Pronation

Pronation—cont'd
   after triangular fibrocartilage complex peripheral tear, 64
   ulnar rotation and, 67
Pronator quadratus, 41
   anterior interosseous nerve and, 42
   innervation of, 6
   median nerve and, 40
Pronator syndrome
   compression sites for, 231-232
   pronator teres and, 231-232
Pronator teres, 41
   median nerve and, 40
   median nerve in forearm and, 48
   tendon transfer for radial nerve palsy and, 174
Propoxyphene, 251
Prostaglandin synthesis, NSAIDs and, 251
ProStep, 254
Prosthetics, 193-203
   above-elbow, terminal device opening, 201
   below-elbow, Muenster socket and, 200
   body-powered terminal device and, 202
   functional use training, 203
   myoelectric, 201-202, 203
   optimal time for fitting, 198
   pediatric cookie crusher, control system for, 201-202
   radioulnar limb-deficient child, optimal fitting time, 198-199
   silicone, radial head fracture and, 58
   terminal devices
      Hosmer-Dorrance voluntary opening hook, 202
      transradial amputation, 203
Protective sensation, 26

Protective sensation—cont'd
  Semmes-Weinstein monofilament classification and, 30
Protective techniques, ulnar nerve repair and, 45
Proximal interphalangeal joint arthroplasty, treatment of, 138
  bony enlargements of, 134
  Bouchard's nodes, 134
  boutonnière deformity and, 16
  camptodactyly and, 196
  central tendon rupture and, 16
  contracture of, 31-32
  dorsal dislocation
    splinting of, 120
    volar plate damage and, 120
  extension of, 16
  fixed contracture of, serial casting for, 185-186
  flexion contracture of, 2
    after proximal phalanx fracture, 115
  flexion of, 16
    longitudinal arch and, 177
  fracture-dislocation of, treatment after arthrodesis, 126-127
  functional flexion of, 116
  intraarticular fracture of, 126
  intrinsic tightness in, 19
  palmar plate stability and, 19-20
  paradoxical extension of, 21
  stiffness of, 114
  torque angle curve of, 31-32
Proximal joints, position during TROM measurement, 32
Proximal phalanx, 17
  comminuted fracture of, treatment for, 126
  complications of fracture, 115
  fracture

Proximal phalanx—cont'd
  fracture—cont'd
    range of motion after fixation of, 121
    treatment options, 138
  oblique fracture of, 125
  ulnar intrinsic rerouting and, 21
Pseudoarthrosis, Suave-Kapandji procedure and, 63
Pseudogout, radiographic evaluation of, 62
Psychological issues, brachial plexus injury and, 48
PT: *see* Pronator teres
Pterygium cubital, 195
Ptosis, 44
Pulley ring splint, 190-191
Pulleys, flexor tendons and, 14
Pulse duration, 213
Pupil contraction, 44
Purdue pegboard, 28
Pus, 100
Pyogenic granuloma, 108
Pyridoxine, 260

Q

Quadrangular space, 7
Quadrigia phenomenon, 9

R

Radial artery
  Allen's test for evaluation, 26-27
  anatomic snuffbox and, 7
Radial deviation, measuring, 27-28
Radial head
  capitulum and, 11
  dislocation, proximal ulna fracture and, 118
  excision, complications after, 128
  fracture
    adjustment after treatment plateau, 128-129

Radial head—cont'd
  fracture—cont'd
    distal radioulnar joint dislocation and, 58
    management of, 58
    silicone prosthesis for, 58
Radial inclination, in wrist, 55
Radial nerve
  anatomy of, 42
  anconeus and, 42
  brachial plexus injury and, 42
  brachioradialis and, 42
  extensor carpi radialis brevis and, 42
  extensor carpi radialis longus and, 42
  extensor indicis proprius innervation by, 27
  in forearm, 42, 48, 225
  function of, triceps reflex testing and, 25
  humerus and, 42
  innervation of, 42
  motor branch of, 42
  palsy
    splinting for, 185, 190-191
    standard tendon transfers for, 174
    supination in, 173-174
    wrist extension restoration after, 174
    wrist extension restoration and, 173
  sensory branch of, 42
  supinator and, 42
  tendon transfer, arm immobilization after, 174
  terminal branches of, 41
  triceps and, 42
  wrist drop and, 173
Radial physis, ulnar impaction syndrome and, 64
Radial sensory nerve entrapment, 226
Radial shaft fracture, distal, 117
  anterior interosseous nerve and, 125
Radial tunnel syndrome, 226
Radian, 168, 170

Radiography
    Barton's fracture and, 56
    gout and, 62
    rheumatoid arthritis and, 62
    soft-tissue calcium deposits and, 62
Radioscapholunate ligament, 55
Radioulnar joint, distal, caput ulnae syndrome and, 135-136
Radius, Lister's tubercle and, 10-11
Radius fracture, distal
    Barton's, 56
    Bower's hemiresection and, 63
    Colles,' 56
    Darrach procedure, 63
    with dorsal displacement, 56
    extensor pollicis longus and, 11
    extensor pollicis longus rupture after, 62
    palmar angulation and, 56
    reverse Colles,' 56
    Smith's, 56
    Suave-Kapandji procedure and, 63
    triangular fibrocartilage complex peripheral tear and, 64
    ulnar abutment after, 63
    ulnar impaction syndrome and, 64
    ulnar resection and, 63
    wrist extension and, 56
Range of motion
    after metacarpophalangeal arthroplasty, 139
    after proximal phalanx fracture fixation, 121
    after wrist ganglion removal, 109
    assessment
        Colles fracture and, 17
        extensor tightness, 17
        flexor tightness, 17
        joint capsular tightness, 17
    exercises

Range of motion—cont'd
    exercises—cont'd
        after biceps tenodesis, 79
        frostbite management, 85
        frozen shoulder and, 76
        reflex sympathetic dystrophy and, 147
        measuring objectivity, 31-32
        passive, after shoulder fracture, 129
        radial deviation, 28
        subacromial decompression and, 74
        torque, 31-32
        total active, 32
        ulnar deviation, 28
        ulnar nerve repair and, 45
        of wrist, 66-67
Raynaud's disease, 84
Raynaud's phenomena
    color response in, 84
    immersion injuries and, 84
    thermal biofeedback for, 84
Raynaud's syndrome, 84
    Nifedipine and, 253
    sympatholytic agents and, 253
Red wounds, 99
Re-education, sensory, treatment modalities in, 46
Reflex sympathetic dystrophy, 143-151
    after Colles' fracture, 150
    amitriptyline and, 253
    burst mode in TENS, 146
    cardinal signs of, 145
    cerebral tumor and, 144
    cerebrovascular accident and, 144
    in children, 150
    conditions associated with, 144
    continuous passive motion in, 148
    diabetes and, 144
    diagnosis of, 144
    dislocation and, 144
    Dupuytren's disease and, 112
    edema prevention in, 147

Reflex sympathetic dystrophy—cont'd
    electrodiagnostic studies of, 144
    forms of, 148
    fractures and, 144
    genetic conditions and, 144
    head injury and, 144
    idiopathic conditions and, 144
    immobilization and, 144
    infection and, 144
    length of stages in, 144
    major traumatic category of, 144-145
    malignancies and, 144
    medications and, 144
    minor traumatic category of, 144-145
    myocardial infarction and, 144
    nerve blocks necessary for, 150
    neuromuscular electrical stimulation and, 146
    Nifedipine and, 253
    osteoporosis detection in, 145
    pain evaluation in, 149
    pain from touch in, 147
    range-of-motion exercises and, 147
    shoulder-hand dystrophy and, 148
    signs of, 112
    soft-tissue injury and, 144
    spinal cord injury and, 144
    splinting in, 146
    stages of, 143
    stellate ganglion nerve block, 149-150
    stress-loading program for, 148
    stress-loading program in, 147
    sympathetic blockade in, 149
    sympatholytic agents and, 253
    thermal biofeedback for vasodilation in, 146

Reflex sympathetic dystrophy—cont'd
   treatment of, 147
   triple-phase bone scan and, 144
Reflex testing
   biceps, 25
   brachioradialis, 25
   C5 assessment, 25
   C6 assessment, 25
   C7 assessment, 25
   nerve supply integrity and, 25
   radial nerve function and, 25
Reflexes
   definition of, 26
   neural pathways and, 26
Regenerating nerves
   connective tissue and, 44
   neuroma and, 44
Regitine, 253
Rehabilitation
   after cubital tunnel release, 228
   after wrist arthroplasty, 142
   BTE tools and, 238
   carpal tunnel syndrome and, 225
   hand, drugs of abuse and, 253-254
   medications used in, 251-258
   postsurgical shoulder, 73
   shoulder impingement, 74
   trigger finger, 220
Reinnervation
   after ulnar nerve injury, 44-45
   Tinel's sign as indicator of, 33
Relafen, 252
Reperfusion, postischemic, 119
Replant failure
   congestion and, 102
   source of, 102
Replantation, 104-105
Research, 245-250
   alternative hypothesis, 250
   clinical services and, 249-250
   confidence level, 250
   correlation coefficient, 248

Research—cont'd
   dependent variables in, 248
   experimental hypothesis and, 249
   interrater variability in, 250
   intrarater variability in, 250
   knowledge base and, 249-250
   null hypothesis, 250
   null hypothesis and, 249
   reliability, 250
   scales of measurement, 245
   standard deviation and, 247
   validity, 250
Resection, ulnar, distal radius fracture and, 63
Reserpine, 253
Residual limb pain, 197-198
Resources
   internet sites, 271-273
   vendors, 265-268
Retinacular ligaments
   oblique: see Oblique retinacular ligament
   transverse: see Transverse retinacular ligaments
Retrograde massage
   edema and, 83
   infection and, 101
Retroposition, 62
Reverse Bennett's fracture, 122-123
Reverse Colles' fracture, 56
Rheobase, 214-215
Rheumatoid arthritis
   adaptive equipment education, 239
   bovine cartilage and, 262
   caput ulnae syndrome and, 135-136
   collapse deformity of thumb, 131
   extensor pollicis longus in, 11
   extensor tendon of little finger in, 135
   extensor tendon rupture in, 136-137
   extensor tendon subluxation in, 136-137

Rheumatoid arthritis—cont'd
   flexor pollicis longus tendon rupture in, 135
   grip strength and, 134-135
   joint protection and, 239
   joint protection principles and, 132
   metacarpophalangeal joint splinting in, 137
   metacarpophalangeal joint treatment in, 137
   NSAIDs and, 252
   pain tolerance in, 132
   pattern of deformity in, 136
   position changes in, 132
   radial nerve palsy and, 136-137
   radiographic evaluation of, 62
   Raynaud's phenomenon and, 84
   resting hand splint positioning, 185
   sleep recommendations in, 132
   synovium and, 131
   total wrist arthrodesis and, 141
   trigger finger and, 219-220
   ulnar drift of fingers, 136
   ulnar intrinsic tightness, 21
   wrist, radial deviation and, 141
Rhomboid major, dorsal subscapular nerve and, 70
Rhomboid minor, dorsal subscapular nerve and, 70
Rhomboids, strengthening, thoracic outlet syndrome and, 80-81
Riboflavin, 260
Riche Cannieu anastomosis, ulnar nerve palsy and, 175
Ringer's solution, lactated, 102
Rocephin, 252
Rolando's fracture, 122
   treatment of, 122

Rolling, 233-234
Rosenbusch test of finger dexterity, 28
Rotation
    forearm, 129
    metacarpophalangeal joint, 44
Rotator cuff
    humeral elevation and, 71
    muscles of, 71
    strengthening
        multidirectional shoulder instability and, 79
        shoulder impingement and, 74
    supraspinatus and, 72
    tear
        acromion shape and, 72-73
        arthroscopy and, 80
        drop-arm test for, 72
        surgical treatment of, 77
        tendon impingement, management of, 74
    weakness, shoulder impingement syndrome and, 73-74
Roxanol, 251
Royle-Thompson tendon transfer, 173
    opposition in median nerve palsy, 176
RSD: see Reflex sympathetic dystrophy
Ruffini corpuscles, 35
Ruffini end organs, 35
    constant touch perception, 36
Rule of nines, 85

S

Safety precautions, sharps disposal, 242
Sagittal plane, definition of, 11-12
Salicylate, 252
Saline, 102
Sarcomas, of wrist, 56
Sarcomere, 168

Sarmiento fracture brace, 187, 190-191
Scalene muscles, stretching of, 39
Scaphoid
    blood supply to, 7
    fracture
        evaluation of, 62
        frequency of, 54
        healing of, 54
        radiographic evaluation, 62
    Preiser's disease and, 66
    trapezium, trapezoid joint, fusion of, 63
Scaphoid tubercle, 1
Scaphoid tuberosity, transverse carpal ligament and, 3
Scapholunate dissociation, dorsal intercalated segment instability and, 57
Scapholunate gap, 57
Scapholunate interosseous ligament, dorsal wrist ganglion and, 56
Scapholunate ligament
    carpal instability dissociative and, 58
    Watson's test for assessment, 61
    wrist ganglion and, 109
Scapula
    coracoclavicular ligament and, 70
    retractors of, 70
    winging of, 69
Scapular rotator, strengthening, shoulder impingement and, 74
Scapulohumeral rhythm, 69
Scar
    elongation, ultrasound frequency for, 208
    hypertrophic, 86
        etiology of, 86-87
    keloid, 86, 99
    maturation, pressure for reduction of, 91

Scar management
    continuous pressure, 239
    otoform, 240
    products for, resource list of vendors, 265-268
    silicone gel sheeting and, 239-240
    Tubigrip and, 239-240
Scar tissue, neuroma development and, 44
Schultz pain assessment questionnaire, 33
Schwann cells
    location of, 38
    nerve growth factor and, 38
Sclerodactyly, postinfarctional, 150-151
Scleroderma
    CREST syndrome and, 132-133
    metacarpophalangeal joint flexion and, 133
    Raynaud's phenomenon and, 84
Scott's grading system, 26
Sea cucumber, 262
Sea mussel, 262
Seddon classification, 43
Self-review, 275
Semipermeable film dressing, 103
Semmes-Weinstein monofilaments, 26
    color coding of, 30
    constant-touch pressure and, 36
    filament thickness and, 30
    threshold testing and, 31
Sensation
    lack of, during nerve regeneration, 34
    loss of
        after digital nerve repair, 46
        after skin graft for burn wound, 90
        C8 nerve root damage and, 50
        Klumpke palsy and, 48

Sensation—cont'd
　loss of—cont'd
　　thumb, after brachial plexus injury, 47
　　protective, Semmes-Weinstein monofilament classification and, 30
　　recovery after brachial plexus injury, 48
Sensibility, Moberg pick-up test and, 29-30
Sensory nerve, kelp and, 262
Sensory neuron, cell body location, 37
Sensory perception
　Dellon two-point discrimination testing, 31
　moving two-point discrimination testing, 31
　neural tension test, 31
　protective, 26
　Semmes-Weinstein monofilaments and, 26
　static two-point discrimination testing, 31
　Weber two-point discrimination testing, 31
Sensory receptors
　Merkel cells and, 36
　Pacinian corpuscle, 35
　sequence of return, 37
Sensory re-education, 26, 35-50
　after ulnar nerve repair, 44-45
　Moberg pick-up test and, 29-30
　treatment modalities for, 46
Sensory return, sequence of, 37
Sepsis, wound, bacterial contamination level, 99-100
Serpasil, 253
Serratus anterior, strengthening of, 39
Sesamoid bone
　patella and, 55
　pisiform and, 55
Shaft fractures, 116
Shark cartilage, 262

Sharps disposal, 242
Shear fractures, serial splinting for joint contractures and, 178
Shear stress, 167, 169
Shortening, ulnar, distal radius fracture and, 63
Shoulder, 69-81
　abduction, glenohumeral joint and, 71
　abduction inhibition, 72
　acromioclavicular joint injury, 76
　adhesive capsulitis of, ultrasound treatment, 76
　Adson maneuver, 80
　amputation at, upper extremity impairment, 197
　anterior inferior glenohumeral ligament and, 75
　anterior instability of, 72
　apprehension test and, 72
　arthrogram evaluation of, 77
　assessment after brachial plexus injury, 47-48
　assessment of, 72
　axillary nerve injury and, 70
　biceps tenodesis, range-of-motion exercises after, 79
　biomechanics of, 71
　capsular pattern for, 75-76
　Codman exercises, 75
　crank test and, 72
　dislocation of, Bankart lesion and, 75
　drop-arm test, 72
　external rotation of, after Bankart lesion repair, 75
　fracture, passive range of motion after, 129
　frozen, 75
　　manipulation of, 76
　　shoulder taping and, 236-237
　　therapy for, 76
　Halstead maneuver, 80

Shoulder—cont'd
　Hawkins-Kennedy impingement test, 72
　home exercise program after, 78
　humeral head depression, 72
　impingement, rehabilitation of, 74
　impingement syndrome, 73-74
　injury, Codman's exercises and, 78
　latissimus dorsi and, 70
　Lippman test and, 72
　multidirectional instability of, nonoperative treatment of, 79
　postsurgical rehabilitation, 73
　primary adhesive capsulitis, 75
　proximal humeral fracture, 78
　scapular winging, 69
　serratus anterior muscle paralysis and, 69
　SLAP lesion repair, 74-75
　stability of, 6
　supraspinatus tendon tear and acromiohumeral impingement, 77
　thoracic outlet syndrome, treatment of, 80-81
Shoulder capsule, suprascapular nerve and, 45
Shoulder girdle muscles, strengthening of, 39
Shoulder taping, goals of, 236-237
Shoulder-hand dystrophy, 148
Shoulder-hand syndrome, 150-151
Shroud fibers/sagittal bands, extensor tendons in metacarpophalangeal joint and, 20
Sigmoid notch, impingement at, Bower's hemiresection and, 63

Silastic arthroplasty, in metacarpophalangeal joint, indications for, 137
Silicon, 261
Silicone gel sheeting, scar management and, 239-240
Silicone prosthesis, radial head fracture and, 58
Silicone tendon implant, 161
Silver nitrate, hypergranulation tissue and, 210
Siris Swan-Neck Silver Ring Splint, 18
Skeletal abnormalities, congenital, 193
Skier's thumb injury, long opponens splint and, 188
Skin
   atrophy, reflex sympathetic dystrophy and, 143
   color, sympathetic nervous system mediation of, 45-46
   color changes, 39
      Raynaud's phenomena and, 84
   discoloration, reflex sympathetic dystrophy and, 145
   full-thickness burns of, 86
   glabrous
      Merkel cells and, 36
      Ruffini end organs and, 36
      sensory receptors in, 35
   graft, dorsal hand reconstruction, 89
   hairy
      constant touch perception, 36
      Ruffini end organs and, 36
   Hansen's disease and, 45
   healed, strength of, 99
   hypertrophic scarring, 86
      etiology of, 86-87
   keloid scar, 86

Skin—cont'd
   lesion, 108
   nonelasticity of, after nerve injury, 45-46
   nonhairy, sensory receptors in, 35
   Pacinian corpuscle and, 35
   pain receptors in, 37
   partial-thickness burns of, 86
   redness after cold therapy, 206-207
   sensory neuron axon and, 37
   superficial burns of, 86
   temperature, sympathetic nervous system mediation of, 45-46
   temperature receptors in, 37
   texture, sympathetic nervous system mediation of, 45-46
   trophic changes, reflex sympathetic dystrophy and, 143
Skin grafts
   allograft, 90
   autograft, 90
   dorsal hand reconstruction, 89
   failure of, 89
   full-thickness
      contracture of, 92
      dermofasciectomy and, 110
      palmar wounds and, 92
   full-thickness groin, 93
   hematoma and, 89
   heterograft, 90
   isograft, 90
   pressure therapy and, 90-91
   splinting for contractures after, 90
   split-thickness, 89
      burn of dorsum of hand, 89
      contracture of, 92
   split-thickness hypothenar, 93
   xenograft, 90
S-L ligament: *see* Scaphoid-lunate ligament

SLAP lesion, 74-75
Sleep, rheumatoid arthritis and, 132
Sling, thoracic outlet syndrome and, 51
Smith's fracture, 56
SNS: *see* Sympathetic nervous system
Snuffbox: *see* Anatomic snuffbox
Sodium, 261
   level in cells, 40
Soft tissue
   atrophy, sympathetic nervous system mediation of, 45-46
   contractures of, static splinting and, 179
   injury, reflex sympathetic dystrophy and, 144
   mobilization, 237
   tumors of, in children, 112
Space of Poirier, 8
Spasticity, manual muscle testing and, 26
Spinal cord
   injury, reflex sympathetic dystrophy and, 144
   kelp and, 262
   ventral horn of, 37
Spinning, 233-234
Splinting, 177-191
   accessory collateral ligament and, 22
   after capsulectomy for metacarpophalangeal joint contractures, 184
   anterior interosseous nerve syndrome, 228-229
   basal joint pain and, 238-239
   boxer's fracture and, 117
   carpal tunnel syndrome and, 224
   collateral ligament injuries, 22
   contractures after skin graft and, 90
   cubital tunnel syndrome, 228
   de Quervain's disease, 222

Splinting—cont'd
  decreasing pressure areas in, 182
  distal palmar crease and, 177-178
  dorsal dislocation, 183
  dorsal dislocation of proximal interphalangeal joint of long finger, 183
  dorsal hand burn, 88
  Dupuytren's contracture and, 108-109
  dynamic
    forces for, 179
    goals of, 179-180
  extension block, 126
  extensor carpi ulnaris subluxation, 224
  extrinsic flexor tightness and, 184
  first web space contracture, 186
  forearm trough length, 178-179
  frostbite management, 85
  golfer's elbow, 186
  high-profile outriggers in, 180
  humeral shaft fracture and, 187
  immobilization
    after flexor tendon repair, 161
    digits after trauma, 182
  lateral epicondylitis, 184-185, 223
  low-profile outriggers in, 180
  medial epicondylitis, 186
  metacarpophalangeal joint, 183
    in rheumatoid arthritis, 137
  metacarpophalangeal joint contractures, 183
  neuromas and, 44
  open-cell padding in, 178
  pressure areas and, 180

Splinting—cont'd
  proper collateral ligament and, 22
  proximal interphalangeal joint contracture, 32
  proximal interphalangeal joint dorsal dislocation, 120
  proximal interphalangeal joint flexion contracture, 181
  proximal interphalangeal joint fracture-dislocation, 126-127
  radial nerve palsy, splinting for, 185
  in reflex sympathetic dystrophy, 146
  securing Velcro in, 179
  serial, stress relaxation and, 178
  skier's thumb injury, 188
  static
    goals of, 179
    MERIT component in, 180
  static progressive, 181
    metacarpophalangeal joint contractures, 183
  tennis elbow and, 184-185
  triangular fibrocartilage complex tear, 67
  triquetral avulsion fracture and, 66
  ulnar nerve injury and, 176
  volar wrist, lateral epicondylitis and, 184-185
  Wartenberg's disease and, 226
Splints: *see also* specific type
  budding strapping, 190-191
  chlorine in cleaning, 179
  cutting away in pressure areas, 181-182
  dorsal finger, 183
  flaring around radial styloid, 180
  Futuro wrist, 62

Splints—cont'd
  Galveston brace, metacarpal shaft fracture and, 182
  long opponens, thumb positioning in, 188
  mallet finger with bone avulsion, 20
  padding of, 180
  pulley ring, 190-191
  radial nerve palsy, 190-191
  redness after removal, 180
  resource list of vendors, 265-268
  resting hand, positioning of for rheumatoid arthritis, 185
  Sarmiento fracture brace, 187, 190-191
  short opponens, 189
  for swan-neck deformity, 18
  thermoplastic figure-of-eight, 18
  ulnar deviation, 190-191
  ulnar nerve injury, 190-191
Sports injuries
  hamate fracture and, 123
  Jersey finger, 163
Sprain, 9
Stabilization, radial head fracture and, 58
Stadol, 251
Standard deviation, 247
Staphylococcus
  cellulitis and, 100
  paronychia and, 100
Static friction, description of, 168
Static two-point discrimination, 31
  constant-touch pressure and, 36
Statistics, 245-250
  β level, 249
  α level, 249
  bell curve in, 247
  central tendency and, 246
  dependent variables in, 248
  experimental hypothesis, 249
  gaussian distribution, 247

Statistics—cont'd
   independent variable and, 249
   normal distribution, 247
   null hypothesis and, 249
   parameter, 249
   parameters and, 248-249
   probability, 249
   range and, 247
   standard deviation, 247
   T test, 249
   type-I error, 249
   type-II error, 249
Stellate ganglion nerve block, therapy after, 149-150
Stener's lesion, 121
Stereognosis, sensory return after nerve injury, 37
Steroid injections, neuromas and, 44
Stiffness, reflex sympathetic dystrophy and, 143
Strain, 9, 169
Strain gauge, torque range of motion and, 32
Strengthening exercises, thoracic outlet syndrome and, 39, 80-81
Stress, 167
   compression, 169
   osteoarthritis and, 133
   shear, 167, 169
   tension, 169
Stress relaxation
   definition of, 169
   serial splinting for joint contractures and, 178
Stress-loading program, in reflex sympathetic dystrophy, 148
Stretching exercises, heat application before, 169-170
Struthers, ligament of, pronator syndrome and, 231-232
STT: *see* Scaphoid, trapezium, trapezoid

Styloid, radial, Chauffeur fracture and, 65
Suave-Kapandji procedure, 63
   pseudoarthrosis and, 63
Subacromial decompression, range of motion after surgery, 74
Subclavius muscle, innervation of, 71
Subluxation, 134
   extensor carpi ulnaris, 224
   of lateral bands, 16
   shoulder taping and, 236-237
   in swan-neck deformity, 18
Subscapular nerve, subscapularis muscle and, 71
Subscapularis
   innervation of, 71
   insertion of, 11
   in rotator cuff, 71
   strengthening, thoracic outlet syndrome and, 80-81
Sudeck's atrophy, 150-151
Sudomotor changes, reflex sympathetic dystrophy and, 145
Sudomotor function, 31, 39
   iodine test and, 33
   sympathetic nervous system mediation of, 45-46
Sulfur, 261
Sulindac, 252
Sunderland's classification, 43
Sunderland's peripheral nerve injury classification, 38
Superficial palmar arch, 6
Superior labrum anterior to posterior lesion, 74-75
Supination
   after triangular fibrocartilage complex peripheral tear, 64
   biceps brachii and, 173-174
   ulnar rotation and, 67
Supinator, 4, 41
   radial nerve and, 42

Supinator—cont'd
   radial nerve in forearm and, 48
Supracondylar fracture, cubitus varus and, in child, 127
Supraganglionic lesion, ipsilateral Horner's syndrome and, 44
Suprascapular nerve
   in brachial plexus, 45
   shoulder abduction and, 72
   shoulder capsule and, 45
Supraspinatus muscle
   insertion of, 11
   in rotator cuff, 71
   rotator cuff and, 72
   suprascapular nerve innervation in, 45
Supraspinatus tendinitis, 72
   ultrasound treatment of, 208
Supraspinatus tendon, tear of, 77
Surgical procedures/techniques
   arthroscopy, subacromial decompression, 74
   Bower's hemiresection, 63
   boxer's fracture and, 113
   compartment syndrome, 103, 119
   crossed-intrinsic transfer, for metacarpophalangeal joint reconstruction, 137
   Darrach procedure, 63
   fasciotomy for compartment syndrome, 119
   high-pressure injection injuries and, 100-101
   Jersey finger, 163
   lunotriquetral fusion, flexion loss after, 67
   proximal interphalangeal joint fracture-dislocation, 126-127
   radius and ulna fractures of forearm, 125
   rotator cuff repair, 80
   rotator cuff tear, 77
   silicone tendon implant, 161

Surgical procedures/techniques—cont'd
 Suave-Kapandji procedure, 63
 triscaphe joint fusion and, 63
 ulnar resection, 63
Swallowtails, 2
Swan-neck deformity
 mallet finger and, 19-20
 metacarpophalangeal arthroplasty and, 138
 splinting, 18
 subluxation of lateral bands in, 18
 transverse retinacular ligament rupture and, 22
Sweat, 39
 loss of, 44
 sympathetic nervous system mediation of, 45-46
Swelling
 psoriatic arthritis and, 135
 reflex sympathetic dystrophy and, 145
Sympathetic blockade, 149
Sympathetic dysfunction, treatment for, 45-46
Sympathetic nervous system
 changes after nerve injury, 45-46
 functions mediated from, 45-46
Sympathetic return, iodine test and, 33
Sympatholytic agents, 253
Syndactyly, 193-194
Synostosis, both bone forearm shaft fractures and, 125
Synovial diffusion, 155
Synovium, rheumatoid arthritis and, 131
Systemic disease, sleep recommendations in, 132

T

T1 nerve root
 brachial plexus traction injury and, 44

T1 nerve root—cont'd
 Horner's syndrome and, 44
T test, 249
Tactile gnosis, 31
 after median nerve injury, 30
Talwin, 251
Taping, shoulder, goals of, 236-237
TCL: *see* Transverse carpal ligament
Tegaderm dressing, 103
Temperature
 changes in, 39
 cumulative trauma disorder and, 229-230
 receptors, location of, 37
 sensory return after nerve injury, 37
 skin, sympathetic nervous system mediation of, 45-46
Tendinitis
 bicipital, 72
 dexamethasone and, 215
 flexor carpi ulnaris, 231
 glucosamine and, 262
 golfer's elbow, splinting for, 186
 shoulder taping and, 236-237
 supraspinatus, 72
 ultrasound treatment, 208
Tendon excursion
 radians and, 170
 wrist motor muscles and, 172
Tendon glide, adhesion prevention and, 155-156
Tendon healing, 154
 extrinsic, 155
 intrinsic, 155
 length of, 154
 manual muscle testing and, 26
 tensile strength and, 154
Tendon movement, neuromas and, 44
Tendon repair
 edema and, 162
 epitenon suture in, 162

Tendon repair—cont'd
 extensor, treatment protocol for, 164-165
 flexor
  finger and wrist positions during active motion, 161-162
  immobilization splinting after, 161
  tenolysis after, 165
 flexor digitorum superficialis, dynamic traction of fingers and, 164
 immediate active motion and, 161
 silicone implant, 161
 suture techniques in, 156
 tensile strength after, 157
Tendon transfer, 167-176
 finger flexion in median nerve palsy and, 172
 flexor pollicis longus after median nerve injury, 173
 manual muscle test after, 171
 opposition, methods of, 172-173
 radial nerve, arm immobilization after, 174
 radial nerve palsy and, 174
Tendons, 153-166
 abductor pollicis longus, 2
  de Quervain's disease and, 220
 adhesions after burn injury, 88
 Camper's chiasm and, 156
 central, extensor tendon subluxation and, 162-163
 exposed, dressings for, 103
 extensor
  closed injury management, 159
  mallet finger and, 20
  nutritional pathway in, 155

Tendons—cont'd
  extensor—cont'd
    subluxation, central tendon involvement and, 162-163
    synovial diffusion in, 155
    wrist ganglion and, 109
  extensor carpi radialis brevis, 2
  extensor carpi radialis longus, 2
  extensor carpi ulnaris, 2
  extensor digiti minimi, 2, 165
  extensor digitorum, 2
  extensor digitorum communis, lumbrical muscles and, 22
  extensor indicis proprius, 2, 165
  extensor pollicis brevis, 2
    de Quervain's disease and, 220
  extensor pollicis longus, 2
  extensor zones in, 153
  flexor, 13
    adhesion prevention after repair, 155-156
    blood supply to, 155
    Duran protocol for passive motion of, 158-159
    "no man's land," 155
    passive motion for treatment, 158-159
    pulleys in, 14
    repair, 158
    vincula and, 155
  flexor carpi radialis, in palmar oblique ligament reconstruction, 140
  flexor digitorum profundus
    full-fist exercise for, 159
    laceration, 158
    lumbrical muscles and, 22
  flexor pollicis longus, rupture in rheumatoid arthritis, 135
  flexor zones in, 154
  long extensor, location of, 15

Tendons—cont'd
  lumbrical muscles and, 22
  passive mobilization programs for, 159
  pulleys in thumb, 154
  supraspinatus, tear of, 77
  tensile strength after repair, 157
  tension stress in, 169
  terminal
    location of, 15
    mallet finger and, 20
    tenotomy for, 18
  triceps, radial nerve assessment and, 25
  in wrist compartment, 2-3
Tennis elbow
  splinting for, 184-185
  testing for, 227
Tenodesis, biceps, range-of-motion exercises after, 79
Tenolysis, after flexor tendon repair, 165
Tenosynovitis
  de Quervain's disease, 220
  of tendon sheath, cardinal signs of Kanavel and, 101
Tenotomy
  active range of motion after, 18
  central tendon, 19-20
  terminal tendon, 18
TENS: see Transcutaneous electrical nerve stimulation
Tensile strength, after tendon repair, 157
Tension band wiring, proximal interphalangeal joint fracture-dislocation, 126-127
Tension stress, 169
Teres major, shoulder extension and, 70
Teres minor
  quadrangular space and, 7
  in rotator cuff, 71
  shoulder extension and, 70

Terminal tendon
  location of, 15
  mallet finger and, 20
  tenotomy for, 18
Terry Thomas sign, 57
Testes, ultrasound and, 207
Testut, ligament of, 55
TFCC: see Triangular fibrocartilage complex
Thenar flaps, 94
Therapy
  after sympathetic nerve injury, 45-46
  hand
    drugs of abuse in, 255-258
    medications encountered in, 255-258
  occupational: see Occupational therapy
  physical: see Physical therapy
  pressure, after skin graft, 90-91
Thermal conditions, 83-95
  burns
    classification of, 85
    excision and grafting for, 93-94
    exercise program after, 87
    joint mobilization after, 88
    pressure therapy after, 91
    "rule of nines" and, 85
    sensory loss after, 90
    superficial heat in treatment of, 87
  chilblains, 84
  cold exposure, Hunting reaction and, 84
  cold injury
    Neoprene glove for, 84
    Raynaud's phenomenon and, 84
  frostbite, 84
    management of, 85
    rewarming after, 84-85
  immersion injuries, 84
  Raynaud's phenomena
    color response in, 84
    thermal biofeedback for, 84

Thermography, reflex sympathetic dystrophy assessment, 144
Thiamine, 260
Thoracic outlet syndrome
　Adson maneuver, 80
　exercise program for, 39
　Halstead maneuver and, 80
　neural gliding and, 50-51
　presenting symptoms of, 80
　symptoms of, 39
　tests for identification of, 80
　treatment in irritable state, 50-51
　treatment of, 80-81
Thoracoabdominal flap, 92-93
Thoracodorsal nerve, latissimus dorsi and, 71
Threshold testing, 31
Thrill, 8
Thrombus, intermittent compression pumps and, 209
Thumb
　boutonnière deformity of, 131
　grind test, 28
　hypoplastic, 197
　osteoarthritis assessment, 28
　pulleys in, 154
　rehabilitation after carpometacarpal joint implant arthroplasty, 140-141
　retroposition, 62
　sensory loss of, 47
Thumb clutched hand, 193
Ticlid, 253
Ticlopidine, 253
Tightness, intrinsic, in proximal interphalangeal joint, 19
Tinel's sign
　regenerating axons and, 46
　regeneration process and, 33
Tingling
　during nerve regeneration, 34
　neural tension test and, 31
Tip pinch, ulnar nerve palsy and, 176

Tissue
　biopsy, wound infection and, 99-100
　connective, regenerating nerves and, 44
　granulating, 104
　repair, growth factors and, 99
　scar
　　neuroma development and, 44
　　regenerating nerves and, 44
Toe, great, gout and, 107-108
Tolazoline, 253
Tomography, ligament injuries in wrist and, 65
Tophus, 108
Toradol, 252
Torque range of motion, 31-32
Touch
　constant, 36
　　after median nerve injury, 36
　　Merkel cells and, 36
　　Ruffini end organs and, 36
　　sensory re-education and, 46
　　sensory return after nerve injury, 37
　　static two-point discrimination and, 36
　light: see Light touch
　moving
　　after median nerve injury, 36
　　sensory re-education and, 46
　　sensory return after nerve injury, 37
Touch localization, sensory return after nerve injury, 37
Traction, dynamic, 126
　comminuted fracture of proximal phalanx, 126
　Kleinert protocol and, 164
　pilon fractures and, 127

Traction lesion, of brachial plexus, 44
Tramadol, 251
Transcutaneous electrical nerve stimulation
　frozen shoulder and, 76
　neuromas and, 44
　during painful procedures, 216
　in reflex sympathetic dystrophy, burst mode and, 146
Transilluminescence, dorsal wrist ganglion and, 56
Transverse carpal ligament
　anatomy of, 3
　attachment sites for, 3
Transverse deficiencies, 193
Transverse plane, definition of, 11-12
Transverse retinacular ligament
　rupture of, 22
　swan-neck deformity and, 18, 22
Trapezium
　excision, pantrapezial arthritis and, 140
　transverse carpal ligament and, 3
Trapezium fracture, frequency of, 54
Trapezium tubercle, 1
Trapezius
　action of, 14
　lower, strengthening of, 39
　middle, strengthening of, 39
　strengthening, thoracic outlet syndrome and, 80-81
　upper, stretching of, 39
Trapezoid, 123
　fracture frequency, 54
Trauma
　cumulative, 219-232
　cumulative trauma disorder: see Cumulative trauma disorder
　intersection syndrome and, 222

Trauma—cont'd
   osteoarthritis and, 133
Treatment modalities, 205-217
   after brachial plexus injury, 48
   antimicrobial therapy, infection and, 101
   cold bath, 205
   cold packs, 205
   cold therapy, 206
      lateral epicondylitis, 213
   conduction and, 205
   continuous passive motion
      contraindications for, 213
      low-load prolonged stress and, 212-213
      musculoskeletal tissue healing, 211-212
   contrast baths, 211
      edema and, 211
   conversion, 205
   electrical stimulation, pain reduction and, 216
   electromyogram feedback, tremor control, 217
   evaporation, 205
   fluidotherapy, 205
      disadvantages of, 207
      temperature of, 209
   Fluori-methane spray, 205, 209-210
   for frozen shoulder, 76
   gate-control theory of pain control, 210
   heat, infection and, 101
   high-voltage galvanic stimulation, 217
   hot pack in hydrocollator, temperature of, 209
   hot packs, 205
   ice massage, lateral epicondylitis and, 213
   immobilization, infection and, 101
   intermittent compression pumps, 206
      contraindications for, 209
   iontophoresis, 215
   paraffin wax, 205
      temperature of, 209

Treatment modalities—cont'd
   phonophoresis, 206
   pulsed ultrasound, 205
   retrograde massage, infection and, 101
   sensory re-education and, 46
   skin redness after cold therapy, 206-207
   stretch-and-spray method, 209-210
   ulnar nerve repair and, 45
   ultrasound, 205
      contraindications for, 207
      gel temperature, 208
      malignant tissue and, 207
      pregnancy and, 207
      supraspinatus tendinitis, 208
      testes and, 207
      thermal effects of, 207
      tissue temperature, 207
   whirlpool, 205
      indications for, 211
      temperature of, 209
      vascular occlusion and, 211
Tremor, electromyogram feedback for control of, 217
Triamcinolone, 252
Triangular fibrocartilage complex
   assessment of, 64
   distal radioulnar joint stability and, 53
   peripheral tear of, 64
      supination/pronation after, 64
   tear, treatment for, 67
Triangular ligament, 219
   boutonniere deformity and, 16, 22
   location of, 15
   rupture of, 22
   swan-neck deformity and, 18
Triceps
   gravity-eliminated plane, 26
   manual muscle testing of, 26
   nerve innervation, 42
   quadrangular space and, 7

Triceps—cont'd
   radial nerve and, 42
   shoulder extension and, 70
Triceps lateral head, 41
Triceps long head, 41
Triceps medial head, 41
Triceps reflex, testing of, 25
Triceps tendon, radial nerve assessment and, 25
Trigger finger, causes of, 219-220
Trigger-points, 237
   scalene, symptoms of, 240
   treatment of, 237
Triphalangism, 193
Triquetral avulsion fracture, splinting, 66
Triquetrum fracture, frequency of, 54
Triscaphe arthritis, triscaphe joint fusion and, 63
Triscaphe joint, fusion of, 63
Trochlea, 11
Trolamine salicylate, phonophoresis and, 206
TROM: see Torque range of motion
Trombly's grading system, 26
Trophic functions, 39
   sympathetic nervous system mediation of, 45-46
Trophic skin changes, reflex sympathetic dystrophy and, 143
Tubercle
   greater: see Greater tubercle
   lesser: see Lesser tubercle
Tubigrip, scar management and, 239-240
Tuft fractures, 116
Tumors, 107-112
   carpometacarpal boss, 108
   cerebral, reflex sympathetic dystrophy and, 144
   enchondroma, 108
   giant cell, 56
   lipomas, 108
      of wrist, 56
   malignant

Tumors—cont'd
   malignant—cont'd
      reflex sympathetic dystrophy and, 144
      of wrist, 56
   nerve, 108
   palmar fibromatosis, 107
   skin, 108
   soft-tissue, in children, 112
   tophus, 108
   vascular, 108
   of wrist, 56
Tuning fork
   Meissner's corpuscles and, 36
   Pacinian corpuscles and, 36
   vibratory perception testing and, 33
Two-point discrimination
   moving, 31
      Meissner's corpuscles and, 36
      sensory return after nerve injury, 37
   static, 31
      constant-touch pressure and, 36
Tylox, 251

U

Ulna
   coronoid process of, brachialis and, 11
   pronation-supination of, 67
Ulna resection, radial head fracture and, 58
Ulnar artery
   Allen's test for evaluation, 26-27
   blood supply to hand and, 6
   evaluation in hand, 26-27
Ulnar collateral ligament, gamekeeper's thumb and, 121
Ulnar deviation
   extensor carpi ulnaris and, 3
   measuring, 27-28

Ulnar deviation—cont'd
   splint for, 190-191
Ulnar drift, 21
   crossed-intrinsic transfer and, 137
Ulnar fracture, proximal, radial head dislocation and, 118
Ulnar head, piano-key sign, 136
Ulnar impaction syndrome, distal radius fracture, 64
Ulnar intrinsics
   rerouting of, 21
   rheumatoid arthritis and, 21
Ulnar nerve
   anatomy of, 42-43
   distal humerus fracture and, 127
   in forearm, 48
   functional outcome after repair, 45
   handlebar palsy and, 227
   injury
      splint for, 190-191
      splinting for, 176
   innervation, 42-43, 43
   laceration
      hook fist after, 42-43
      regeneration after, 42-43
   Martin-Gruber anastomosis and, 3
   modalities after repair, 45
   palsy
      Froment's sign and, 175
      function loss after, 176
      intrinsic minus hand deformity and, 175-176
      key pinch loss after, 176
      lasso technique for clawing in, 176
      lateral pinch loss after, 176
      proficient grip loss after, 176
      Riche Cannieu anastomosis and, 175
      tip pinch loss after, 176
   paralysis

Ulnar nerve—cont'd
   paralysis—cont'd
      Andre-Thomas sign and, 44
      Duchenne sign and, 44
      Egawa sign and, 44
      Froment sign and, 44
      Jeanne sign and, 44
      Masse sign and, 44
      Wartenberg sign and, 44
   protective techniques after repair, 45
   range of motion after repair, 45
   repair, immobilization after, 44-45
   sensory re-education after repair of, 44-45
   splinting after repair, 45
   terminal branches of, 41
   testing status of, 27
Ulnar sensory fibers, Martin-Gruber anastomosis and, 3
Ulnar variance, measuring, 58
Ultram, 251
Ultrasonography
   adhesive capsulitis of shoulder and, 76
   ligament injuries in wrist and, 65
Ultrasound, 205
   contraindications for, 207
   frequency for scar elongation, 208
   frozen shoulder and, 76
   gel temperature, 208
   malignant tissue and, 207
   neuromas and, 44
   pregnancy and, 207
   pulsed, 205
   supraspinatus tendinitis, 208
   testes and, 207
   thermal effects of, 207
   tissue temperature, 207
Unasyn, 252
Unipen, 252
Universal Precautions, 242
Uric acid, gout and, 107-108

V

Vanadium, 261
Vaplar work samples, 238
VAS: *see* Visual analog scale
Vascular compromise, replant failure and, 102
Vascular insufficiency, white finger and, 232
Vascular occlusion, whirlpool and, 211
Vasoconstriction, nicotine and, 253-254
Vasodilation, in reflex sympathetic dystrophy, thermal biofeedback for, 146
Vasomotor function, 39
  sympathetic nervous system mediation of, 45-46
Vasomotor instability, reflex sympathetic dystrophy and, 145
Vasospasm, 102
Veins: *see also* specific vein
  axillary, formation of, 10
  basilic
    axillary vein and, 10
    in forearm, 8
Velcro, securing in splints, 179
Velocity production, lumbrical muscles, 22
Vendors, resource list of, 265-268
Venous grafts, arterial reconstruction and, 10
Venous insufficiency, 14
  replant failure and, 102
Venous occlusion, anticoagulants and, 252
Ventral horn of spinal cord, cell body of motor neuron in, 37
Vibramycin, 252
Vibration, cumulative trauma disorder and, 221
Vibratory perception testing, tuning fork and, 33
Vibratory trauma

Vibratory trauma—cont'd
  digital, Raynaud's phenomenon and, 84
  white finger and, 232
Vicodin, 251
Vincula, flexor tendon blood supply and, 155
Viscoelasticity, 170
  serial splinting for joint contractures and, 178
VISI: *see* Volar intercalated segment instability
Visual analog scale, disadvantages of, 33
Vitamins, 260
Vocational rehabilitation, McCarron-Dial system for, 238
Volar flexion, after Colles' fracture, 56-57
Volar intercalated segment instability, scapholunate dissociation and, 57
Volar interosseous, first, description of, 4
Volar metacarpophalangeal joint capsulectomy, indications for, 118-119
Volar plate, 2
  accessory collateral ligament and, 22
  of metacarpophalangeal joint, 20
  posterior interphalangeal joint and, 22
  proximal interphalangeal joint, attenuation of, 18
  proximal interphalangeal joint dorsal dislocation and, 120
Volar wrist capsule, anterior interosseous nerve and, 42
Voltaren, 252
Volumeter, edema assessment, 30

Volumetry, water temperature, 33

W

Wad of Henry, muscles in, 11
Wallerian degeneration, 43
  digital nerve repair and, 46
Warfarin, 253
Wart, 108
Wartenberg sign, 44
Wartenberg's disease, 226
Waste, biomedical, 242
  contaminated dressings as, 242
Watson's test, scaphoid-lunate ligament tear, 61
Wave forms, 214
Webbed fingers, 193
Weber two-point discrimination test, 31, 32
Whirlpool, 205
  frostbite management, 85
  indications for, 211
  temperature of, 209
  vascular occlusion and, 211
White finger, vibration and, 232
Wigraine, 254
Windblown hand, 195
Work
  definition of, 169
  sustained, extensor carpi radialis longus and, 171
Work conditioning, software products for, resource list of vendors, 265-268
Wound care
  products for, resource list of vendors, 265-268
  whirlpool and, 211
Wound healing
  Adaptic dressing and, 102
  bovine cartilage and, 262
  Coban dressing and, 102
  collagen synthesis and, 98-99
  dressings for, 102
  dry sterile dressing and, 102

Wound healing—cont'd
  exudative stage of, 97
  growth factors in, 99
  high-voltage galvanic stimulation, 217
  honey and, 262
  inflammatory stage, length of, 97-98
  inflammatory stage of, 97
  lactated Ringer's solution and, 102
  lag stage of, 97
  macrophages and, 99
  nicotine and, 253-254
  platelets and, 99
  pus and, 100
  saline and, 102
  stages of, 97
  substrate stage of, 97
  wet-to-dry dressing and, 102
Wounds, 97-105
  black, 99
  chemotaxis and, 98
  classification of, 99
  collagen and, 98
  collagen synthesis after, 98-99
  dehiscence and, 98
  exudate in, 98, 99
  granulating tissue and, 104
  healed skin strength, 99
  healing of: see Wound healing
  high-level, 98
  honey and, 262
  infected, dressings for, 103-104
  infection of: see Infection; Sepsis
  keloid scar and, 99
  low-level, 98
  necrotic tissue, 99
  open, antibiotics and, 98
  open crush injury, 98
  red, 99
  replantation and, 104-105
  sepsis in: see Infection; Sepsis
  serosanguinous drainage, 99
  surgical débridement of, 99
  tidy, 98

Wounds—cont'd
  untidy, 98
  yellow, 99
Wrist, 53-67
  Andre-Thomas sign and, 44
  carpal instability, triscaphe joint fusion and, 63
  carpal instability dissociative and, 58
  carpal instability nondissociative and, 58
  Chauffeur fracture and, 65
  Colles' fracture of, 56
  distal radius fracture
    extensor pollicis longus rupture after, 62
    ulnar impaction syndrome and, 64
  dorsal compartments of, 2
  dorsal wrist ganglion in, 56
  dorsiflexion instability of, 57
  Essex-Lopresti fracture-dislocation and, 58
  extension restoration
    after radial nerve palsy, 174
    in radial nerve palsy, 173
  extensor tightness in, 17
  extensors, 3
  flexor tightness in, 17
  force at joints of, 54
  functional range of motion, 66-67
  ganglion, 109
  ganglion of, range of motion after removal, 109
  hypomobile, dorsiflexion in, 236
  instability, Darrach resection and, 63
  intersection syndrome and, 222
  joint capsular tightness, 17
  Kienböck's disease
    signs of, 59
    treatment options for, 60
    triscaphe joint fusion and, 63
  Kienböck's disease and, 58
  ligament injuries of

Wrist—cont'd
  ligament injuries of—cont'd
    arthrography, 65
    diagnosing, 65
  lipomas of, 56
  lunotriquetral fusion, flexion loss after, 67
  lunotriquetral ligament, ballottement test for, 60
  Madelung's deformity, 194
  malignant tumors of, 56
  median nerve in, 40
  median nerve innervation in, 40
  motor muscle tendinous excursion, 172
  nerve repair at, assessment of recovery after, 47
  pain, after radial head excision, 128
  palmar tilt in, 55
  palmarflexion instability of, 57
  position, during Jamar dynamometry, 29
  posterior interosseous nerve injury and, 60
  Preiser's disease and, 66
  radial deviation of, 27-28
  radial inclination in, 55
  reverse Colles' fracture of, 56
  scaphoid fracture, evaluation of, 62
  Smith's fracture of, 56
  space of Poirier and, 8
  sprain
    evaluation of, 62
    splinting, 67
    triangular fibrocartilage complex tear and, 67
  triangular fibrocartilage complex peripheral tear, 64
  supination/pronation after, 64
  triquetral avulsion fracture, splinting of, 66
  ulnar deviation, 27-28
    carpal row in, 65

Wrist—cont'd
  ulnar pronation-supination, 67
  volar flexion, 44
    after Colles' fracture, 56-57
  weakness, Darrach resection and, 63
Wrist capsule, volar, anterior interosseous nerve and, 42
Wrist drop, radial nerve injury and, 173

X

Xanthoma, 111
Xenograft, 90
Xylocaine, corticosteroids and, 252

Y

Yellow wounds, 99
Yergason test, biceps head stability and, 32-33

Z

Zancolli technique, clawing in ulnar nerve palsy and, 176
Zinc, 261
Zithromax, 252
Zostrix, 253

Chapter 1
Anatomy Extravaganza

Topics to be reviewed in random order are:

- **Origins and insertions**
- **Nerve innervations**
- **Anatomic terms**
- **Interesting anatomy facts**
- **Arteries and veins of the arm**
- **Key terms for vascularity**

1. Which structures run through the carpal tunnel? (Pick the most complete answer.)

A. Median nerve, flexor digitorum profundus, flexor digitorum superficialis
B. Median nerve, palmaris longus, flexor digitorum profundus, flexor digitorum superficialis
C. Median nerve, flexor pollicis longus, flexor digitorum profundus, flexor digitorum superficialis
D. Median nerve, flexor pollicis longus, palmaris longus, flexor digitorum profundus, flexor digitorum superficialis

The carpal tunnel contains ten structures: the median nerve, four flexor digitorum profundus tendons, four flexor digitorum superficialis tendons, and the flexor pollicis longus tendon. The carpal tunnel lies deep to the palmaris longus. Its borders are the pisiform, the scaphoid tubercle, the hook of the hamate, and the trapezium tubercle.

Answer: **C**
Hoppenfeld, p. 83
Refer to Fig. 1-1.

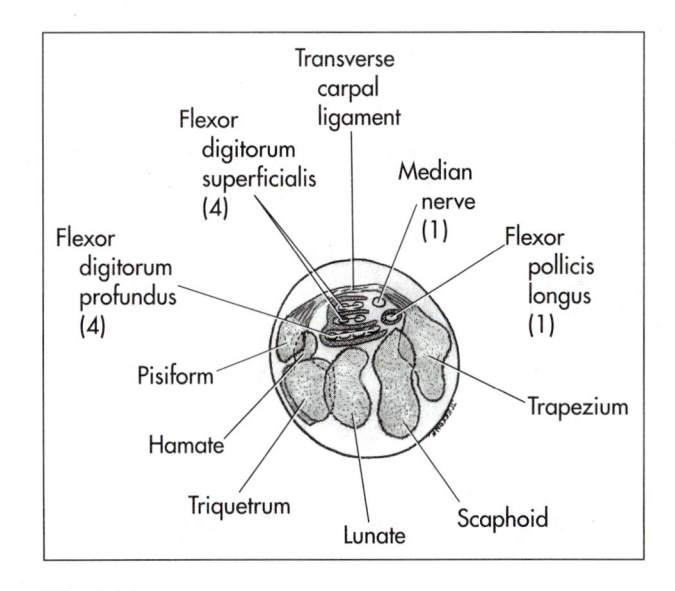

Fig. 1-1

2. An anatomic interconnection between the flexor pollicis longus and the index finger flexor digitorum profundus is called:

A. Egawa's sign
B. Linburg's sign
C. Reiter's syndrome
D. None of the above

An anatomic interconnection between the flexor pollicis longus and the index flexor digitorum profundus is present in approximately 31% of the population. The connection may be through an anomalous tendon, musculotendinous slip, or an adherence to the tenosynovium. This anatomic variation is called Linburg's **sign**.

Linburg's **syndrome** can occur when this interconnection leads to pain and aggravation with activity. The discomfort is located over the radiopalmar aspect of the distal forearm and thumb. A relationship between carpal tunnel syndrome and Linburg's syndrome has been noted in some patients.

Answer: **B**
Cooney, Linscheid, Dobyns, p. 1194

> **Clinical Gem:**
> To assess for Linburg's sign, have the patient actively flex the thumb interphalangeal joint and look for involuntary motion at the index finger distal interphalangeal joint.

3. What are the primary pathological structures that produce proximal interphalangeal joint flexion contractures?

A. Collateral ligaments of the proximal interphalangeal joint
B. Lateral bands
C. Check rein ligaments
D. Oblique retinacular ligaments

Contractures of the proximal interphalangeal joints occur after an unspecified period of time in a negative hand position (intrinsic minus). Thin fibers referred to as "swallowtails" are extensions of the volar plate at the proximal interphalangeal joint. When these swallowtails become hypertrophied and shortened, they are termed check rein ligaments. Check rein ligaments can develop rapidly after edema occurs, or progressively, as in Dupuytren's contracture.

Answer: **C**
Green, p. 550
Refer to Fig. 1-2.

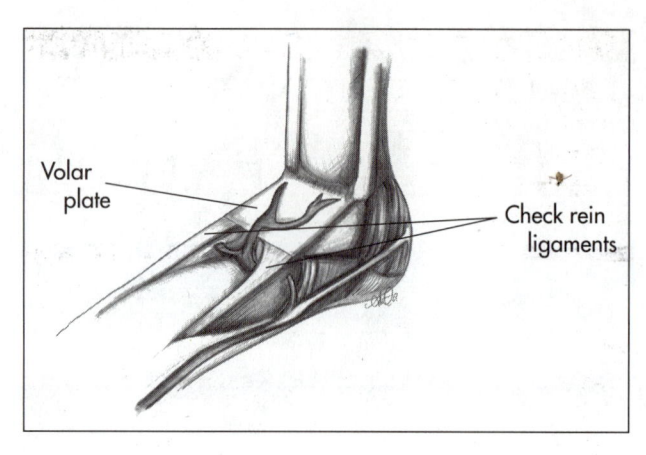

Fig. 1-2

4. Match the following dorsal wrist compartment with the tendon(s) residing in each compartment:

Compartment

1. First dorsal wrist compartment
2. Second dorsal wrist compartment
3. Third dorsal wrist compartment
4. Fourth dorsal wrist compartment
5. Fifth dorsal wrist compartment
6. Sixth dorsal wrist compartment

Tendon(s)

A. Abductor pollicis longus (APL), extensor pollicis brevis (EPB)
B. Extensor digiti minimi (EDM)
C. Extensor carpi ulnaris (ECU)
D. Extensor pollicis longus (EPL)
E. Extensor digitorum (ED); extensor indicis proprius (EIP)
F. Extensor carpi radialis longus (ECRL); extensor carpi radialis brevis (ECRB)

Answers: **1. A; 2. F; 3. D; 4. E; 5. B; 6. C**
Stanley, Tribuzi, p. 9

> **Clinical Gem:**
> To remember the dorsal compartments, it is helpful to recall the numbers 22, 12, and 11. These numbers correlate with the numbers of tendons in each of the six dorsal compartments.

Compartment	1	2	3	4	5	6
Number to recall	22	12	11			
Tendons	EPB APL	ECRL ECRB	EPL	EDC EIP	EDM	ECU

CLINICAL GEM:
To avoid confusing the fifth and sixth compartments, remember that the tendon to the fifth digit is the extensor digiti minimi (fifth digit equals fifth compartment).

5. The extensor carpi radialis brevis is the strongest wrist extensor. True or False?

The extensor carpi radialis brevis (ECRB) originates from the lateral epicondyle of the humerus and inserts onto the base of the third metacarpal. The ECRB has the longest extension moment arm, the largest cross-section, and is the strongest and most efficient wrist extensor. The extensor carpi radialis longus, in contrast, has the longest muscle fibers and the largest mass, and therefore has a greater capacity for sustained work. The extensor carpi ulnaris (ECU) has the longest moment arm for ulnar deviation. The ECU becomes a more efficient wrist extensor when the forearm is supinated.

Answer: **True**
Hunter, Mackin, Callahan, p. 523

6. All of the following serve as attachment sites for the transverse carpal ligament, except:

A. Scaphoid
B. Trapezium
C. Hamate
D. Triquetrum
E. Pisiform

The transverse carpal ligament (TCL) attaches to the scaphoid tuberosity, the crest of the trapezium, the pisiform, and the hook of the hamate. The TCL forms the roof of the carpal canal and ranges in thickness from 1 to 3.5 mm. The TCL prevents the long flexors of the fingers from bowstringing when the wrist flexes and serves as an attachment site for thenar and hypothenar muscles.

Answer: **D**
Hunter, Mackin, Callahan, pp. 905-906

7. A Martin-Gruber anastomosis is present in 35% to 45% of the population. True or False?

This anomaly is present in 15% to 20% of the population. The Martin-Gruber anastomosis is between the median nerve and the ulnar nerve at the forearm level. The anastomosis usually consists of median-nerve innervated motor fibers supplying the typically ulnar innervated intrinsics. Ulnar sensory fibers also may be innervated by the median nerve when this anastomosis exists. Refer to Figure 1-3 for a clinical example.

Answer: **False**
Kimura, p. 418
Tubiana, Thomine, Mackin, p. 277

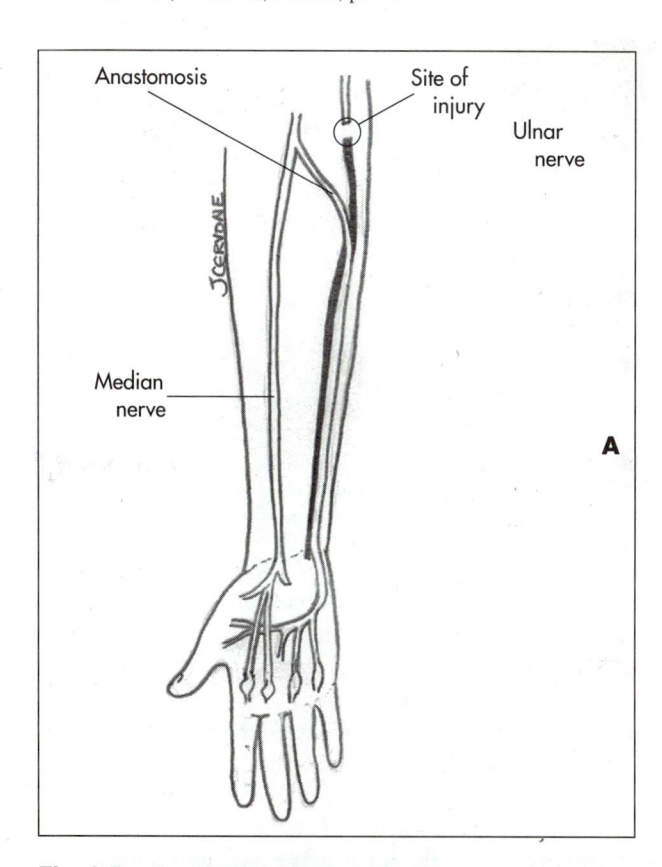

Fig. 1-3 ■ **A,** Indicates a high ulnar nerve lesion in which the anastomosis from the median to ulnar nerve occurs distal to the injury and prevents paralysis of the ulnar innervated intrinsics.

Continued

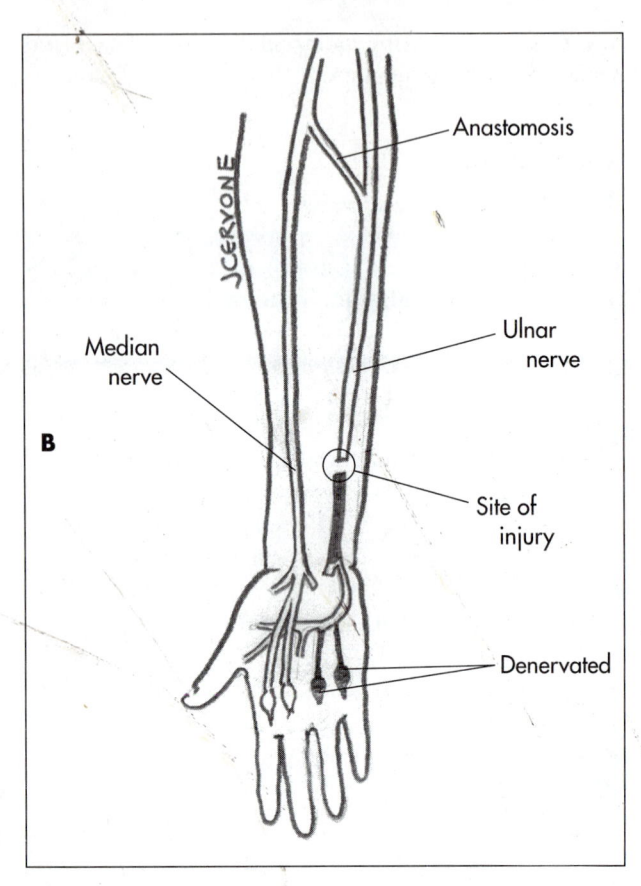

Fig. 1-3, cont'd ■ **B,** Indicates a low ulnar nerve injury distal to the anastomosis, which causes paralysis of the ulnar innervated digits.

8. Match each muscle to the correct description:

Muscle

1. Abductor pollicis brevis
2. Extensor carpi radialis brevis
3. Extensor carpi ulnaris
4. Supinator
5. Extensor pollicis longus
6. Adductor pollicis
7. First volar interosseous
8. First dorsal interosseous

Description

A. Strong finger abductor that inserts into the base of the proximal phalanx of the index
B. Innervated by the median nerve and originates from transverse carpal ligament
C. Innervated by the ulnar nerve and inserts into ulnar side of the proximal phalanx of the thumb and the extensor expansion of the thumb
D. Inserts into the base of the third metacarpal
E. Innervated by the posterior interosseous nerve (PIN) and inserts into the base of the fifth metacarpal
F. Originates from the lateral epicondyle of the humerus and the adjacent portion of the ulna and inserts into the upper one third of the radius
G. Innervated by the posterior interosseous nerve and inserts into the first distal phalanx
H. Originates from the length of the second metacarpal and adducts the index finger

Answers: 1. B; 2. D; 3. E; 4. F; 5. G; 6. C; 7. H; 8. A
Malick, Kasch, pp. 57, 58, 66

CLINICAL GEM:
The APB is the strongest muscle of anteposition (opposition). In 1867, Duchenne called the APB muscle the opposing phalangeal muscle of the thumb because of its action on the tip.

9. What is the major arterial supply to the forearm and hand?

A. Radial artery
B. Brachial artery
C. Median artery
D. Interosseous artery

The brachial artery continues from the axillary artery and travels distally along the medial arm with the median nerve nearby. At the antecubital fossa it dives below the lacertus fibrosis and splits into the radial and ulnar arteries. The brachial artery is the major inflow vessel to the forearm and hand.

Answer: **B**
Spinner, p. 203
Refer to Fig. 1-4.

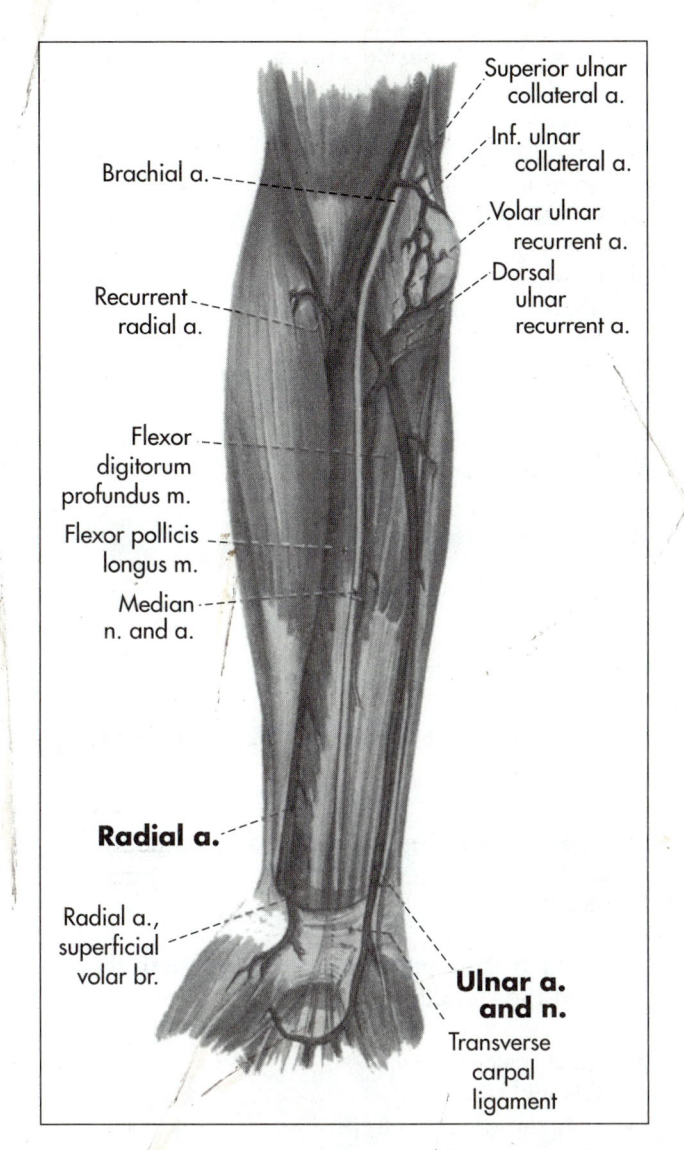

Fig. 1-4 ■ From Hunter JM, Mackin EJ, Callahan AD: *Rehabilitation of the hand: surgery and therapy,* ed 4, St. Louis, 1995, Mosby-Year Book.

10. Blood vessels require protection after surgical repair for how long?

A. 1 to 5 days
B. 7 to 14 days
C. 14 to 21 days
D. 21 to 28 days

Blood vessels require 1 to 2 weeks of protection. This is generally provided by the immobilization needed to protect other structures that are repaired.

Answer: **B**
Hunter, Mackin, Callahan, p. 1059

11. What is the combined function of Cleland's and Grayson's ligaments?

A. Prevents Dupuytren's contracture
B. Stabilizes the metacarpophalangeal joint
C. Stabilizes the basal joint
D. Prevents rotary movements of the skin around the fingers

Grayson's ligament originates from the volar aspect of the flexor tendon sheath, runs volar to the neurovascular bundle, and inserts into the skin. Cleland's ligament passes dorsal to the neurovascular bundle and inserts into the skin. According to Hoppenfeld, both Grayson's and Cleland's ligaments prevent rotary movement of the skin around the fingers, allowing the ability to grasp objects. Grayson's ligament may contribute to a proximal interphalangeal joint flexion contracture in Dupuytren's disease.

Answer: **D**
Hoppenfeld, p. 65
Green, pp. 564-565
Refer to Fig. 1-5.

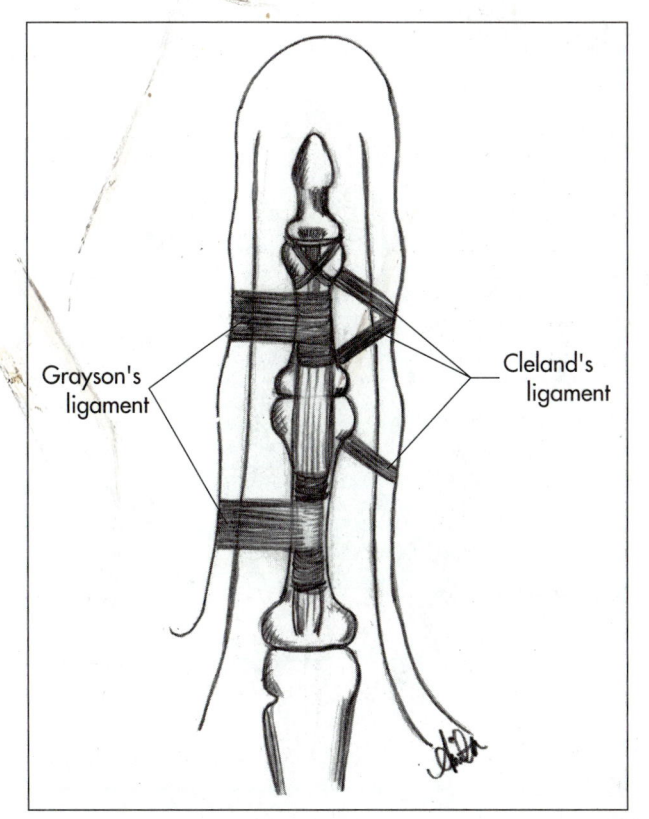

Fig. 1-5

CLINICAL GEM:
Cleland's ligaments are **d**orsal to the neurovascular bundle. One way to remember this is to recall that "C" for **C**leland precedes "D" for **d**orsal.

12. Which artery provides the primary blood supply to the hand?

A. Radial artery
B. Ulnar artery
C. Persistent median artery
D. All above arteries supply the hand equally

The ulnar artery is larger than the radial artery and usually is the primary contributor, supplying 60% of blood to the hand. This artery supplies the superficial palmar arch in most hands and the radial artery usually supplies the deep palmer arch. The median artery contributes to the superficial palmar arch in approximately 10% of the population. There is greater variation in the superficial arch whereas the deep palmar arch is more consistent. In general, arterial variations occur in up to one third of the population.

Answer: **B**
Anderson, Sec. 6-78
Refer to Fig. 1-6.

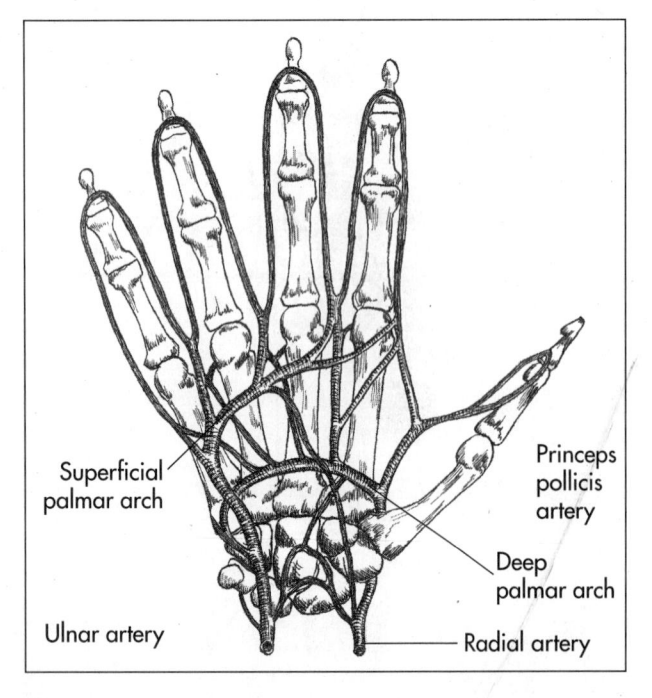

Fig. 1-6 ■ From Smith AA, Lacey SH: *Hand surgery review,* St. Louis, 1996, Mosby-Year Book.

13. Match each muscle with its innervation:

Muscle

1. Adductor pollicis
2. Brachioradialis
3. Extensor indicis proprius
4. Palmaris brevis
5. Abductor pollicis brevis
6. Pronator quadratus

Innervation

A. Superficial branch of ulnar nerve
B. Deep branch of ulnar nerve
C. Posterior interosseous nerve
D. Anterior interosseous nerve
E. Median nerve
F. Radial nerve

Answers: **1. B; 2. F; 3. C; 4. A; 5. E; 6. D**
Hunter, Mackin, Callahan, Appendix pp. A1-A40
Malick, pp. 57-66

14. Which structure plays a critical role in the stability of the shoulder?

A. Teres major
B. Glenoid labrum
C. Long head of the biceps
D. Coracoacromial ligament

The stability of the glenohumeral joint is sacrificed because of its great freedom of movement. The humeral head articulates against the glenoid cavity of the scapula. The labrum is important because it gives the glenoid a deeper cavity, allowing for increased surface area and stability. The head of the humerus is held in the glenoid cavity by the rotator cuff muscles. The glenoid labrum is a fibrocartilaginous rim attached around the margin of the glenoid process.

Answer: **B**
Netter, p. 34
Refer to Fig. 1-7.

CHAPTER 1 Anatomy Extravaganza   7

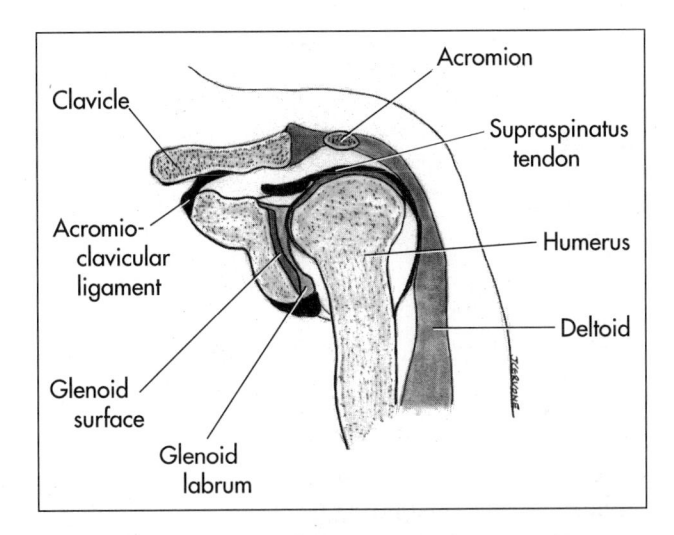

Fig. 1-7

15. Which pole of the scaphoid has a generous blood supply?

A. Distal pole
B. Waist
C. Proximal pole
D. All of the above have excellent vascularity

The scaphoid most often receives its arterial blood supply from the radial artery through ligamentous attachments. The distal pole has a rich blood supply and tends to heal promptly, whereas the proximal pole has poor vascularity and may result in avascular necrosis or nonunion after fracture.

Answer: **A**
Taleisnik, p. 67
Green, p. 824

16. Which nerve and artery pass through the quadrangular space?

A. Musculocutaneous nerve and posterior circumflex artery
B. Axillary nerve and posterior circumflex artery
C. Musculocutaneous nerve and anterior circumflex artery
D. Axillary nerve and anterior circumflex artery

The quadrangular space is bordered by the teres minor superiorly, the teres major inferiorly, the humerus laterally, and the triceps medially. The axillary nerve and posterior circumflex artery pass through this space.

Answer: **B**
Netter, p. 24
Refer to Fig. 1-8.

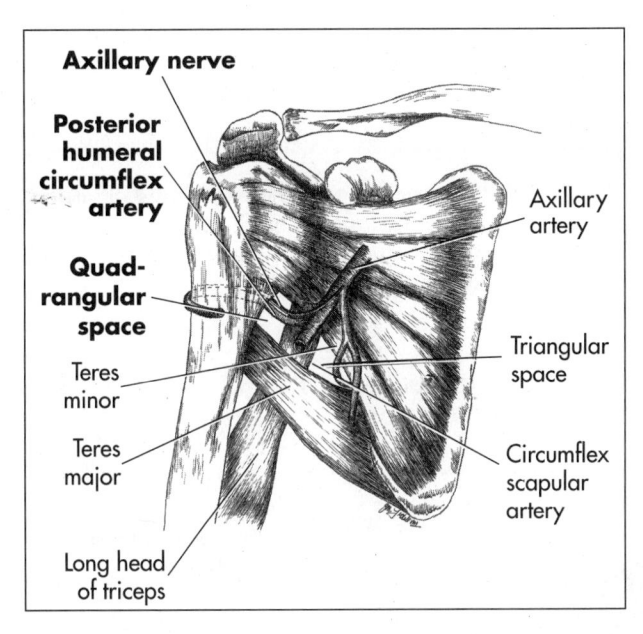

Fig. 1-8 ■ From Smith AA, Lacey SH: *Hand surgery review*, St. Louis, 1996, Mosby-Year Book.

17. Which artery passes over the floor of the anatomic snuffbox?

A. Radial artery
B. Ulnar artery
C. Median artery
D. Anterior interosseous artery

The anatomic snuffbox is a concave space made by the convergence of the extensor pollicis longus tendon with the extensor pollicis brevis and the abductor pollicis longus tendons. On the floor, the radial artery passes toward the back of the hand to the dorsal carpal branch.

Answer: **A**
Netter, p. 60

8 CHAPTER 1 Anatomy Extravaganza

> **CLINICAL GEM:**
> Tenderness in the snuffbox may be indicative of a scaphoid fracture.

18. In the forearm, at the level of the elbow, which three veins make the "M" shape?

A. Median cubital vein, basilic vein, and lateral cutaneous vein
B. Basilic vein, cephalic vein, and median cubital vein
C. Cephalic vein, lateral cutaneous vein, and basilic vein
D. None of the above

The cephalic vein running on the lateral (radial) aspect of the upper extremity and the basilic vein coursing the medial (ulnar) upper extremity form an "M" shape with the median cubital vein at the elbow.

Answer: **B**
Hunter, Mackin, Callahan, p. A-17
Refer to Fig. 1-9.

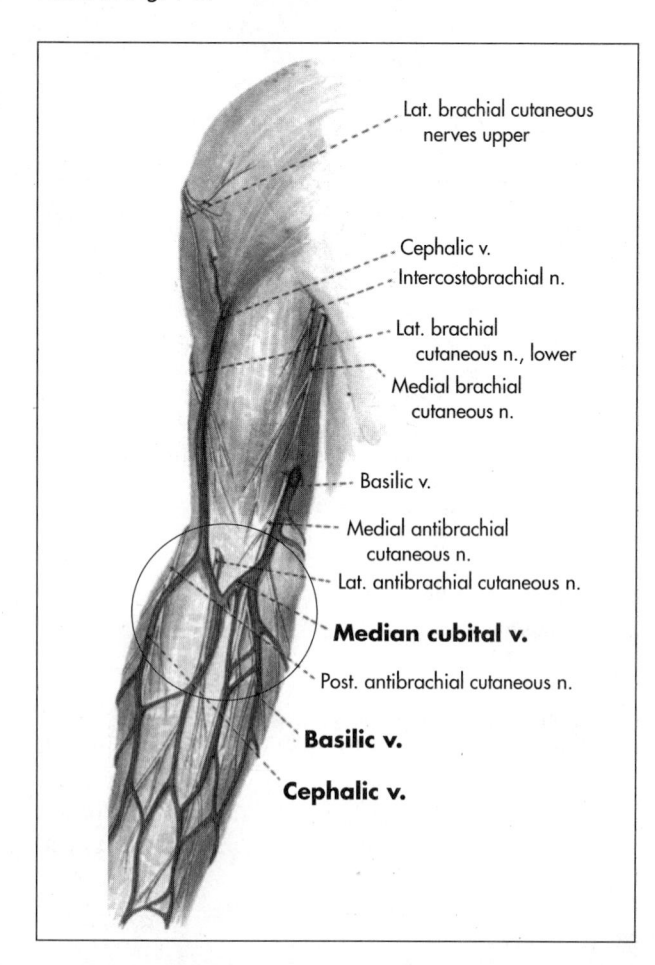

Fig. 1-9 ■ From Hunter JM, Mackin EJ, Callahan AD: *Rehabilitation of the hand: surgery and therapy*, ed 4, St. Louis, 1995, Mosby-Year Book.

19. Match the following vascular terms with the correct definitions:

Terms

1. Thrill
2. Bruit
3. Aneurysm
4. Doppler echocardiography
5. Hemangioma

Definitions

A. An adventitious sound of venous or arterial origin heard on auscultation
B. An abnormal tremor accompanying a vascular or cardiac murmur felt on palpation
C. Localized abnormal dilation of a blood vessel, usually an artery
D. A benign tumor of dilated blood vessels
E. A sensitive noninvasive technique for determining blood-flow

---

Answers: **1. B; 2. A; 3. C; 4. E; 5. D**
Taber's

20. What is the "space of Poirier"?

A. A gap between the scaphoid and lunate bones
B. An area of avascularity in the scaphoid
C. Weakness from an absence of ligamentous support
D. T-shaped ligaments over the hamate and triquetrum

The volar wrist capsule frequently contains an area of weakness referred to as the "space of Poirier." This weakness is caused by the absence of a volar lunocapitate ligament. Some authors report wrist instability caused by this lack of ligamentous support.

Answer: **C**
Taleisnik, p. 25
Refer to Fig. 1-10.

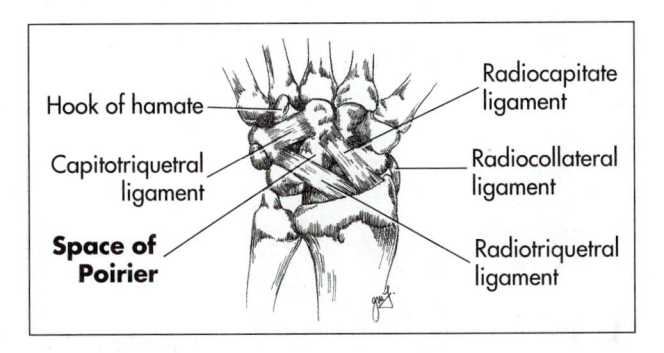

Fig. 1-10 ■ From Smith AA, Lacey SH: *Hand surgery review*, St. Louis, 1996, Mosby-Year Book.

21. You are treating a patient status post (following) flexor digitorum profundus repair to the ring finger. You note that he has a significant reduction of finger flexion force in the digits adjacent to the ring finger. You also recognize a flexion contracture of the ring finger. What might this patient be experiencing?

A. Lumbrical-plus phenomenon
B. Quadrigia phenomenon
C. Linburg's sign
D. Egawa's sign

When a quadrigia phenomenon occurs, the patient exhibits a decreased amount of flexion force in the digits next to the injured finger, as well as a flexion contracture of the involved digit. The quadrigia effect can occur if the flexor digitorum profundus is advanced more than 1 cm during repair, resulting in limited proximal excursion of the remaining flexor digitorum profundus tendons. To prevent a quadrigia effect, advancement should be used only for the flexor pollicis longus.

Answer: **B**
Hunter, Schneider, Mackin, pp. 423, 428, 595
Ejeskar, p. 63
Hunter, Mackin, Callahan, pp. 423, 428

22. What is the lacertus fibrosus?

A. Part of the arcade of Frohse
B. Continuation of the arcade of Struthers
C. The ligament of Struthers
D. Synonymous with the bicipital aponeurosis

The lacertus fibrosus is another name for the bicipital aponeurosis. It is a fibrous band originating from the tendon of biceps brachii. The lacertus fibrosus is tightened with pronation. Active flexion of the elbow in conjunction with pronation may contribute to compression of the median nerve at the lacertus fibrosus.

Answer: **D**
Green, pp. 1342-1343
Refer to Fig. 1-11.

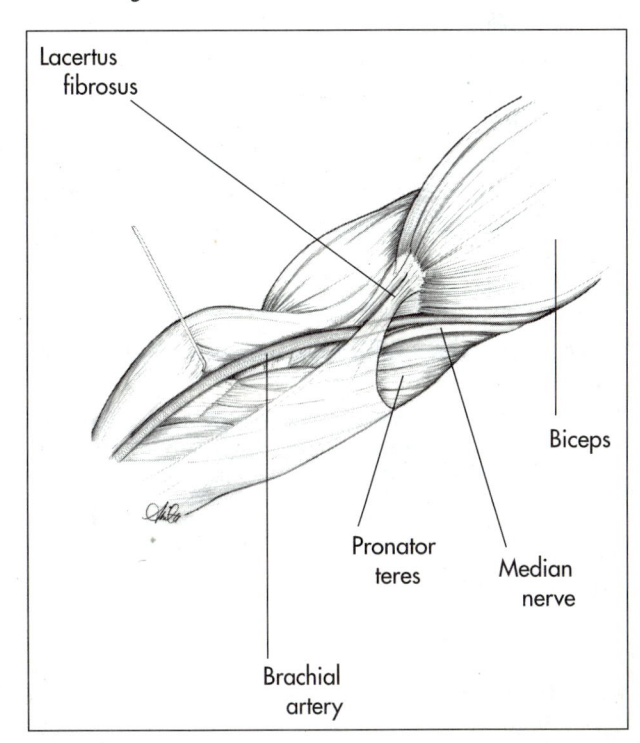

Fig. 1-11

23. Match the following terms with the correct definitions:

Terms

1. Fascia
2. Muscle
3. Sprain
4. Strain
5. Erythematous

Definitions

A. Injury to the joint with ligamentous damage
B. Injury to the muscle or musculotendinous unit
C. A fibrous membrane covering, supporting, and separating muscles
D. A type of tissue composed of contractile fibers
E. Dry, pink patches of skin that are itchy and burn

Answers: 1. C; 2. D; 3. A; 4. B; 5. E
Taber's

24. Which of the following muscles does not originate from the common flexor origin on the medial epicondyle of the humerus?

A. Pronator quadratus
B. Flexor carpi radialis
C. Flexor digitorum superficialis
D. Flexor carpi ulnaris
E. Pronator teres

Muscles originating from the common flexor origin include pronator teres, flexor carpi radialis, flexor digitorum superficialis, palmaris longus, and flexor carpi ulnaris. Pronator quadratus is a distal forearm muscle originating from the distal ulna.

Answer: **A**
Hoppenfeld, de Boer, p. 102

25. The basilic vein and the brachial vein form which vein?

A. Axillary vein
B. Cephalic vein
C. Thoracoepigastric vein
D. Thoracodorsal vein

The basilic vein joins the brachial vein at the lower border of the teres major and goes on to form the axillary vein. The axillary vein is termed the subclavian vein at the first rib.

Answer: **A**
Hunter, Mackin, Callahan, p. A12
Refer to Fig. 1-12.

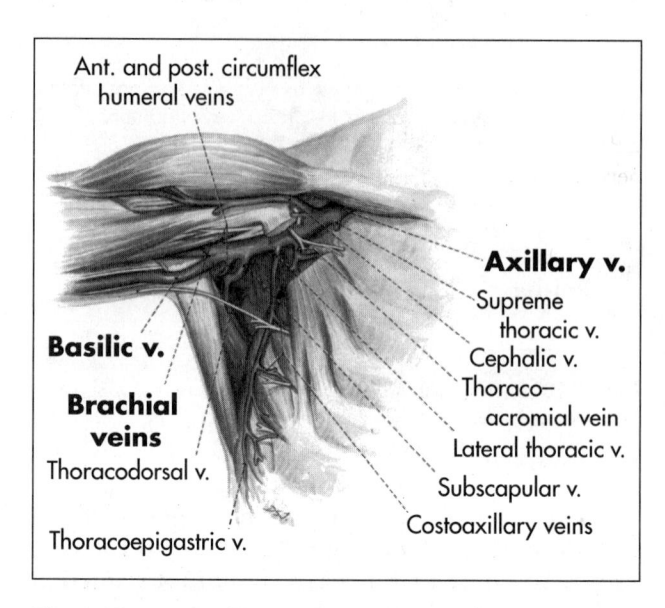

Fig. 1-12 ■ From Hunter JM, Mackin EJ, Callahan AD: *Rehabilitation of the hand: surgery and therapy,* ed 4, St. Louis, 1995, Mosby-Year Book.

26. All vein grafts should be marked and reversed when used in arterial reconstruction. True or False?

Both veins and arteries have been used for interposition grafts and microsurgery but venous grafts are more readily available and appear to have the highest patency rate. All vein grafts should be marked and reversed when used in arterial reconstruction because it has been shown that even the smallest digital vessels contain valves. Veins have valves preventing backward circulation; therefore, if veins are not reversed, blood will not flow properly.

Answer: **True**
Green, p. 1061

27. Lister's tubercle is a bony prominence located on the:

A. Scaphoid
B. Proximal ulna
C. Distal radius
D. Distal ulna

Lister's tubercle is located on the distal radius. The extensor pollicis longus (EPL) takes a 45-degree turn around Lister's tubercle, which acts as a pulley on its course to the thumb. It is not uncommon for the EPL to rupture in patients with rheumatoid arthritis. The EPL may rupture after a distal radius fracture if the tubercle is disrupted.

Answer: **C**
Hoppenfeld, p. 78

28. Which structure articulates with the cupped surface of the proximal radius?

A. Trochlea
B. Coronoid
C. Capitulum
D. Medial epicondyle

The capitulum is spherical in shape and smaller than the trochlea. The capitulum articulates with the cupped surface of the radius (radial head). The trochlea is shaped like a spool and superior to the coronoid fossa.

Answer: **C**
Netter, p. 31
Refer to Fig. 1-13.

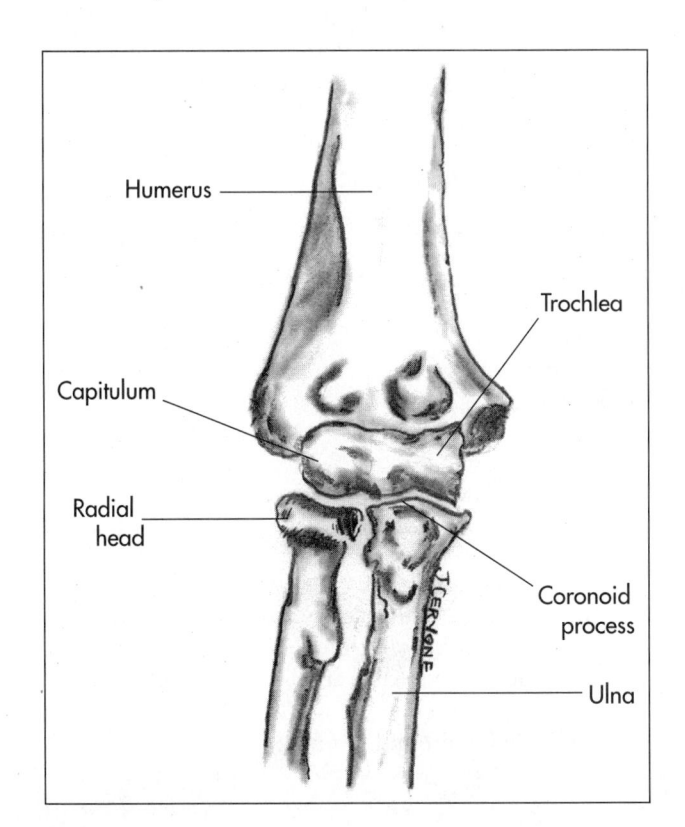

Fig. 1-13

29. Match each muscle with the correct insertion:

Muscle

1. Subscapularis
2. Pectoralis major
3. Coracobrachialis
4. Brachialis
5. Supraspinatus

Insertion

A. Bicipital groove
B. Coronoid process of ulna
C. Greater tubercle of humerus
D. Shaft of humerus
E. Lesser tubercle of humerus

Answers: **1. E; 2. A; 3. D; 4. B; 5. C**
Hunter, Mackin, Callahan, pp. 16-18

30. Which muscle is NOT included in the "wad of Henry"?

A. Brachioradialis
B. Supinator
C. Extensor carpi radialis brevis
D. Extensor carpi radialis longus

Hoppenfeld describes the brachioradialis, extensor carpi radialis brevis, and extensor carpi radialis longus as "the mobile wad of Henry" or "mobile wad of three." It is best to palpate these muscles as a unit, which is easily held and moves between the fingers. You can assess this group of muscles when the forearm and wrist are in the neutral position.

Answer: **B**
Hoppenfeld, p. 47

31. Match each plane with the correct definition:

Plane

1. Coronal plane
2. Frontal plane
3. Sagittal plane
4. Transverse plane

Definition

A. Another name for coronal plane
B. Divides the body into superior and inferior portions at right angles to the long axis of the body
C. Divides the body into right and left parts; referred to as the median plane
D. Divides the body into front and back portions

Answers: **1. D; 2. A or D; 3. C; 4. B**
Putz-Anderson, p. 116

32. Landsmeer's ligament is another term for which structure?

A. The oblique retinacular ligament
B. The transverse retinacular ligament
C. The triangular ligament
D. Cleland's ligament

The oblique retinacular ligament (ORL) was described by Landsmeer in 1949. This ligament coordinates the movement of the interphalangeal joints. The functional value of this ligament is controversial in normal fingers but evident in pathological conditions. The ORL is taut in distal interphalangeal joint flexion; therefore, if this ligament is contracted in extension, the distal interphalangeal joint is not able to fully flex. When the ORL is contracted, it contributes to the boutonniere deformity.

Answer: **A**
Hunter, Mackin, Callahan, p. 65
Tubiana, Thomine, Mackin, p. 103
Refer to Fig. 1-14.

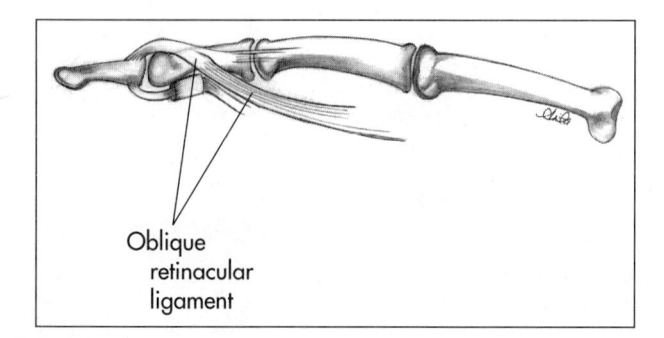

Fig. 1-14

33. A ligament attaches a muscle to a bone. True or False?

A ligament is a band or sheet of strong, fibrous, connective tissue connecting the articular ends of bones; it binds them together and facilitates or limits motion. A tendon is a fibrous, connective tissue that attaches muscle to bone.

Answer: **False**
Taber's

34. A fingerprint is made from:

A. Reticular dermis
B. Skin bulging
C. Papillary ridges
D. Oil in the fingertips

Fingerprints are formed from cutaneous striations that are reflective of organized papillary ridges in the underlying dermis. The reticular dermis is incorrect because it is a deeper layer, consisting of collagen and elastic fibers.

Answer: **C**
Tubiana, Thomine, Mackin, p. 131

35. Which of the following is the term for the white area at the base of the nail?

A. Hyponychium
B. Eponychium
C. Paronychia
D. Lunula

The lunula is the white convex area seen at the base of the nail. The hyponychium is under the nail bed. The eponychium is the embryonic structure from which the nail develops. A paronychia is an acute or chronic infection around the nail.

Answer: **D**
Tubiana, Thomine, Mackin, p. 151
Taber's

36. Label Figure 1-15.

1. Distal phalanx
2. Hyponychium
3. Nail bed
4. Eponychium
5. Nail plate

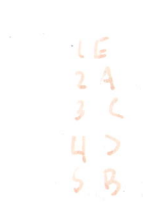

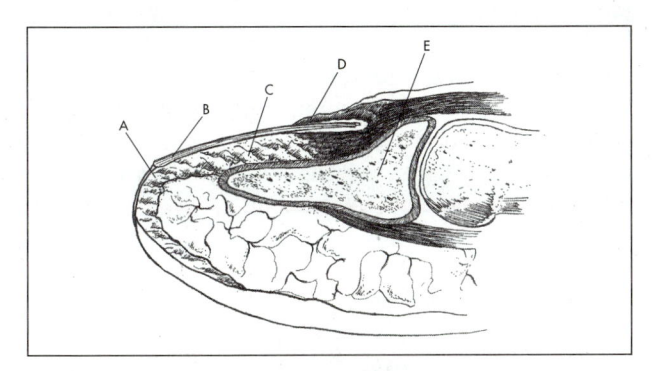

Fig. 1-15 ■ Modified from Smith AA, Lacey SH: *Hand surgery review*, St. Louis, 1996, Mosby-Year Book.

Answers: **1. E; 2. A; 3. C; 4. D; 5. B**
Green, p. 1283

37. The palmaris longus is absent in what percent of the population?

A. 30% to 40%
B. 5% to 8%
C. 13% to 20%
D. 75% to 85%

The palmaris longus is absent in 13% to 20% of the population. It originates from the medial epicondyle of the humerus and inserts into the palmar aponeurosis. The palmaris longus tendon is easily detected as it courses over the transverse carpal ligament. This tendon often is sacrificed when performing tendon transfers.

Answer: **C**
Hunter, Mackin, Callahan, p. 26

38. The fingernails of digits two and three receive their sensation from which nerve?

A. Median nerve
B. Ulnar nerve
C. Radial nerve
D. Anterior interosseous nerve

As the proper digital nerves pass toward their destination in the pad of the finger, they give off branches for the innervation of the skin on the dorsum of the fingers and matrices of the fingernails. Digital nerves for the first, second, third, and one half of the fourth fingers are median-nerve innervated.

Answer: **A**
Netter, p. 58

39. The "attitude" of the hand in Figure 1-16, *A* depicts a:

A. Position of rest
B. Lumbrical plus position
C. Intrinsic minus position
D. Intrinsic plus position

The "attitude" of the hand is an important factor to assess during evaluation. The "position of rest" occurs when the metacarpophalangeal joints and the interphalangeal joints are slightly flexed and the fingers line up almost parallel to each other (Fig. 1-16, *A*). If one finger is extended (perpendicular to the others), its flexor tendon may have been damaged (Fig. 1-16, *B*).

Answer: **A**
Hoppenfeld, p. 61

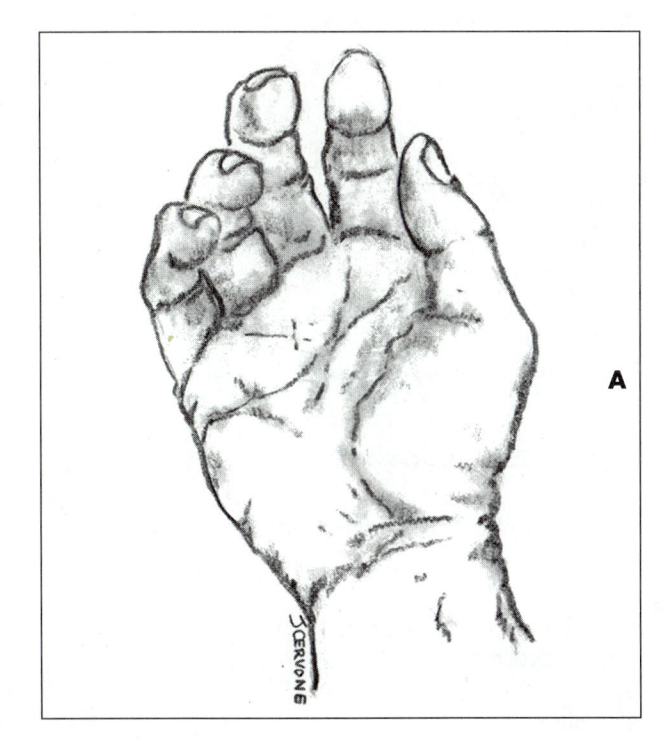

Fig. 1-16

Continued

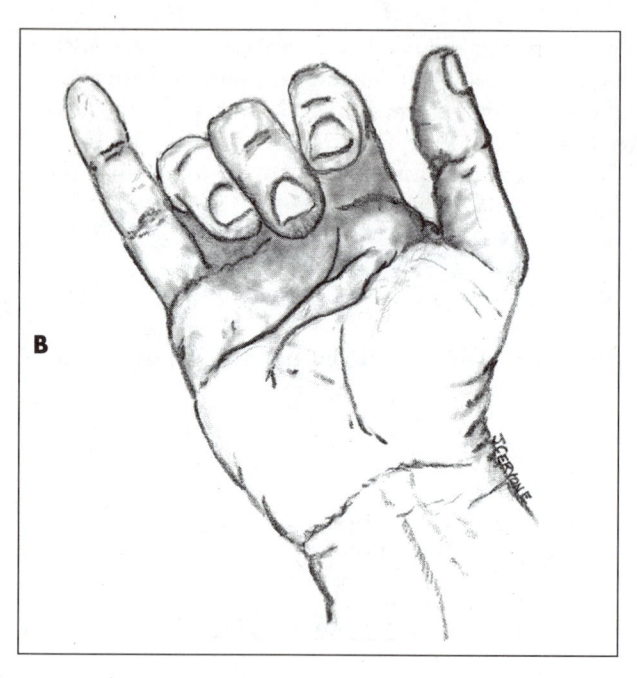

Fig. 1-16, cont'd

40. Match the following muscles with their actions:

Muscle

1. Middle deltoid
2. Upper trapezius
3. Latissimus dorsi
4. Coracobrachialis
5. Pectoralis minor

Actions

A. Protraction, depression, and downward rotation of the scapula
B. Flexion and adduction of the humerus
C. Elevation and upward rotation of scapula
D. Extension, internal rotation, and adduction of the humerus
E. Abduction of humerus to 90 degrees

Answers: **1. E; 2. C; 3. D; 4. B; 5. A**
Sieg, Adams, p. 30

41. All of the following are signs of arterial insufficiency, except:

A. Pallor
B. Decreased temperature
C. Sluggish capillary refill
D. Cyanosis

Arterial insufficiency results in pallor (lack of color), decreased temperature, increased pain, slow capillary refill, and loss of pulse. Venous insufficiency is recognized by cyanosis (bluish discoloration of the skin caused by reduced amounts of hemoglobin in the blood) and abnormal capillary refill. Excessive elevation above the level of the heart can stress the arterial system during the acute phase and should be avoided. Elevation at the level of the heart is the recommended position. In general, slight elevation above the heart is beneficial for venous stasis and slight lowering below the heart is helpful for arterial system management.

Answer: **D**
Hunter, Mackin, Callahan, pp. 1059, 1092

42. The most important pulleys in the flexor tendon system are A3 and A5. True or False?

Pulleys ensure biomechanical efficiency of the flexor tendons. Their role is to prevent bowstringing of the tendons and to allow the flexors to work efficiently. Five annular pulleys and three cruciate pulleys are in each finger. A2 and A4 are the most important pulleys in the flexor tendon system.

Answer: **False**
Malick, p. 43
Refer to Fig. 1-17.

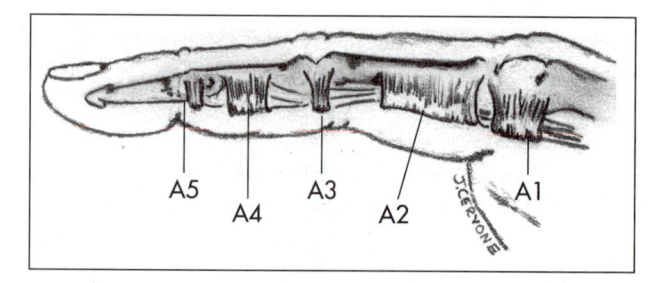

Figure 1-17

> **CLINICAL GEM:**
> An easy way to remember the pulleys is to recall that the odd numbers for the annular pulleys correlate with finger joints:
> MPJ - A1
> PIPJ - A3
> DIPJ - A5

Chapter 2

Intrinsic Mechanism

Topics to be reviewed in random order are:

- **Structures of the intrinsic mechanism**
- **Swan-neck deformity**
- **Boutonniere deformity**
- **Mallet finger**
- **Intrinsic/extrinsic tightness**
- **Collateral ligaments**
- **Therapy treatment for the intrinsic mechanism**
- **Surgical considerations**

1. Match the following numbers with the corresponding letters in Figure 2-1.

   1. Triangular ligament
   2. Dorsal hood
   3. Terminal tendon
   4. Lateral bands
   5. Interosseous muscle
   6. Lumbrical muscle
   7. Long extensor tendon

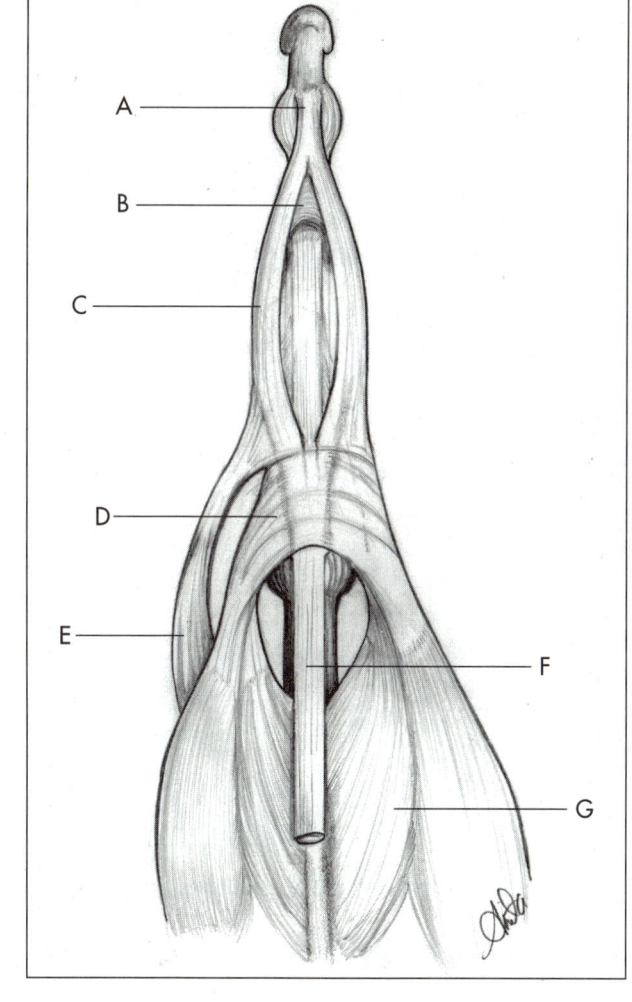

Fig. 2-1

Answers: **1. B; 2. D; 3. A; 4. C; 5. G; 6. E; 7. F**
Hunter, Schneider, Mackin, p. 549

16 CHAPTER 2 Intrinsic Mechanism

2. **A boutonnière deformity presents with:**

   A. Metacarpophalangeal joint extension with interphalangeal joint flexion
   B. Flexion of the proximal interphalangeal joint with hyperextension of the distal interphalangeal joint
   C. Hyperextension of the proximal interphalangeal joint with flexion of the distal interphalangeal joint
   D. Hyperextension of the proximal interphalangeal joint with distal interphalangeal joint flexion

A boutonnière deformity is caused by an injury to the complex extensor mechanism of the digit. The central tendon is ruptured or interrupted at the proximal interphalangeal joint (zone III) level, contributing to a loss of function of the triangular ligament. The rupture of the central slip causes proximal displacement of the extensor mechanism and a palmar subluxation of the lateral bands. The extensor force is therefore concentrated on the distal interphalangeal joint, resulting in hyperextension and loss of flexion at the distal interphalangeal joint. The flexor digitorum superficialis is unopposed, causing increased proximal interphalangeal joint flexion. As the lateral bands sublux further, the proximal interphalangeal joint is unable to achieve full extension actively or passively.

Answer: **B**
Hunter, Mackin, Callahan, p. 536
Blair, p. 610
Refer to Fig. 2-2.

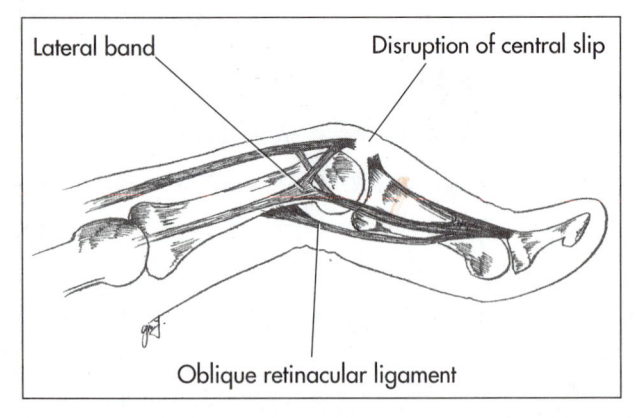

Fig. 2-2 ■ From Smith AA, Lacey SH: *Hand surgery review,* St. Louis, 1996, Mosby-Year Book.

3. **Which exercise is most important for a patient who is developing boutonnière deformity to perform?**

   A. Isolated distal interphalangeal joint flexion
   B. Isolated proximal interphalangeal joint flexion
   C. Proximal interphalangeal joint extension
   D. Composite digital extension

Active and passive flexion exercises of the distal interphalangeal joint (Fig. 2-3) prevent oblique retinacular ligament (ORL) tightness, centralize the lateral bands, and advance the central slip. It is important to note that the most disabling element of the boutonnière deformity is the limitation of distal interphalangeal joint flexion, not the lack of proximal interphalangeal joint motion. Patients often complain of a weak grip and an inability to grasp and manipulate small objects with the tip of the digit.

Answer: **A**
Blair, p. 614

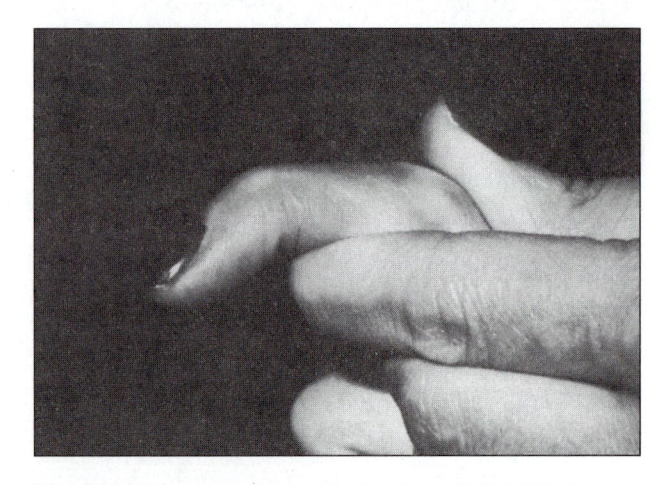

Fig. 2-3 ■ From Hunter JM, Mackin EJ, Callahan AD: *Rehabilitation of the hand: surgery and therapy,* ed 4, St. Louis, 1995, Mosby-Year Book.

> **CLINICAL GEM:**
> Remember, the most disabling element of the boutonnière deformity is the loss of prehension caused by decreased distal interphalangeal joint flexion.

4. **You are treating a patient in the clinic 8 weeks after a middle phalanx fracture and you observe the following:**

When the proximal interphalangeal joint is passively flexed at 90°, the distal interphalangeal joint can achieve 50° flexion; however, when the proximal interphalangeal joint is placed at 0°, the distal interphalangeal joint can achieve only 25° of flexion. This is caused by:

A. Intrinsic tightness
B. Extrinsic tightness
C. Oblique retinacular ligament tightness
D. Extensor tendon adherence
E. Triangular ligament tightness

If distal interphalangeal joint flexion is more limited when the proximal interphalangeal joint is passively extended than when it is flexed, a tightness of the oblique retinacular ligament (ORL) results. To treat this condition, the therapist should perform ORL stretches (passive distal interphalangeal joint flexion with the proximal interphalangeal joint held in extension), joint blocking exercises, or apply a dynamic distal interphalangeal joint flexion splint with a P2 block.

Answer: **C**
Hunter, Mackin, Callahan, p. 65
Walters, pp. 116-123

> **CLINICAL GEM:**
> P1 refers to the proximal phalanx, P2 refers to the middle phalanx, and P3 refers to the distal phalanx.

5. You are treating a patient who sustained a Colles fracture 4 months ago. The following is noted during the re-evaluation:

Range-of-motion assessment:

	Active (degrees)	Passive (degrees)
Metacarpophalangeal	0/70	0/75
Proximal interphalangeal	0/85	0/90
Distal interphalangeal	0/55	0/60

(Note: Wrist is at neutral during active and passive measures.)

However, when the fist is fully flexed in the available range of motion and the wrist is passively flexed to 25°, tension is felt in the digits as they pull into extension and are unable to maintain their flexed position. What might cause this patient to experience this tension?

A. Flexor tightness distal to the wrist
B. Flexor tightness proximal to the wrist
C. Joint capsular tightness
D. Extensor tightness distal to the wrist
E. Extensor tightness proximal to the wrist

During ongoing assessments of patients, it is important to determine the origin of the limitation and treat it accordingly. Therefore, it is necessary to observe the surrounding joints and their impact on range of motion. The following definitions describe various levels of tightness patients may have:

EXTENSOR TIGHTNESS PROXIMAL TO THE WRIST: To test, passively hold the digits in composite flexion while passively flexing the wrist. If the digits are pulled into extension as the wrist is passively flexed, extrinsic tightness proximal to the wrist exists. Note the position of the wrist when the extensor tension is first detected to document stiffness.

EXTENSOR TIGHTNESS DISTAL TO THE WRIST: To test, passively hold the proximal interphalangeal and distal interphalangeal joints in flexion and passively flex the metacarpophalangeal joint. If the proximal interphalangeal joint and distal interphalangeal joint are pulled into extension when the metacarpophalangeal joint is passively flexed, extensor tightness distal to the wrist exists.

FLEXOR TIGHTNESS DISTAL TO THE WRIST: To test, passively hold the proximal interphalangeal and distal interphalangeal joints in extension and passively extend the metacarpophalangeal joint. If the proximal interphalangeal and distal interphalangeal joints are pulled into flexion as the metacarpophalangeal joint is passively extended, flexor tightness distal to the wrist exists.

FLEXOR TIGHTNESS PROXIMAL TO THE WRIST: To test, passively maintain digits in full extension and passively extend the wrist. If flexor tension develops and the digits are pulled into flexion as the wrist is extended, extrinsic flexor tightness proximal to the wrist exists. Note the position of the wrist when the flexor tightness is first detected to document stiffness.

JOINT CAPSULAR TIGHTNESS: To test, measure active range of motion and passive range of motion. If the measurements are the same regardless of the position of the proximal and distal joints, joint capsular tightness is present.

CHAPTER 2 Intrinsic Mechanism

Answer: **E**
Hunter, Mackin, Callahan, p. 1148
Walters, pp. 116-123

6. Terminal tendon tenotomy (for treating a Boutonnière deformity) restores:

A. Proximal interphalangeal joint flexion
B. Complete proximal interphalangeal joint extension
C. Distal interphalangeal joint flexion
D. Partial distal interphalangeal joint extension

A terminal tendon tenotomy is performed primarily to improve distal interphalangeal joint flexion; secondarily, the proximal interphalangeal joint extensor deficit may show improvement. Distal interphalangeal joint extension is provided by the oblique retinacular ligament through a static tenodesis effect. Patients can begin active range of motion immediately after tenotomy. If after surgery extensor deficits at the distal interphalangeal joint are greater than 10° to 15°, some surgeons recommend splinting the proximal and distal interphalangeal joints in full extension for 10 days. The distal interphalangeal joint must be monitored closely for extensor lags, with appropriate splinting adjustments made.

Answer: **C**
Blair, pp. 610-614
Hunter, Mackin, Callahan, pp. 549, 1318

7. In a swan-neck deformity, the lateral bands sublux volarly. True or False?

A swan-neck deformity presents with hyperextension of the proximal interphalangeal joint and flexion of the distal interphalangeal joint. This deformity is caused by an imbalance of forces in the digit. This imbalance is summarized as follows: the transverse retinacular ligaments stretch, the triangular ligament fibers shorten, and the lateral bands sublux dorsally, causing attenuation of the proximal interphalangeal joint volar plate.

Answer: **False**
Hunter, Mackin, Callahan, pp. 549, 1318
Refer to Fig. 2-4.

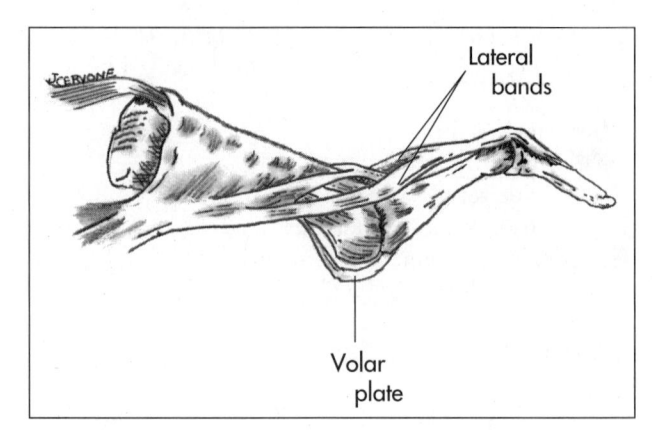

Fig. 2-4

8. Which splint is most appropriate for a swan-neck deformity?

A. Silver ring to the proximal interphalangeal joint
B. Stack splint
C. Gutter splint to the proximal interphalangeal and distal interphalangeal joints
D. No splint will help

A Siris Swan-Neck Silver Ring Splint or a thermoplastic figure-of-eight splint at the proximal interphalangeal joint reduces or eliminates proximal interphalangeal joint hyperextension and decreases the imbalance of the lateral bands. It is important to understand that swan-neck deformity splints do not permanently correct the imbalance; after they are removed, the deformity will reoccur.

Answer: **A**
Silver Ring Splint Company Catalog
Malick, Kasch, p. 132
Refer to Fig. 2-5.

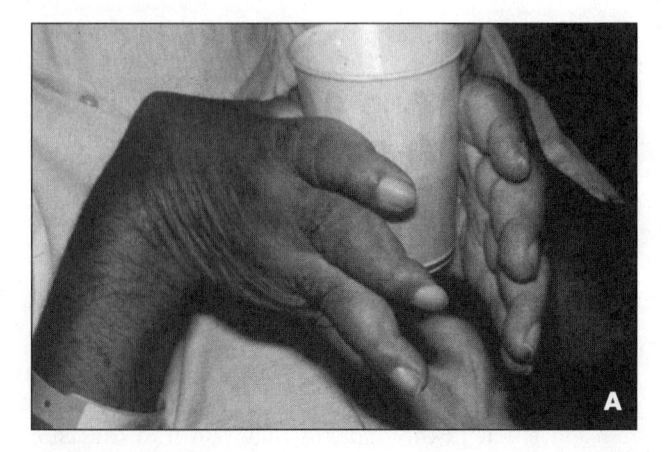

Fig. 2-5 *Continued*

CHAPTER 2 Intrinsic Mechanism 19

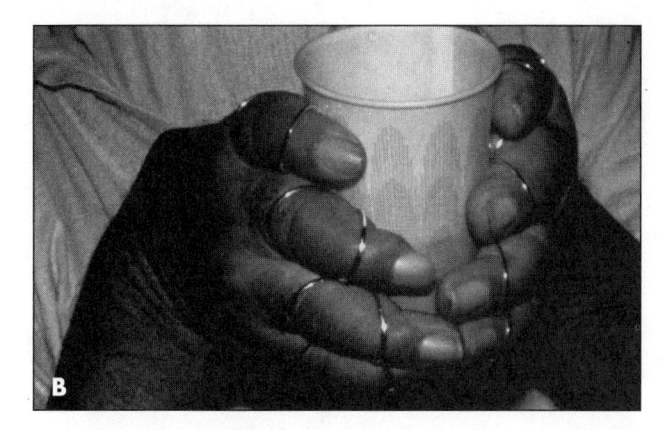

Fig. 2-5, cont'd ■ With permission from the Silver Ring Splint Company.

> ✦ CLINICAL GEM:
> Siris Silver Ring Splints are durable, attractive, and functional. Patients may choose to have gems inserted into these rings; the rings also are available in gold.

9. If a patient has intrinsic tightness, which of the following is true about the proximal interphalangeal joint?

A. Flexes more when the metacarpophalangeal joint is in flexion
B. Flexes more when the metacarpophalangeal joint is extended
C. Flexes the same degree regardless of the position of the metacarpophalangeal joint
D. Does not flex at all

When testing for intrinsic tightness, the metacarpophalangeal joint is held in extension while the proximal interphalangeal joint is passively stretched in flexion (Fig. 2-6, *A*). Next, the metacarpophalangeal joint is placed in flexion while the proximal interphalangeal joint is again passively stretched in flexion (Fig. 2-6, *B*). If the proximal interphalangeal joint can be passively flexed to a greater extent when the metacarpophalangeal joint is flexed than when it is extended, there is intrinsic tightness.

If the proximal interphalangeal joint flexes more when the metacarpophalangeal joint is extended, as in *answer B*, extrinsic extensor tightness exists.

Answer: **A**
Hunter, Mackin, Callahan, pp. 66, 1148

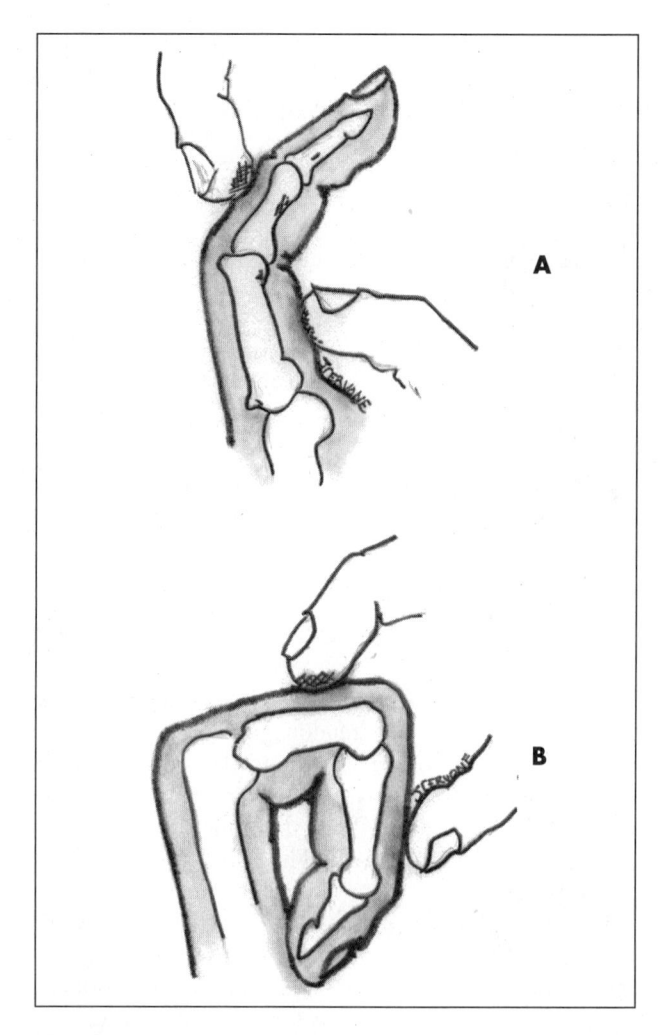

Fig. 2-6

10. The mallet finger can progress to which type of deformity if untreated?

A. Boutonnière
B. Jersey finger
C. Hyperplasia
D. Swan-neck

A swan-neck deformity can occur from a mallet lesion. The severity of the deformity is proportional to the stability of the palmar plate at the proximal interphalangeal joint. If the proximal interphalangeal joint palmar plate is lax, swan-neck deformity increases and the flexor digitorum profundus flexes the distal interphalangeal joint, contributing to the deformity. If the possibility of surgery is entertained, the finger can be rebalanced with tenotomy of the central tendon at the proximal interphalangeal joint. It also can be treated with reconstruction of the oblique retinacular ligament using a free tendon graft (see Fig. 2-4).

Answer: **D**
Hunter, Mackin, Callahan, p. 544

11. A mallet deformity with bone avulsion should be splinted for:

A. Four to 6 weeks, with distal interphalangeal joint in full extension
B. Four to 6 weeks, with distal interphalangeal joint in slight flexion
C. Six to 8 weeks, with distal interphalangeal joint in full extension
D. Six to 8 weeks, with distal interphalangeal joint in slight flexion

A mallet finger occurs when the extensor tendon is disrupted at the terminal tendon. The patient presents with an inability to actively extend the distal interphalangeal joint. Conservative management is recommended for the patient if less than one third of the articulating surface is avulsed. The distal interphalangeal joint is splinted at 0° to 15° of hyperextension (the proximal interphalangeal joint is free) for 6 to 8 weeks (Fig. 2-7). Immobilization for 8 weeks is indicated in injuries that are more than 3 weeks old. An additional 2 weeks is indicated in a patient who loses extension quickly when the splint is weaned at 6 weeks. Studies have shown excellent results with compliant patients.

Answer: **C**
Malick, Kasch, p. 62
Grothe, pp. 21-24

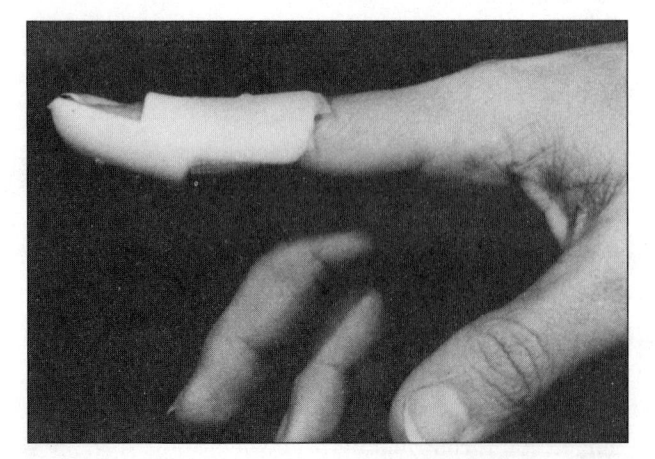

Fig. 2-7 ■ Reprinted with permission from Evans RB: Therapeutic management of extensor tendon injuries, *Hand Clin* 2:157, 1986.

12. Which structure(s) maintains the central position of the extensor tendon over the metacarpophalangeal joint?

A. Collateral ligaments
B. Shroud fibers/sagittal bands
C. Central slip
D. Lumbricals

The shroud fibers/sagittal bands stabilize the extensor tendons over the metacarpophalangeal joint. They arise from the extrinsic extensors and insert into the volar plate of the metacarpophalangeal joint. When these structures becomes attenuated, the patient is unable to extend the metacarpophalangeal joint from the flexed position. However, the patient is able to hold the finger at zero when placed there as the tendon relocates over the metacarpophalangeal joint. Nonoperative management involves splinting the metacarpophalangeal joint at zero for 3 to 4 weeks while allowing proximal interphalangeal joint motion. If this does not work, surgical repair is indicated.

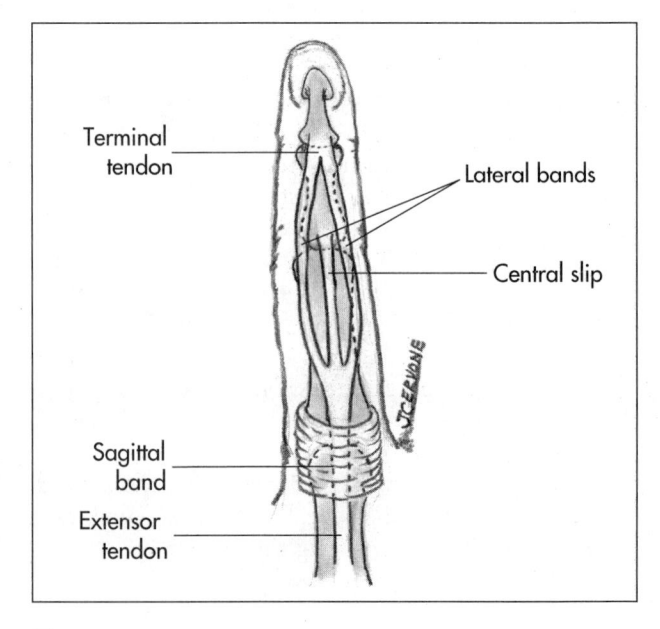

Answer: **B**
Green, pp. 1964-1965
Refer to Fig. 2-8.

Fig. 2-8

13. You are treating a patient 3 months after a flexor digitorum profundus tendon graft to the ring finger. You notice that every time he attempts to make a fist the interphalangeal joints extend rather than flex. Why might this be happening?

A. Quadrigia
B. Paradoxical extension
C. The tendon graft has ruptured
D. The patient is not giving full effort

Normally, flexion of the interphalangeal joints is dependent on contraction of the profundus and relaxation of the lumbricals. In contrast, paradoxical extension is an abnormal phenomenon that occurs when the patient attempts to contract the profundus; but instead the lumbrical is pulled proximally, resulting in proximal interphalangeal and distal interphalangeal joint extension rather than flexion. Tendon laxity after a tendon graft can cause this phenomenon because the profundus contraction may have a greater effect on the lumbrical than on the graft. Paradoxical extension may also occur if the lumbrical is fibrotic or contracted and the profundus force is transmitted to the lumbrical tendon and not the distal phalanx during muscle contraction.

Answer: **B**
Green, p. 623

> **CLINICAL GEM:**
> The involved finger will assume an intrinsic plus position when paradoxical extension occurs.

14. In a patient with rheumatoid arthritis, the ulnar intrinsics become tighter than the radial intrinsics. True or False?

The ulnar intrinsics become contracted because of a variety of dynamic and anatomic factors occurring in the rheumatoid hand, which can result in ulnar drift (Fig. 2-9, *A*). Cross intrinsic transfers can be performed by resecting the ulnar intrinsics and rerouting them to the radial side of the proximal phalanx (Fig. 2-9, *B*). These transfers can be performed in a patient exhibiting early rheumatoid arthritis or in conjunction with metacarpophalangeal joint arthroplasty in an attempt to rebalance the hand.

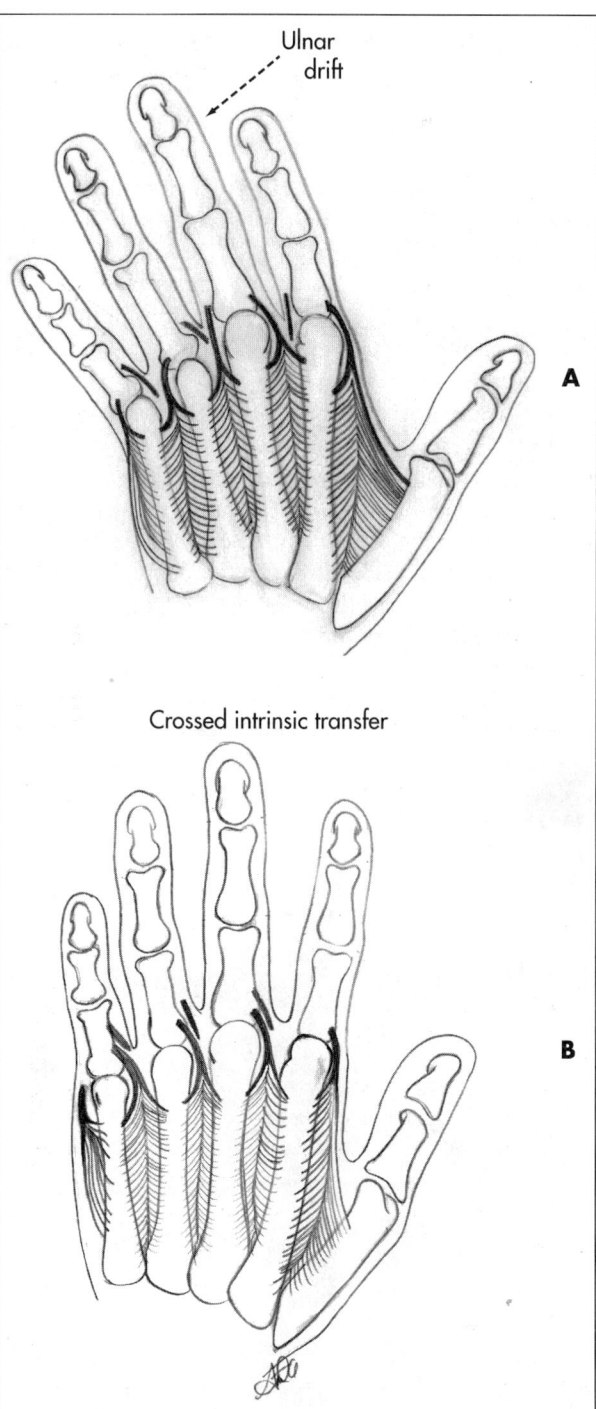

Answer: **True**
Green, pp. 617-618

Fig. 2-9

CHAPTER 2 Intrinsic Mechanism

15. What is the only muscle that arises from and inserts into tendon?

A. Dorsal interosseous
B. Volar interosseous
C. Lumbricals
D. Abductor digiti minimi quinti

The lumbrical muscles are the only muscles that arise and insert into tendon. They arise from the flexor digitorum profundus tendons and insert into the extensor expansion of the extensor digitorum communis. The lumbricals are known as the "workhorses" of the hand; however, a consensus about the actual role of the lumbricals has not been reached. Jacobsen et al have shown that the lumbricals are designed for high excursion and velocity production. Backhouse and Catton have indicated that the primary action of the lumbricals is to extend the interphalangeal joints and that they are weak flexors of the metacarpophalangeal joint. Brand and Hollister have indicated that the lumbricals ensure that the metacarpophalangeal joints flex ahead of the interphalangeal joints, allowing the hand to grasp a large object. The lumbricals have fascinated researchers for years and will require further research before their role is fully understood.

Answer: **C**
Schreuders, Stam, pp. 303-305
Brand, Hollister, p. 330
Refer to Fig. 2-10.

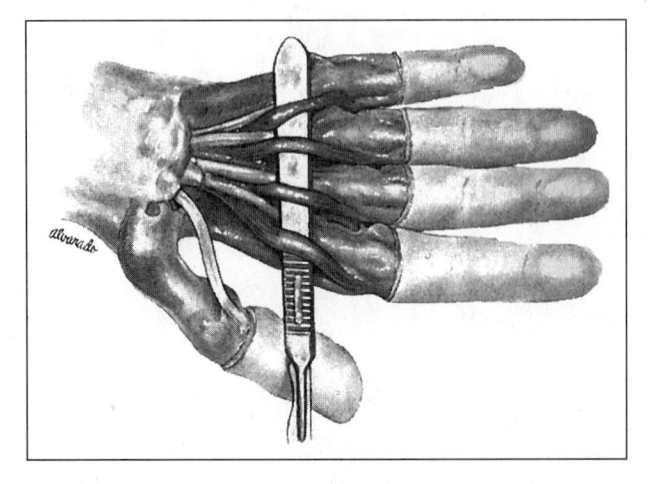

Fig. 2-10 ■ The four lumbrical muscles. (From Brand PW, Hollister A: *Clinical mechanics of the hand,* ed 2, St. Louis, 1993, Mosby-Year Book.)

16. If the transverse retinacular ligament is ruptured, the result is the development of a swan-neck deformity. True or False?

The transverse retinacular ligament encircles the proximal interphalangeal joint. This ligament restrains dorsal displacement of the lateral bands. If the transverse retinacular ligament is injured, the lateral bands bowstring dorsally and contribute to the development of a swan-neck deformity (see Fig. 2-4). In contrast, the triangular ligament holds the lateral bands dorsally and loss of this ligament results in the development of a boutonnière.

Answer: **True**
Hunter, Mackin, Callahan, p. 530

17. Which of the following does not apply to the accessory collateral ligament at the proximal interphalangeal joint?

A. It is a stabilizer of the proximal interphalangeal joint
B. It is taught in extension
C. It inserts into the volar plate
D. It is taught in flexion

The proper collateral ligament (PCL) and accessory collateral ligament (ACL) are primary stabilizers of the proximal interphalangeal joint. The ACL is an anterior continuation of the joint capsule and attaches to the volar plate. In full extension, the ACL becomes taut; the PCL is taut in flexion. These ligamentous structures must be considered when splinting. Splinting the proximal interphalangeal joint at 0° to 15° flexion is recommended when treating collateral ligament injuries.

Answer: **D**
Hunter, Mackin, Callahan, p. 378
Refer to Fig. 2-11.

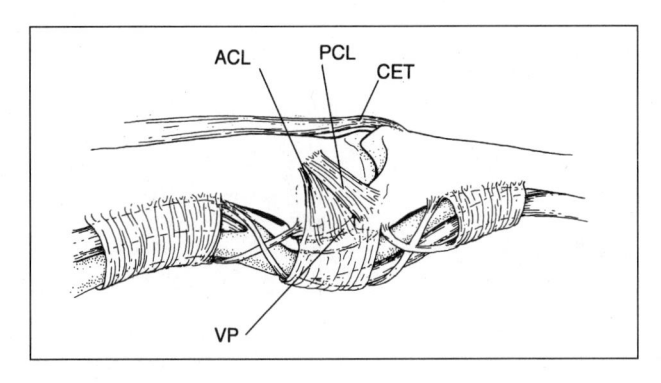

Fig. 2-11 ■ Posterior interphalangeal (PIP) joint. The major retaining ligaments of the PIP joint include the proper and accessory collateral ligaments (*PCL* and *ACL*), the volar plate (*VP*), and the dorsal capsule, with its central extensor tendon (*CET*). The VP acts as a gliding surface for the flexor tendon. (From Hunter JM, Mackin EJ, Callahan AD: *Rehabilitation of the hand: surgery and therapy,* ed 4, St. Louis, 1995, Mosby-Year Book.)

Chapter 3
Evaluation

Topics to be reviewed in random order are:
- Manual muscle testing
- Goniometry
- Dynamometer use
- Dexterity testing
- Sensibility testing
- Coefficient of variation
- Volumetric measurement
- Various other tests and signs
- Reflex testing

1. Reflex testing is used to evaluate the integrity of nerve supply. The triceps reflex frequently is evaluated to assess radial nerve function. This reflex is largely a function of what neurological level?

A. C5
B. C6
C. C7
D. C8

The triceps is innervated by the radial nerve. This reflex is largely a function of the C7 neurological level. To assess the triceps, place the patient's arm over your opposite arm so that it rests on your forearm. Hold the patient's arm under the medial epicondyle. Have the patient put his or her arm in a slightly flexed position, with the arm relaxed. Tap the triceps tendon where it crosses the olecranon fossa with the narrow end of a reflex hammer. You should be able to see the reflex or feel it slightly as the patient's arm jerks your supporting arm.

Answer: **C**
Hoppenfeld, p. 55
Refer to Fig. 3-1.

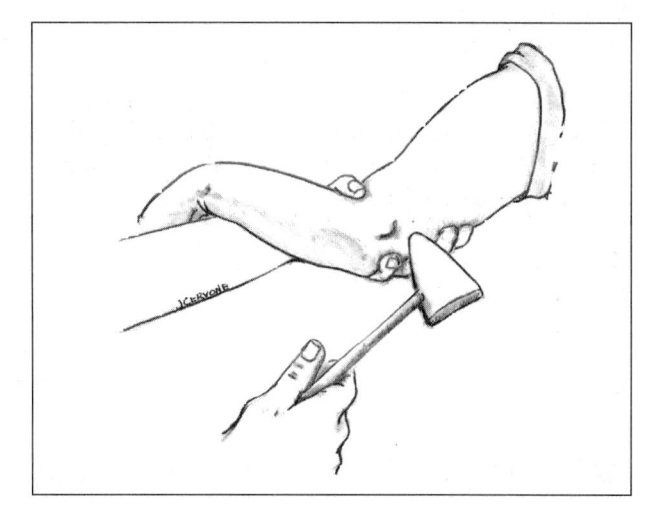

Fig. 3-1

CLINICAL GEM:
To assess C5, perform a biceps reflex test. To assess C6, perform a brachioradialis reflex test.

CLINICAL GEM:
A reflex is an involuntary response to a stimulus. Reflexes depend on intact neural pathways.

2. For optimal results when performing discriminative sensory re-education, certain requirements must be met. A specific level of return in touch perception must be present for successful retraining. With Semmes-Weinstein monofilaments, the patient must be able to perceive:

A. 6.65 monofilament
B. 5.07 monofilament
C. 4.56 monofilament
D. 4.31 monofilament

A patient must have protective sensation (4.31) on the fingertips with monofilament testing before discrimination retraining can be initiated. If discriminative sensory re-education is begun before this sensibility is obtained, the treatment will not be beneficial and the patient may become discouraged.

Answer: **D**
Hunter, Mackin, Callahan, p. 706

3. You are manual muscle testing the triceps muscle and note that the patient can achieve full active range of motion in the gravity-eliminated plane. The triceps should be rated:

A. Poor minus
B. Poor
C. Poor plus
D. Fair minus
E. Fair

Manual muscle testing (MMT) involves observing, palpating, and manually resisting muscles or groups of muscles to determine the quality and quantity of muscle contraction. Contraindications to MMT include spasticity and situations in which active range of motion or resistance is not allowed, such as during the healing of bone, muscle, and tendon. Several grading scales have been noted in the literature and are used in academic programs.

Following are the classifications and definitions from Trombly and Scott's grading system.

Word	Number	Definition
Zero (0)	0	No contraction palpable; no movement at joint
Trace (T)	1	Contraction/tension palpated in the muscle or tendon; no movement at joint
Poor − (P−)	2−	Part moves through only a portion of range of motion on a gravity-eliminated plane
Poor (P)	2	Part moves through full range of motion on a gravity-eliminated plane with no added resistance
Poor + (P+)	2+	Part moves through full range of motion on a gravity-eliminated plane; takes minimal resistance and then "breaks"
Fair − (F−)	3−	Part moves through less than full range of motion against gravity
Fair (F)	3	Part moves through full range of motion against gravity with no added resistance
Fair + (F+)	3+	Part moves through full range of motion against gravity with minimal resistance
Good − (G−)	4−	Part moves through full range of motion against gravity with less than moderate resistance
Good (G)	4	Part moves through full range of motion against gravity with moderate resistance
Normal (N)	5	Part moves through full range of motion against gravity with maximum resistance

Answer: **B**
Clinical Assessment Recommendations, pp. 47-52
Trombly, Scott, p. 174

4. Which is the most useful and widely known noninvasive test for evaluating the contribution of the radial and ulnar arteries to the hand?

A. Allen's test
B. Plethysmography
C. Arteriography
D. Radionuclide studies

The Allen's test is used to assess both ulnar and radial arteries of the hand. The examiner performs this test by compressing the arteries at the patient's wrist (Fig. 3-2, *A*) and asking the patient to make a fist several times to exsanguinate the blood (Fig. 3-2, *B*). Next, the patient is asked to open the hand approximately 90% while one artery is released and the refill time is noted (Fig. 3-2, *C*); the patient should not open the hand forcefully. The test is performed again with the other artery. The test is positive if there is no arterial flush in 5 to 15 seconds. This is a modification of the test originally described by Allen.

Answer: **A**
Green, p. 2254
Hunter, Mackin, Callahan, p. 74

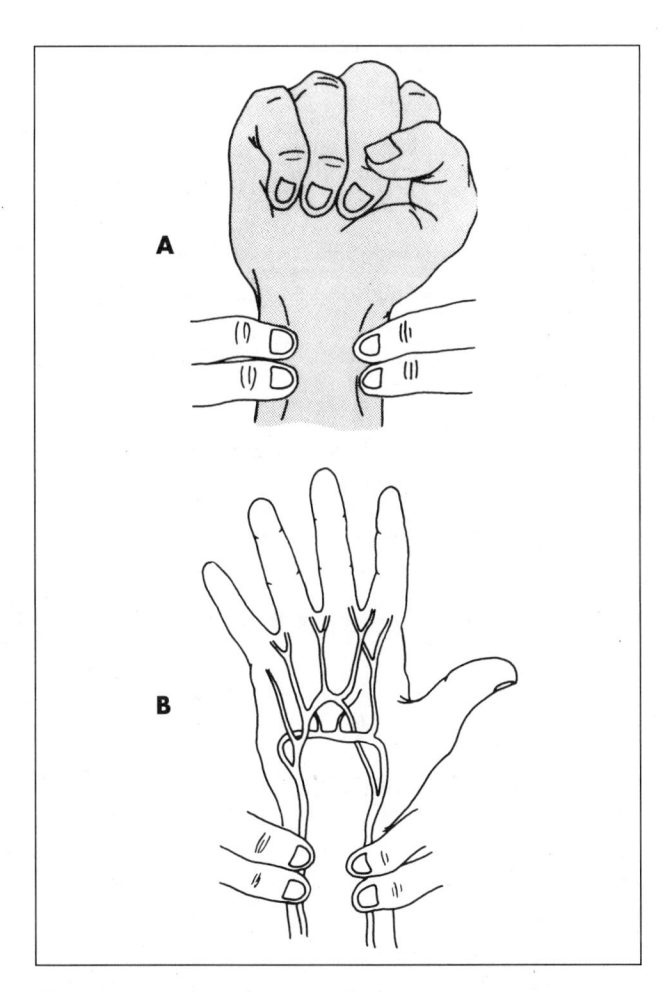

Fig. 3-2 ■ Redrawn from American Society for Surgery of the Hand: *The hand, examination and diagnosis,* Aurora, Colo., 1978, The Society.

Continued

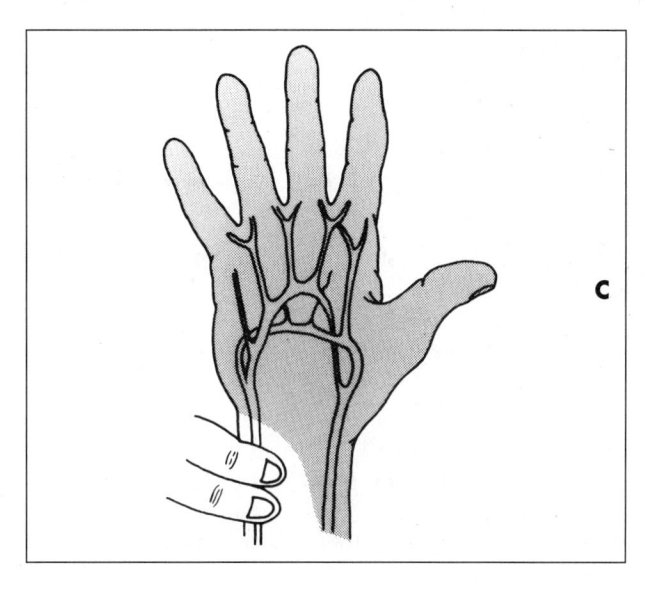

Fig. 3-2, cont'd

5. For a quick check of ulnar-nerve status, which muscle would you test?

A. Abductor pollicis brevis
B. Extensor indicis proprius
C. First dorsal interosseous
D. Palmaris longus

Assessment of the dorsal interossei, which abduct the digits, is a quick test for ulnar nerve function. The extensor indicis proprius is innervated by the radial nerve and the abductor pollicis brevis and palmaris longus are innervated by the median nerve.

Answer: **C**
Hoppenfeld, p. 95

> **CLINICAL GEM:**
> To remember the actions of the interossei, remember **PAD** and **DAB**. **PAD** refers to **P**almar interossei—**AD**duct and **DAB** refers to **D**orsal interossei—**AB**duct.

6. When measuring radial and ulnar deviation of the wrist, the axis of the goniometer is placed at the:

A. Scaphoid
B. Lunate

28 CHAPTER 3 Evaluation

C. Triquetrum
D. Capitate
E. Distal radius

When measuring wrist deviation, the goniometer is positioned so that the stationary arm is aligned with the forearm, the axis is at the capitate, and the moveable arm is placed along the third metacarpal. Wrist flexion and extension should be avoided during the assessment. Normal range of motion is: radial deviation, 0° to 20°; ulnar deviation, 0° to 30°.

When assessing range of motion, the therapist should indicate whether active, passive, or torque range of motion is being measured. Joints typically are measured on the dorsal aspect, with the axis of the goniometer lining up with the axis of the joint. It is imperative to record any deviations in the method of assessing range of motion to allow for accurate future comparisons.

Answer: **D**
Clinical Assessment Recommendations, p. 57
Hunter, Mackin, Callahan, pp. 102-103

> **CLINICAL GEM:**
> A quick way to find the capitate is to slide your finger down the patient's middle finger until you feel a divot in the wrist. The waist of the capitate lies beneath your finger.

7. A grind test on the thumb is performed to assess:

A. Osteoarthritis
B. Tenosynovitis
C. Rheumatoid arthritis
D. Ligament weakness

The grind test is performed by applying mild axial compression and gentle rotation of the thumb. If osteoarthritis is present, this test will cause pain at the first carpometacarpal joint.

Answer: **A**
Hunter, Mackin, Callahan, p. 72
Refer to Fig. 3-3.

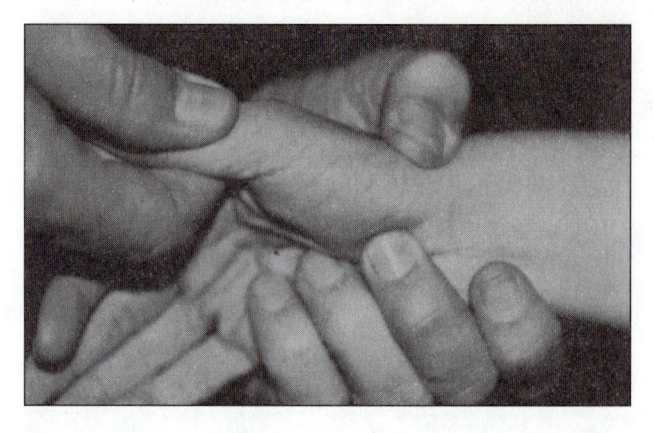

Fig. 3-3 ■ From Hunter JM, Mackin EJ, Callahan AD: *Rehabilitation of the hand: surgery and therapy,* ed 4, St. Louis, 1995, Mosby-Year Book.

8. Match the following test to the correct description:

Test

1. Jebsen hand function test
2. Crawford small parts dexterity test
3. Rosenbusch test of finger dexterity
4. Purdue pegboard
5. Minnesota rate of manipulation test

Description

A. Fine-motor coordination test using tweezers and screwdrivers
B. Gross-motor coordination test that addresses bilateral turning and placing
C. Test that focuses on the ability to simultaneously hold, manipulate, and place small objects
D. Test involving the manipulation of washers, small pins, and collars
E. Test used to assess activities-of-daily-living skills

Answers: **1. E; 2. A; 3. C; 4. D; 5. B**
Hunter, Mackin, Callahan, p. 211

9. What does a coefficient of variation of 20% refer to?

A. A good level of effort
B. Consistent effort
C. Inconsistent effort
D. Malingering

A coefficient of variation (COV) provides a percentage of variation between trials of a test. This information can be used to assess a patient's level of effort during testing. Factors that may interfere with a patient's performance include anxiety, fear of pain or re-injury, difficulty understanding the testing procedures, and other impairments. According to an accepted standard, a COV of 15% or less means that the patient's performance is at a good level of effort; a COV of greater than 15% is considered inconsistent. The authors believe that COV results should be interpreted with caution.

Answer: **C**
Hunter, Mackin, Callahan, pp. 1739-1774

10. Which handle position on the Jamar dynamometer is widely accepted when testing only one-handle span?

A. Handle position I
B. Handle position II
C. Handle position III
D. Handle position IV
E. Handle position V

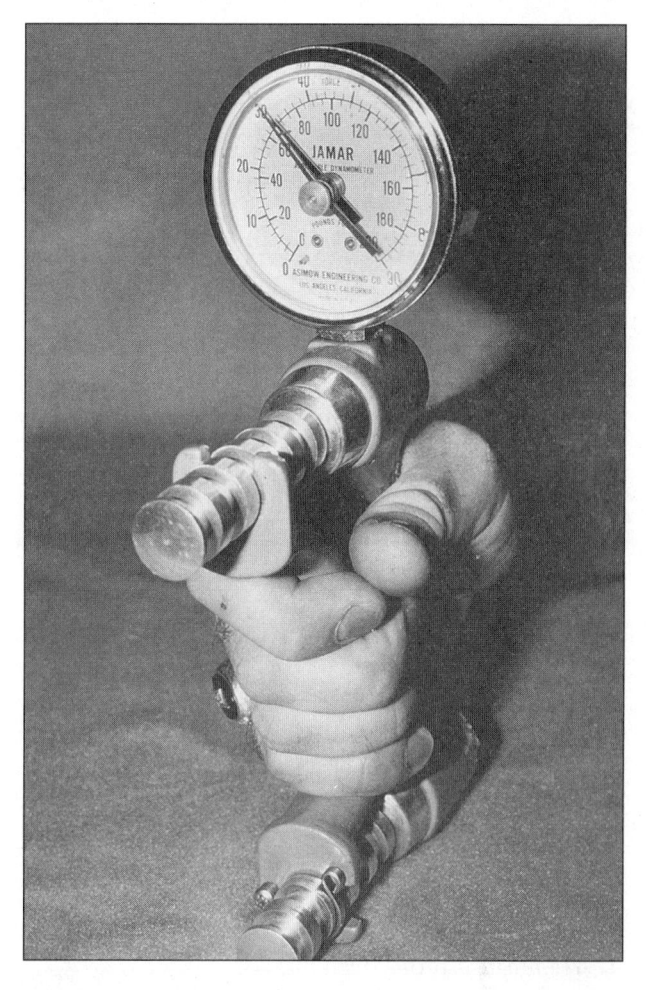

Fig. 3-4 ■ From Pedretti LW: *Occupational therapy: practice skills for physical dysfunction,* ed 4, St. Louis, 1996, Mosby-Year Book.

The Jamar dynamometer (Fig. 3-4) is a standardized instrument used for grip testing. It has five adjustable settings. The American Society of Hand Therapists (ASHT) recommends that the patient be seated comfortably during testing, with the shoulder adducted, the elbow flexed to 90°, and the forearm and wrist in neutral positions. There is controversy regarding the optimal wrist position. Most authors report that the wrist should be positioned between 0° and 30°. If wrist extension exceeds 30°, this should be noted. Both the American Society of Surgery of the Hand (ASSH) and ASHT recommend testing in the second-handle position (if only one handle span is used), as well as obtaining three grip trials.

Answer: **B**
Clinical Assessment Recommendations, pp. 41-44

11. A five-year-old girl is referred to you for evaluation of her sensibility 3 months after a median nerve repair. Which test would best determine her status of sensibility?

A. Two-point discrimination (2PD)
B. Semmes-Weinstein monofilament testing
C. Moberg pick-up test
D. O'Connor tweezer dexterity test

The Moberg pick-up test is the best choice for testing a child's functional level of sensibility because other sensory tests may be confusing and easily misunderstood by the child. The Moberg test is a nonstandardized test that consists of picking up everyday objects and placing them in a container. One may choose to use this as a clinical tool for sensory and motor re-education; however, if the Moberg test is used in this manner, it should not be used for testing.

Answer: **C**
Dellon, pp. 86-104

> **CLINICAL GEM:**
> When addressing tactile gnosis after a median nerve injury, sensory input to the ulnar-nerve-innervated digits should be decreased to ensure that object recognition is being determined by the median-nerve-innervated digits. One way to ensure this is to modify a glove by cutting away the median-innervated digits (index, thumb, and long) and keeping ring and little finger glove material intact.

12. Match each Semmes-Weinstein monofilament classification with the correct filament thickness:

Classification

1. Normal
2. Diminished light touch
3. Diminished protective sensation
4. Loss of protective sensation
5. Not testable

Filament Thickness

A. 3.22
B. Greater than 6.65
C. 5.46
D. 2.44
E. 4.08

Color key to correlate with monofilament results

Green: Normal sensation	1.65 - 2.83
Blue: Diminished light touch	3.22 - 3.61
Purple: Diminished protective sensation	3.84 - 4.31
Red: Loss of protective sensation	4.56 - 6.65
Red-lined: Not testable	Greater than 6.65

Answers: **1. D; 2. A; 3. E; 4. C; 5. B**
Hunter, Mackin, Callahan, pp. 120-121

> **CLINICAL GEM:**
> When assessing with the Semmes-Weinstein monofilament (SWM) classification, remember to bowstring the monofilament at a perpendicular angle to the finger. Monofilaments 1.65 through 4.08 are applied three times per targeted area. One out of three quantifies as a correct response; larger monofilaments are applied only one time to each targeted area.

> **CLINICAL GEM:**
> Each monofilament thickness has a range of numbers that correlates with a specific color (see question 12). When the Semmes-Weinstein monofilament results are completed, a hand diagram is color-coded. Color coding provides a quick reference to the person's level of sensibility. Repeat mappings should be performed to determine sensory recovery.

13. A 36-year-old man presents with "balloon" edema in the right, dominant hand. You choose to test the edema using a volumeter. When this test is performed, the patient should lower his hand until the stop dowel rests at which web space?

A. Web one
B. Web two
C. Web three
D. Web four

In a hand volumeter test, water is poured into the volumeter until overflow occurs and the overflow is discarded. Next, the patient slowly lowers his palm in the anatomic position (palms up) until the third web rests on the stop dowel (the third web is between digits three and four) (Fig. 3-5). The patient's hand is removed and water is measured in the graduated cylinder.

Answer: **C**
Hunter, Mackin, Callahan, p. 81

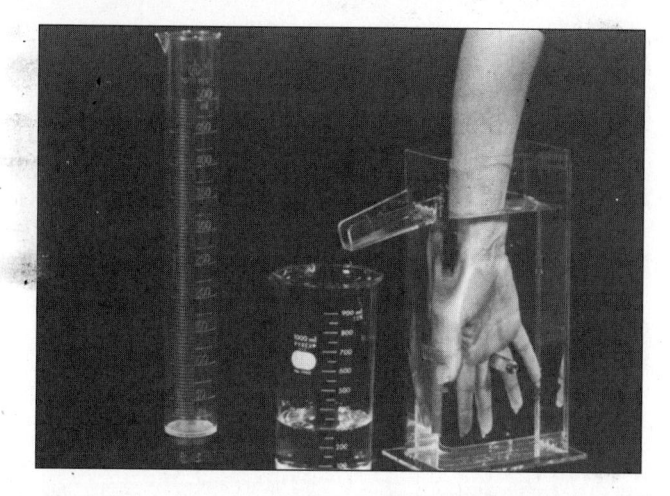

Fig. 3-5 ■ From Hunter JM, Mackin EJ, Callahan AD: *Rehabilitation of the hand: surgery and therapy*, ed 4, St. Louis, 1995, Mosby-Year Book.

> **CLINICAL GEM:**
> When testing, remember that the hand is lowered into the volumeter with the thumb facing the spout. If the patient cannot perform the test in the anatomic position, the test can be performed with the arm in pronation. This often is more comfortable.

14. A neural tension test is positive if a patient feels any tingling or discomfort during the test. True or False?

A neural tension test, according to Butler, is positive when it reproduces the patient's symptoms or current complaints. One must realize that in "normal" people tension testing may cause some discomfort or numbness. Clinicians should familiarize themselves with the expected responses.

Answer: **False**
Butler, p. 162

15. A safety pin is a good way to assess pain perception. True or False?

A sharp/dull test is used to assess pain perception. According to Waylett-Rendall, a sterile needle should be used instead of a safety pin because denervated skin lacks calluses for protection and is more susceptible to damage. The test is performed to slight blanching to prevent puncture.

According to Moberg, Dellon, and others, pinprick (sterile needle) is not recommended because of discomfort and poor correlation with functional sensation. However, if sensibility return is absent, it may be used to determine when protective sensation is intact.

Answer: **False**
Clinical Assessment Recommendations, p. 73
Hunter, Mackin, Callahan, p. 144

16. Match each test with the correct description/names:

Test

1. Ninhydrin test
2. Semmes-Weinstein
3. Moving two-point
4. Static two-point
5. Moberg pick-up test

Description/Names

A. Weber
B. Dellon
C. Threshold testing
D. Sudomotor function
E. Functional test for tactile gnosis

Answers: **1. D; 2. C ; 3. B; 4. A; 5. E**
Clinical Assessment Recommendations, pp. 71-77

17. Which of the curves in Figure 3-6 represents a treatable torque angle curve for a 50-degree proximal interphalangeal joint contracture? A or B?

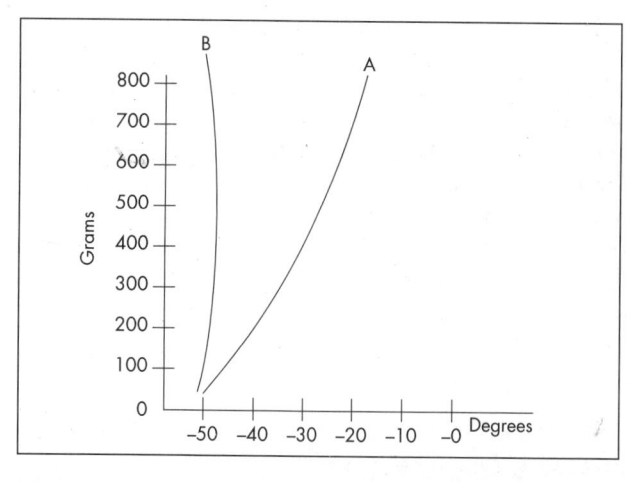

Fig. 3-6

Brand and Hollister have suggested the use of torque range of motion (TROM) to improve objectivity in measuring range of motion. TROM can be performed in the clinic using a goniometer, a strain gauge, and a finger cuff. Force is applied at a right angle to the digit that is to move. One must remember to note the position of the proximal joints. A curve with a soft slope, such as curve A, changes rapidly with increased gram load and indicates that the joint should respond to treatment. However, if the joint is in a fixed joint contracture, the slope (curve B) is steep with increased loading. This may indicate that conservative treatment (e.g., splinting) may not be effective.

Answer: **A**
Hunter, Mackin, Callahan, pp. 170-174
Brand, Hollister, pp. 115-119

18. You are testing a patient with median nerve damage using the Weber test. The resulting score is a 12 on digits one through three. According to the normative scale, this would be rated:

A. Normal
B. Fair
C. Poor
D. Protective

The Weber two-point discrimination test assesses innervation density and can be used to determine tactile gnosis. Testing should begin with the discriminator 5 mm apart. The patient responds as to whether one or two points is perceived. Seven out of ten correct responses must be obtained to receive a score. Categories are as follows:

Normal: 0 to 5 mm
Fair: 6 to 10 mm
Poor: 11 to 15 mm
Protective: One point perceived
Anesthetic: No points perceived

Answer: **C**
Clinical Assessment Recommendations, p. 79

19. Total active motion is derived by:

A. Summation of fixation minus the summation of the extension deficits
B. Summation of extension minus the summation of flexion
C. Summation of flexion and extension
D. All of the above are acceptable ways to calculate TAM

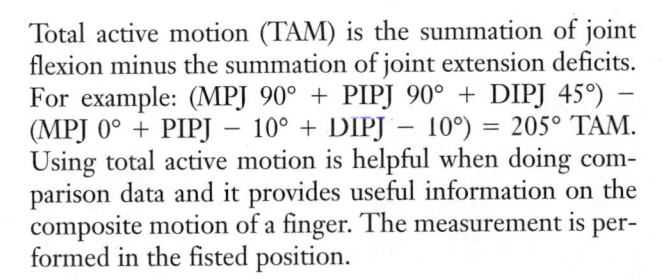

Total active motion (TAM) is the summation of joint flexion minus the summation of joint extension deficits. For example: (MPJ 90° + PIPJ 90° + DIPJ 45°) − (MPJ 0° + PIPJ − 10° + DIPJ − 10°) = 205° TAM. Using total active motion is helpful when doing comparison data and it provides useful information on the composite motion of a finger. The measurement is performed in the fisted position.

Answer: **A**
Clinical Assessment Recommendations, p. 68

20. To determine whether the biceps head is stable in the bicipital groove, which of the following should be performed?

A. Roos test
B. Wright's maneuver
C. Yergason test
D. Elbow flexion test
E. Valgus/Varus test

The Yergason test (Fig. 3-7) is performed by having the patient fully flex the elbow. The examiner grasps the flexed elbow with one hand while using the other hand to hold the wrist. The patient should be instructed to resist motion while the examiner externally rotates the arm. At the same time, the examiner pulls the patient's elbow into extension. This test will determine whether the head of the biceps is stable in the bicipital groove. If the tendon is not stable, the patient may experience pain or the tendon may pop out.

Answer: **C**
Hoppenfeld, p. 32

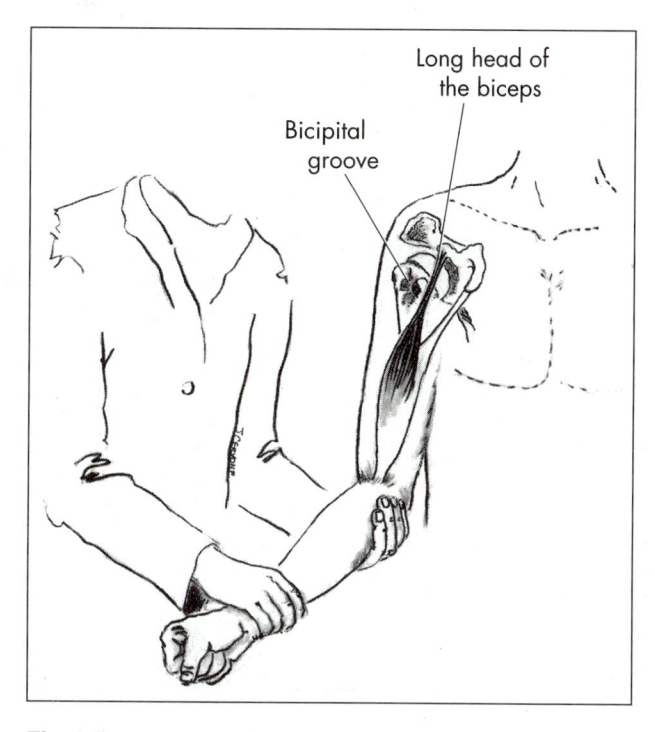

Fig. 3-7

21. What is a disadvantage of using the visual analog scale?

A. It is a highly sensitive test.
B. It is difficult and awkward to use.
C. It has a high failure rate because patients have difficulty interpreting the instructions.
D. Examiners must have experience using the test.

The visual analog scale (VAS) is performed by drawing a 10-cm line horizontally or vertically, with the ends labeled "no pain" and "pain as bad as it could be." The patient marks the line to indicate his or her current level of pain. The test may have a high failure rate because patients may have difficulty interpreting the instruc-

tions. It is recommended that the pain assessment be completed with supervision to ensure proper patient understanding. Answer A is an advantage of this test but answers B and D do not apply. Other pain tests include an array of rating scales and pain questionnaires such as the McGill or Schultz pain assessment.

Answer: **C**
Clinical Assessment Recommendations, p. 100

22. The temperature of the water has no effect on the results of volumetric measurements. True or False?

According to a study by Theodore King in 1993, water temperature should be controlled. His study revealed statistical significance related to variation in temperature. Therefore, cool or "tepid" water is recommended for accurate results (see Fig. 3-5).

Answer: **False**
King, p. 203

23. The presence of axons in the process of regeneration can be detected by a (an):

A. 256-Hz tuning fork
B. Phalen's sign
C. Iodine test
D. Tinel's sign

A Tinel's sign assists in predicting distal reinnervation after nerve repair. Percussion is applied along the nerve and is positive at the most distal point at which the patient has a tingling sensation.

A tuning fork is used for vibratory perception testing. The iodine assessment tests the sudomotor function of a nerve to assess sympathetic return. The Phalen's sign is a test performed to assist in the diagnosis of median nerve compression at the wrist.

Answer: **D**
Clinical Assessment Recommendation, p. 71
Dellon, pp. 44-45
Refer to Fig. 3-8.

34 CHAPTER 3 Evaluation

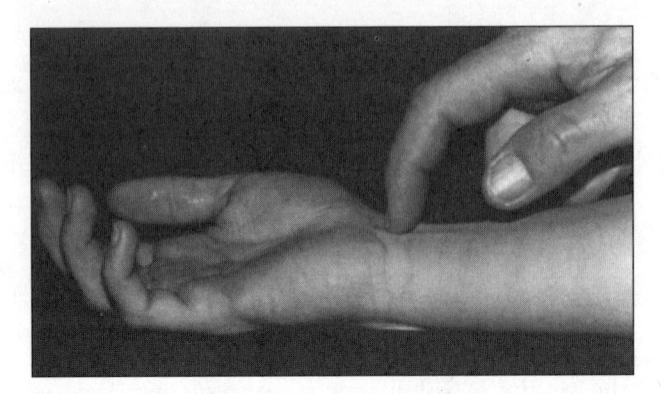

Fig. 3-8

> **CLINICAL GEM:**
> Sensations during nerve regeneration may include sharp pain, shooting pain, hot and cold flashes, the sensation of water running down the arm, numbness, tingling, or no sensation at all.

Chapter 4
Neuroanatomy and Sensory Re-education

Topics to be reviewed in random order are:

- Sensory receptors
- Sensory re-education
- Order of sensory recovery
- Sunderland and Seddon classification systems
- Neuroanatomy terms
- Sympathetic nervous system
- Brachial plexus anatomy, pathology, and therapy
- Horner's syndrome
- Hansen's disease
- Nerve regeneration

1. Which sensory receptor is responsible for detecting a sensation of a gentle breeze blowing against the skin?

A. Pacinian corpuscle
B. Merkel cell
C. Ruffini end organs
D. None of the above

The Pacinian corpuscle is a sensory receptor that is innervated by a single, quickly adapting nerve fiber. The Pacinian corpuscle is large and located in subcutaneous tissue. It is extremely sensitive to mechanical stimuli and therefore is responsible for detecting a very gentle breeze blowing across the skin.

Answer: **A**
Dellon, p. 20
Refer to Fig. 4-1.

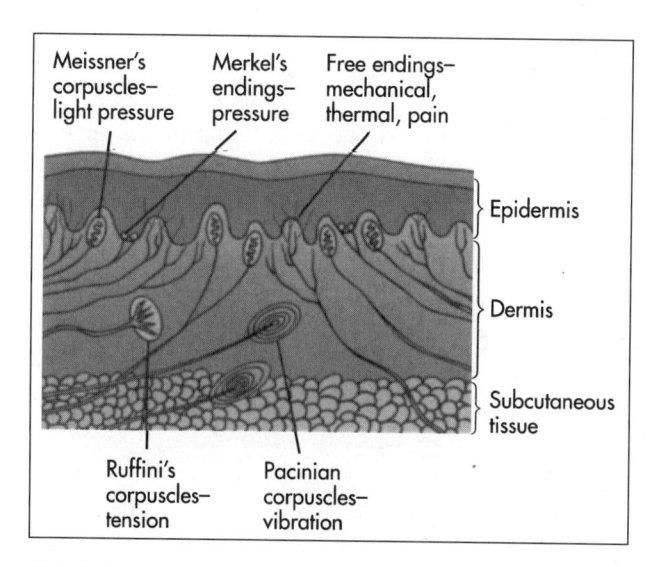

Fig. 4-1 ■ From Lindsay DT: *Functional human anatomy*, St. Louis, 1996, Mosby-Year Book.

2. **Thirty-Hertz vibration is perceived by:**

A. Quickly adapting Meissner corpuscles
B. Quickly adapting Pacinian corpuscles
C. Slowly adapting Merkel cells
D. Slowly adapting Ruffini end organs

Thirty-Hertz (Hz) vibration and movement are perceived by quickly adapting A-β fibers known as Meissner corpuscles. Two hundred fifty six-Hz vibration and movement are perceived by the quickly adapting A-β fibers known as Pacinian corpuscles. Both receptors are found in glabrous (nonhairy) skin and are encapsulated (see Fig. 4-1).

Answer: **A**
Dellon, pp. 10, 11

3. Constant-touch pressure is perceived by:

A. Large myelinated A-β fibers quickly adapting
B. Large myelinated A-δ fiber quickly adapting
C. Large myelinated A-α fibers slowly adapting
D. Large myelinated A-β fibers slowly adapting

A-β fibers are referred to as neuroreceptive afferents, which may be either slowly or quickly adapting nerve fibers. Constant-touch pressure is perceived by slowly adapting, large, myelinated A-β fibers. Constant touch is perceived by the Merkel cells found in the glabrous skin and the Ruffini end organs in hairy skin.

Answer: **D**
Dellon, p. 10

> **CLINICAL GEM:**
> Following is a quick reference chart to correlate receptors, functions, and applicable tests:
>
> | Specialized Receptors | Functions | Applicable Tests |
> |---|---|---|
> | Merkel cell | Constant-touch pressure | Semmes-Weinstein monofilament
Static two-point discrimination |
> | Pacinian corpuscle | 256-Hertz Movement and vibration | Tuning fork |
> | Meissner corpuscle | 30-Hertz Movement and vibration | Tuning fork; moving two-point discrimination |

4. When you put on a pair of gloves, which receptor perceives stimuli until the glove is removed?

A. Pacinian corpuscles
B. Merkel cells
C. Meissner corpuscles
D. Free nerve endings

The large, myelinated, A-β slowly adapting fibers perceive the constant touch of your gloves. The Merkel cells begin to transmit impulses immediately and continue to transmit them until you remove the gloves.

Answer: **B**
Dellon, p. 10

5. You are treating a 41-year-old woman who sustained a median nerve injury at the wrist level. A nerve repair was performed. The patient's repair was protected for 3 weeks; next, range of motion and early sensory re-education were initiated. You would like to progress to object recognition or late-phase sensory re-education. Which would be the best screening test for determining whether your patient is ready to start late-phase re-education?

A. 30-Hertz vibration
B. Perception of pinprick
C. 256-Hertz vibration
D. Detection of hot or cold

The recovery sequence begins with pain and temperature because these sensations are perceived through unmyelinated and thinly myelinated fibers. Next, the large myelinated fibers begin to receive 30 Hertz (Hz) by the Meissner corpuscles, which are easy to reinnervate because any of the nine different nerves may innervate this receptor from any direction. After this, moving touch is perceived, followed by constant touch. Next, a 256-Hz stimulus is perceived by means of a single, quickly adapting nerve fiber, which can enter through either end of the large, football-shaped Pacinian corpuscle. When your patient can detect 256 Hz, she is ready for object recognition or late-phase re-education. If you begin object recognition before the detection of 256 Hz, it will most likely be uneventful, and you and the patient will become frustrated.

Answer: **C**
Dellon, pp. 20, 249-250, 262

> ★ **CLINICAL GEM:**
> Following is a quick reference list of the order of sensory return:
>
> - Pain and temperature
> - 30-Hz vibration
> - Moving touch
> - Constant touch
> - 256-Hz vibration
> - Touch localization
> - Two-point discrimination
> - Stereognosis

6. After an anterolateral surgical approach to the forearm, a patient experiences numbness on the lateral (radial) aspect of his forearm. The structure most likely affected is the:

A. Axillary nerve
B. Posterior interosseous nerve
C. Lateral antebrachial cutaneous nerve
D. Anterior interosseous nerve

The lateral antebrachial cutaneous nerve crosses the elbow and enters the forearm between the biceps and the brachialis. This nerve is at risk in the anterolateral and anterior surgical approaches to the forearm.

Answer: **C**
Hoppenfeld, deBoer, pp. 93, 96

7. Pain receptors are in encapsulated cells. True or False?

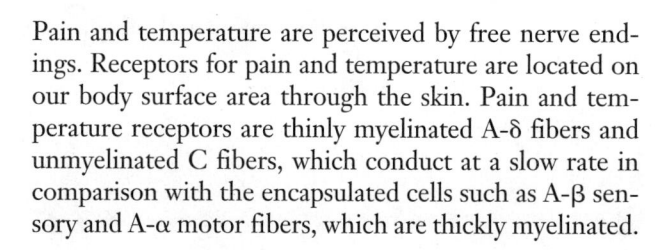

Pain and temperature are perceived by free nerve endings. Receptors for pain and temperature are located on our body surface area through the skin. Pain and temperature receptors are thinly myelinated A-δ fibers and unmyelinated C fibers, which conduct at a slow rate in comparison with the encapsulated cells such as A-β sensory and A-α motor fibers, which are thickly myelinated.

Answer: **False**
Dellon, pp. 6, 9-13

8. The cell body of the sensory neuron is located in the _____:

A. Brain
B. Spinal cord
C. Dorsal root ganglion
D. A and B are correct
E. All are correct

The most basic unit of the nervous system is the neuron. The neuron is the functional and structural unit that initiates and conducts impulses. In the peripheral nervous system, there are motor and sensory neurons. The cell body of the motor neuron is located in the ventral horn of the spinal cord. The cell body of the sensory neuron is located in the dorsal root ganglion, outside the central nervous system. The sensory neuron's axon extends to skin.

Answer: **C**
Dellon, p. 2
Refer to Fig. 4-2.

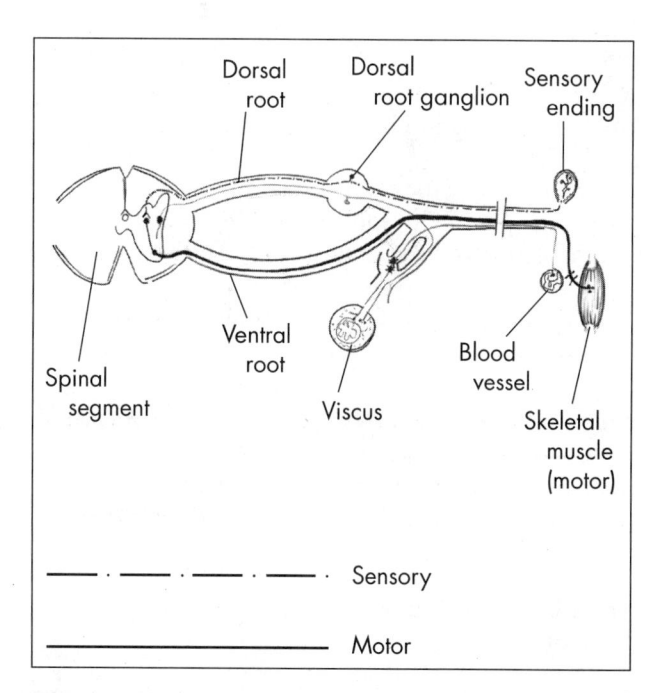

Fig. 4-2

9. Schwann cells are located in the central nervous system. True or False?

Schwann cells are located in the peripheral nervous system and create the myelin sheath around the axon. For axons to conduct fast impulses, an insulation or myelin is required. Myelin is a lipoprotein. The slower conducting axons within the peripheral nervous system are not myelinated. Schwann cells serve an extremely important functional role for the peripheral nervous system. They make nerve growth factor, which enables the peripheral nerve to regenerate. The central nervous system does not have Schwann cells; the analogous cells in this system are oligodendrocytes and astroglia.

Answer: **False**
Dellon, p. 4

10. Match Sunderland's five numerical classifications of peripheral nerve injury with their definitions.

Degree

1. First
2. Second
3. Third
4. Fourth
5. Fifth

Definition

A. Transection of the entire trunk
B. Local conduction block with minimal structural disruption
C. Disruption of the axon, endoneurium, and perineurium. The epineural tissue is spared.
D. Disruption of axon only, leaving the endoneurium intact; a neuroma-in-continuity.
E. An intact perineurium surrounding a disruption of the axon and endoneurium.

Answers: **1. B; 2. D; 3. E; 4. C; 5. A**
Hunter, Mackin, Callahan, p. 610
Butler, p. 176

11. The epineurium surrounds the entire nerve. True or False?

A nerve is composed of nerve fibers found together in bundles or fascicles. The perineurium is the connective tissue layer surrounding the fascicle. The endoneurium is the space within the fascicle. The internal (interfascicular) epineurium is the connective tissue lying between the fascicles facilitating gliding. The structure that surrounds the entire nerve is referred to as the external epineurium.

Answer: **True**
Dellon, p. 6
Green, p. 1317
Butler, p. 8
Refer to Fig. 4-3.

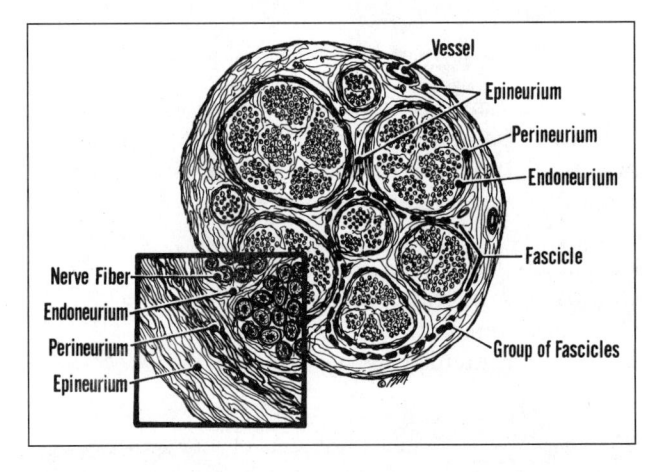

Fig. 4-3 ■ Cross-section of normal peripheral nerve. Peripheral nerve fibrosis of the epineurium constricts the nerve anatomy and metabolism of the axon flow, resulting in altered functional and sensory patterns. (Copyright, Elizabeth Roselius, 1993. From Wilgis EFS, Brushart TM: *Nerve repair and grafting*. In Green DP, Hotchkiss RN, editors: *Operative hand surgery*, vol 2, ed 3, New York, 1993, Churchill Livingstone, with permission.)

CLINICAL GEM:
The fascicle is the smallest unit of nerve structure that can be manipulated surgically.

12. The perineurium has the following function:

A. Protects the contents of the endoneural tubes
B. Surrounds each fascicle
C. Acts as a diffusion barrier
D. All of the above

The perineurium is a strong, elastic tissue that surrounds each fascicle and protects the contents of the endoneural tubes. It has an important role as a diffusion barrier. The perineurium aids in keeping certain substances out of the intrafascicular environment (see Fig. 4-3).

Answer: **D**
Butler, pp. 8, 23-24

13. Match the medical terminology with the sympathetic function for that term.

Terminology

1. Vasomotor
2. Sudomotor
3. Pilomotor
4. Trophic

Sympathetic Function

A. Gooseflesh response
B. Hair growth and nail changes
C. Skin color and skin temperature changes
D. Sweat

Answers: **1. C; 2. D; 3. A; 4. B**
Malick, Kasch, p. 19

14. A 29-year-old woman who is a professional flute player is referred to you for evaluation and treatment. Her complaints range from aching shoulders to coldness and numbness in the whole hand and occasional tingling in the little and ring fingers. The evaluation reveals no intrinsic wasting. The referring physician has ruled out carpal tunnel syndrome, cubital tunnel syndrome, tumors, temporomandibular joint pathology, and cervical disc disease. Which exercise program would you choose?

A. Stretching the wrist and elbow muscles and strengthening the pectoralis minor and scalene muscles.
B. Stretching the middle and lower trapezius and strengthening the pectoralis major and minor muscles.
C. Stretching the pectoralis minor, upper trapezius, and scalene muscles and strengthening the middle and lower trapezius, serratus anterior, and levator scapulae muscles.
D. A and B are correct.
E. B and C are correct.

After careful examination and discussion with the referring physician, you would conclude that this patient has thoracic outlet syndrome. If the word "thoracic outlet" is taken literally, confusion may occur. Some authors and clinicians refer to thoracic outlet syndrome as brachial plexus compression in the thoracic inlet; thoracic outlet syndrome, by name, implies that the diaphragm is restricted because the thoracic outlet is the region between the thorax and the abdomen.

Thoracic outlet syndrome is accepted among surgeons and neurologists in the following two situations: (1) when the patient presents with a cervical rib, which can cause either subclavian artery or vein occlusion; or (2) when the patient presents with intrinsic muscle wasting and numbness of the little finger. The latter is confirmed with electromyography. These two conditions are uncommon and require surgical intervention. Fortunately, the majority of cases do not fall into these categories and can be managed conservatively.

In this case study, the therapist should observe the patient playing her flute, adjust her practice schedule, change her positioning, and teach exercises to strengthen the patient's shoulder girdle muscles and to relax or stretch the other musculature. The therapist should design a program to strengthen the middle and lower trapezius, serratus anterior, and levator muscles while stretching or relaxing the pectoralis minor, upper trapezius, and scalene muscles. One way to stretch the pectoralis minor and strengthen the serratus is to perform wall push-ups while facing a corner, using both walls.

Answer: **C**
Dellon, pp. 506-539

> **CLINICAL GEM:**
> A helpful reference book to recommend to musicians with musculoskeletal pathologies is Richard Norris: *The musician's survival manual: a guide to preventing and treating injuries in instrumentalists*, St. Louis, 1993, International Conference of Symphony and Opera Musicians.

CHAPTER 4 Neuroanatomy and Sensory Re-education

15. The concentration of potassium is higher on the inside of a cell in normal muscle and nerve tissue. True or False?

To understand the physiology of normal cell excitability, it is important to understand active and passive diffusion through the cell membrane. Muscle and nerve cells are encased in a membrane that separates a charge from the inside and the outside of a cell. This charge has a resting membrane state of approximately −60 millivolts (MV). The inside of the cell is negative compared with the outside of the cell. In normal muscle and nerve tissue, potassium (K+) ions are higher on the inside of the cell and sodium (Na+) is higher on the outside of the cell.

The concentration differences are maintained by an active pump across the membrane. This pump helps the cell eliminate sodium ions while receiving potassium ions. In addition, a passive diffusion of ions across the membrane attempts to equalize the ion concentration.

Answer: **True**
Hunter, Mackin, Callahan, pp. 1508,1509
Refer to Fig. 4-4.

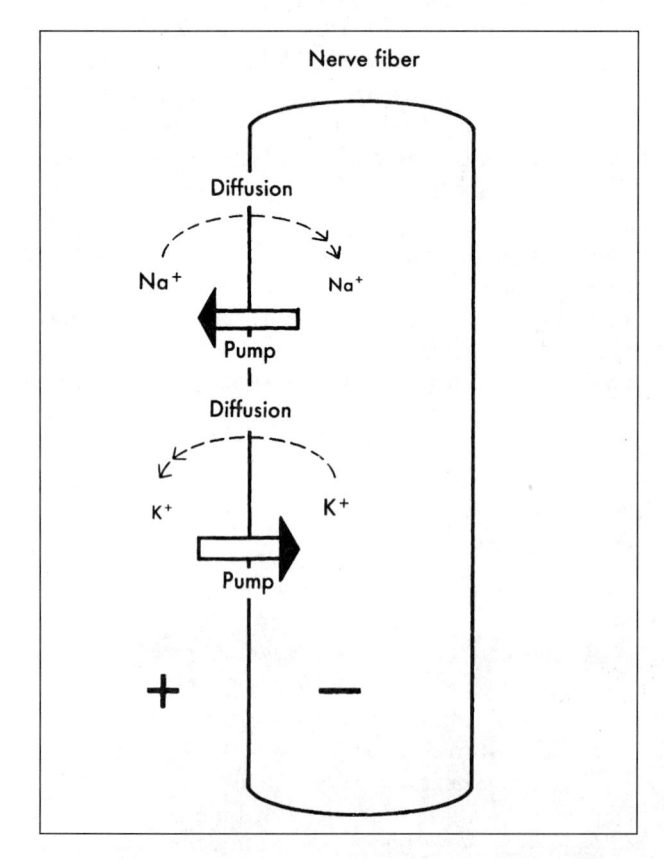

Fig. 4-4 ■ From Hunter JM, Mackin EJ, Callahan AD: *Rehabilitation of the hand: surgery and therapy*, ed 4, St. Louis, 1995, Mosby-Year Book.

16. A 32-year-old male sustained a median nerve laceration at the level of the elbow 6 months ago. The nerve was repaired. Manual muscle testing revealed a 4+/5 for the pronator teres and a 3/5 for the flexor digitorum superficialis. Which muscle would you expect to return next?

A. Palmaris longus
B. Palmaris brevis
C. Flexor digitorum profundus to the first and second digits
D. Flexor digitorum profundus to the second and third digits
E. Pronator quadratus

The median nerve (Fig. 4-5, *B*) arises from the lateral cord (C6, C7) and the medial cord (C8, T1) of the brachial plexus. The median nerve enters the forearm between the two heads of the pronator teres, innervating them, and then innervates the flexor carpi radialis. The next muscle innervated along the course of the median nerve is the palmaris longus, followed by the flexor digitorum superficialis, the flexor digitorum profundus to the index and middle finger (second and third digits), the flexor pollicis longus, and the pronator quadratus. The first muscle that the nerve innervates after crossing the wrist is the abductor pollicis brevis, followed by the opponens pollicis and the flexor pollicis brevis; the nerve terminates in the first and second lumbricals. Answer C, the first and second digits, refers to the thumb and index fingers.

Answer: **D**
Hunter, pp. 70,765

> **CLINICAL GEM:**
> Following is a quick reference to median nerve innervation:
>
> | Number of Muscles per Group | Specific Muscles | Anatomical Location |
> |---|---|---|
> | Four muscles | 1. Pronator teres
2. Flexor carpi radialis
3. Palmaris longus
4. Flexor digitorum superficial | Forearm |

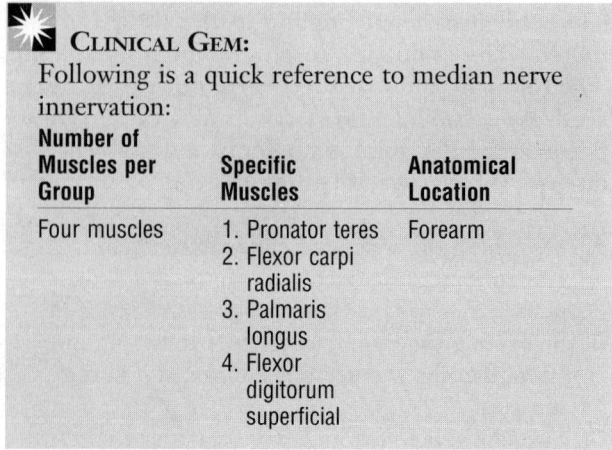

Continued on page 42

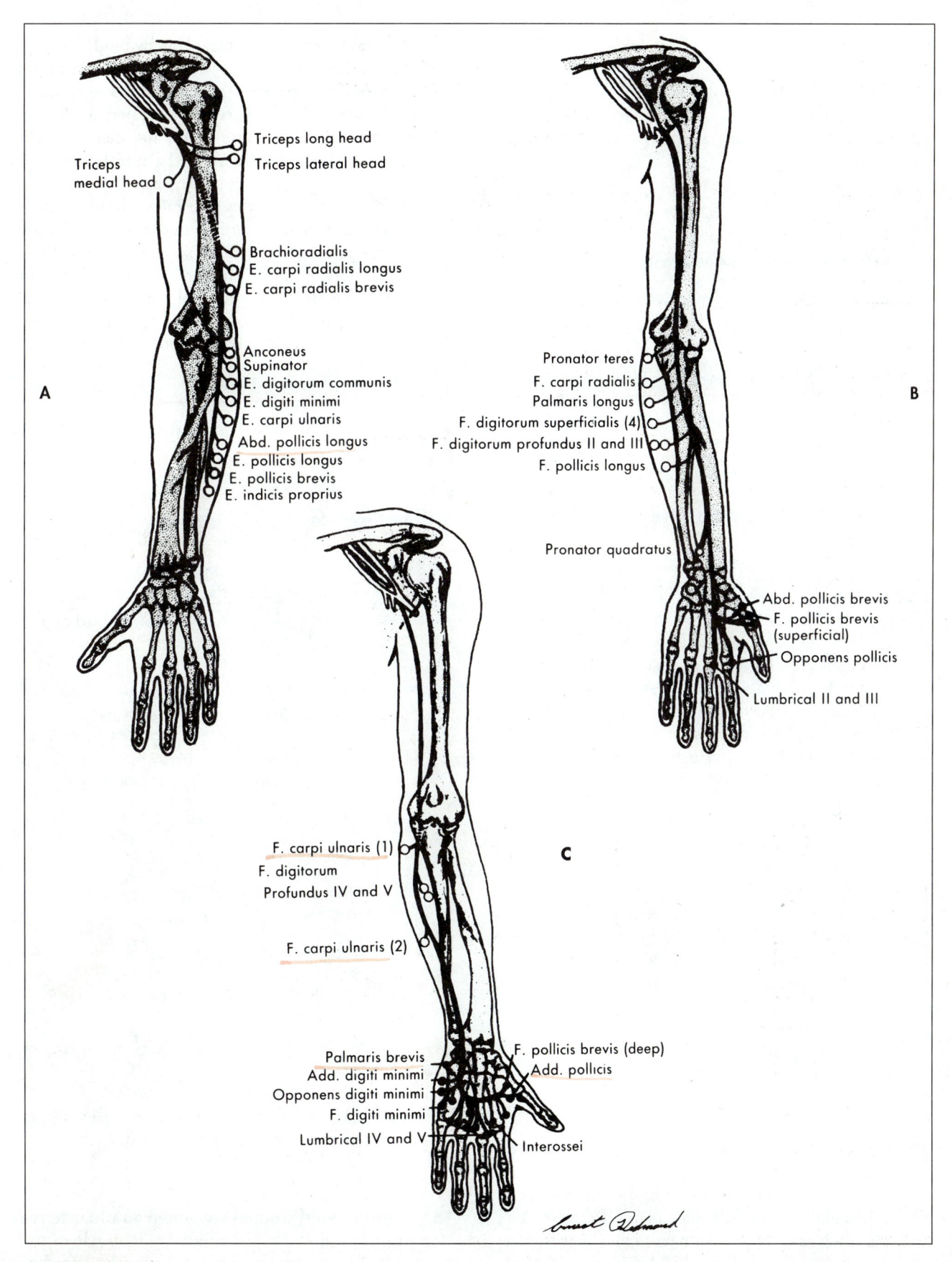

Fig. 4-5 ■ Terminal branches of the **A**, radial, **B**, median, and **C**, ulnar nerves. (Redrawn from the American Society for Surgery of the Hand: *The hand, examination and diagnosis,* Aurora, Colo., 1978, The Society.)

CLINICAL GEM—CONT'D

Number of Muscles per Group	Specific Muscles	Anatomical Location
Three muscles	1. Flexor digitorum profundus (index and middle) 2. Flexor pollicis longus 3. Pronator quadratus	Forearm (anterior interosseous nerve)
Four muscles	1. Abductor pollicis brevis 2. Opponens pollicis 3. Flexor pollicis brevis (superficial head) 4. Lumbricals (one and two)	Wrist; Hand

CLINICAL GEM:
At the mid-forearm, the median nerve branches into the anterior interosseous nerve (AIN). The AIN innervates the flexor digitorum profundus to the index and middle fingers, the flexor pollicis longus, and the pronator quadratus, and then innervates the volar wrist capsule. When the AIN is damaged, a patient cannot form an "O" with the thumb and index fingers (see Fig. 18-12).

17. **An 18-year-old male sustained an injury to the posterior cord of the brachial plexus. Initially, return of the triceps was observed. Eight months later the patient is able to radially deviate his wrist and slight forearm supination is observed. Which muscle would you expect to return next?**

A. Brachioradialis
B. Extensor carpi ulnaris
C. Extensor digitorum communis
D. Extensor indicis

The radial nerve is a continuation of the posterior cord of the brachial plexus. Its roots emerge from C6, C7, C8, and T1 levels. The radial nerve innervates the triceps, anconeus, and brachioradialis as it winds posteriorly on the humerus. Next, the motor branch innervates the extensor carpi radialis longus and extensor carpi radialis brevis, and enters the forearm between the two heads of the supinator. At this point, there is a division of the motor and sensory nerves. They divide into the superficial sensory branch and the deep branch. There is controversy as to when the radial nerve becomes termed the posterior interosseous nerve (PIN). In about 55% of extremities, the radial nerve supplies the extensor carpi radialis brevis; in the other 45%, the extensor carpi radialis brevis is supplied by the PIN. The PIN supplies the supinator, extensor digitorum communis, extensor digiti minimi, extensor carpi ulnaris, abductor pollicis longus, extensor pollicis longus, extensor pollicis brevis, and extensor indicis proprius (see Fig. 4-5, *A*).

Answer: **C**
Tubiana, Thomine, Mackin, p. 266

CLINICAL GEM:
Following is a quick reference to radial nerve innervation:

Muscle	Nerve
Triceps Anconeus Extensor carpi radialis longus	Radial nerve
Extensor carpi radialis brevis	Radial nerve or posterior interosseous nerve
Supinator Extensor digitorum communis Extensor digiti minimi Extensor carpi ulnaris Abductor pollicis longus Extensor pollicis longus Extensor pollicis brevis Extensor indicis proprius	Posterior interosseous nerve

CLINICAL GEM:
With respect to nerve innervation order, some authors place the anconeus muscle after the triceps and others place it after the extensor carpi radialis brevis.

18. **A 56-year-old woman sustained an ulnar nerve laceration just distal to the medial epicondyle of the humerus. The patient presented 2 months after her initial injury. You noted full wrist flexion and ulnar**

deviation with gravity eliminated. The patient was unable to flex the wrist against gravity and no other ulnar-innervated muscles were functioning. A month later you note that the patient can ulnarly deviate the wrist and flex the wrist against gravity and can tolerate minimal resistance. Knowing the course of the ulnar nerve, what is the next activity or position that would lead you to believe that the ulnar nerve is regenerating?

A. Having the patient pinch a piece of paper
B. Having the patient spread the fingers apart
C. Having the patient bring fingers back together
D. Having the patient perform a hook fist

The ulnar nerve arises from the medial cord of the brachial plexus. Its roots emerge from C7, C8, and T1. The ulnar nerve does not innervate any part of the upper extremity until it crosses the elbow and enters the forearm between the two heads of the flexor carpi ulnaris, followed by the flexor digitorum profundus to the fourth and fifth digits. If your patient is able to perform a hook fist (flexing the tips of the fingers), this would indicate regeneration of the ulnar nerve to the flexor digitorum profundus.

The ulnar nerve then crosses the wrist and innervates the following: the abductor digiti minimi, the opponens digiti minimi, the flexor digiti minimi, the third and fourth lumbricals, the palmar interossei, the dorsal interossei, the deep head of the flexor pollicis brevis, and the adductor pollicis. The order of innervation after the ulnar nerve crosses the wrist varies according to different authors (see Fig. 4-5, C).

Answer: **D**
Tubiana, Thomine, Mackin, p. 275
Hunter, Mackin, Callahan, p. 70

CLINICAL GEM:
Following is a quick reference to ulnar nerve innervation:

Flexor carpi ulnaris	Forearm
Flexor digitorum profundus (fourth and fifth digits)	
Abductor digiti minimi	Wrist and hand muscle (order varies)
Opponens digiti minimi	
Flexor digiti minimi	NOTE: Hunter, Mackin, and Callahan indicate that the first dorsal interosseus is the last muscle to be innervated.
Lumbricals (three and four)	
Interossei (palmar and dorsal)	
Flexor pollicis brevis (deep)	
Adductor pollicis	

19. In 1943, Seddon introduced a three-part classification of the injured peripheral nerve. The mildest form of nerve injury in Seddon's categorization is referred to as a neurotmesis. True or False?

The first part of Seddon's three-part classification is the neuropraxic injury, which is the mildest form of nerve injury. The neuropraxic injury is a local conduction block; with this injury the prognosis is excellent because the axonal continuity and nerve conduction is preserved proximal and distal to the injury. The second part, called axonotmesis, is more severe because axonal disruption leads to Wallerian degeneration of the distal axon. Wallerian degeneration is a degeneration of the distal axon taking place over a period of 1 to 2 months. Recovery time varies with axonotmesis and prognosis is good. The most severe type of injury is the third part, referred to as neurotmesis, which involves complete transsection of the entire nerve trunk. Prognosis is poor, unless surgical repair is performed.

Answer: **False**
Hunter, Mackin, Callahan, p. 609
Butler, p. 176

CLINICAL GEM:
Following are nerve injury correlations between Seddon's classification (as described in question 19) and Sunderland's classification (a frequently referenced peripheral nerve injury classification):

Sunderland's Classification	Seddon's Classification	Injury	Recovery Potential
I	Neuropraxia	Axon maintained; stimulation can occur distal to lesion; possible segmental demyelinization	Full
II	Axonotmesis	Loss of axonal integrity with distal axonal degeneration (Wallerian degeneration); endoneurial tube intact	Full
III	Axonotmesis	Endoneurial tube torn; perineurium intact	Slow; incomplete
IV	Axonotmesis	Only epineurium intact	Neuroma-in-continuity is common
V	Neurotmesis	Complete transection of the nerve	None

20. Scar tissue may be the culprit in neuroma development. True or False?

A neuroma is a result of a blocked regenerating nerve. This block may have various causes, one of which may be scar tissue. The block causes the regenerating sprouts to become trapped and surrounded by connective tissue. By definition, a neuroma is not painful. When a neuroma is in a vulnerable environment related to tendon or joint movement, the entrapped ends of the failed regenerating axons send painful messages when stimulation occurs from the motion of surrounding tissues. The diagnosis of a neuroma is easy to make because direct tapping over the nerve elicits a painful paresthesia. Conservative treatment consists of iontophoresis, desensitization, protective splinting, ultrasound, transcutaneous electrical nerve stimulation, or steroid injection.

Answer: **True**
Dellon, pp. 44, 45
Green, pp. 1387-1400

> **CLINICAL GEM:**
> The term "neuroma-in-continuity" refers to a neuroma in a nerve that has not been completely severed.

21. Match the following signs with their corresponding descriptions. Note that all relate to ulnar nerve paralysis.

Signs

1. Froment
2. Jeanne
3. Wartenberg
4. Duchenne
5. Egawa
6. Andre-Thomas
7. Masse

Descriptions

A. Clawing of the ring and little finger
B. Hyperextension of the metacarpophalangeal joint of the thumb in pinch grip
C. Pronounced flexion of the thumb interphalangeal joint during adduction toward the index finger (key pinch)
D. Flattening of the metacarpal arch
E. Wrist falls into volar flexion during action of the extensors to the middle finger
F. Inability to adduct the extended little finger to the extended ring finger
G. Inability of the flexed middle finger to abduct radially and ulnarly and to rotate at the metacarpophalangeal joint

Answers: **1. C; 2. B; 3. F; 4. A; 5. G; 6. E; 7. D**
Tubiana, Thomine, Mackin, p. 280

22. The presence of an ipsilateral Horner's syndrome in a patient with a traction lesion of the brachial plexus indicates:

A. Infraganglionic lesion involving C8
B. Supraganglionic lesion involving T1
C. Dorsal root injury at C8
D. Cervical stenosis at C8-T1

Horner's syndrome is contraction of the pupil, partial ptosis (drooping), enophthalmos (recession of eyeball into orbit), and sometimes loss of sweating over the affected side of the face. An ipsilateral Horner's syndrome in a patient with a brachial plexus traction injury indicates a supraganglionic lesion involving the T1 nerve root, through which sympathetic fibers enter the plexus. A poor prognosis is associated with root damage at this level.

Answer: **B**
Hunter, Mackin, Callahan, p. 363

23. You are treating a patient following ulnar nerve repair at the wrist; no tendons were involved. How long should the nerve be protected by immobilization?

A. 1 day
B. 7 to 10 days
C. 4 weeks
D. 6 to 8 weeks

After nerve repair, immobilization should be required for approximately 7 to 10 days. However, some authors promote 3 weeks of protection after nerve repair before mobilization is initiated. During the period of nerve regeneration, therapy should focus on keeping the affected area supple, mobile, and ready to accept the growing axons. Sensory re-education programs should be initiated when appropriate reinnervation occurs. It is the therapist's responsibility to ensure end organ protection through splinting, gentle range of motion, massage, modalities, and protective techniques to maximize functional outcome.

Answer: **B**
Hunter, Mackin, Callahan, p. 622

24. The suprascapular nerve arises from the middle trunk of the brachial plexus. True or False?

The suprascapular nerve arises from the upper trunk, from C5 and C6 nerve roots. The suprascapular nerve innervates the supraspinatus and infraspinatus muscles, and sensation to the shoulder capsule (see Fig. 4-7).

Answer: **False**
Hunter, Mackin, Callahan, pp. 652, 1876, 1883

25. Hansen's disease belongs in the family of peripheral nerve diseases and disorders. True or False?

Hansen's disease, also known as leprosy, is an infectious bacterial disease. This disease damages the nerves (especially in the limbs and facial areas) and can cause skin damage. If the disease is caught early, severe deformity can be prevented. Damage occurs to the peripheral nerves and this causes most of the deformities seen in patients with Hansen's disease.

Answer: **True**
Bell-Krotoski, p. 133

26. The lower two thirds of the dermatome that covers the deltoid muscle is derived from which nerve root?

A. C4
B. C5
C. C6
D. C7
E. C8

The deltoid is motored by the axillary nerve, which is derived from the brachial plexus roots C5 and C6. The cutaneous nerve supplying sensory innervation to the skin over the lower two thirds of the deltoid is derived from the superior lateral brachial cutaneous nerve (C5 nerve root), branching from the axillary nerve.

Answer: **B**
Hunter, Mackin, Callahan, p. 1876
Butler, p. 111
Refer to Fig. 4-6.

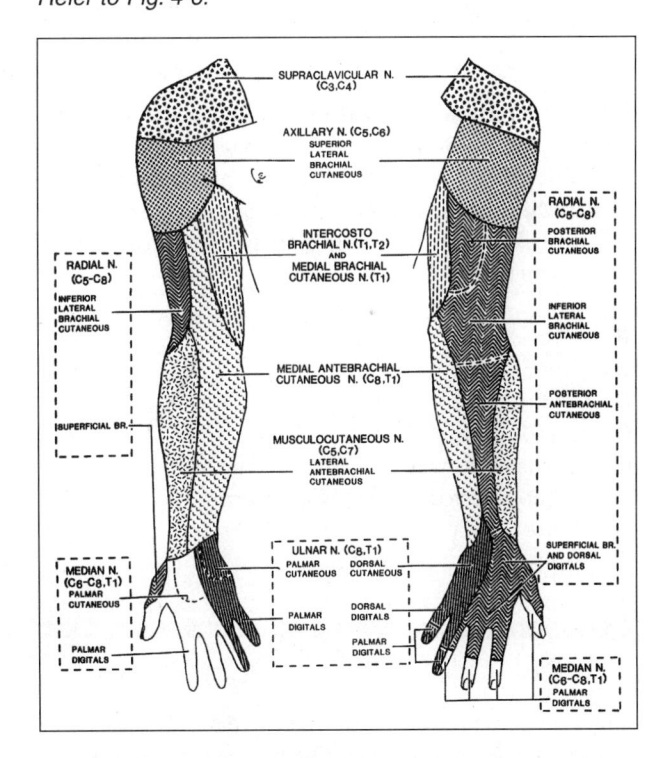

Fig. 4-6 ■. Adapted with permission from Netter FH: *The atlas of human anatomy*, Summit, NJ, 1989, CIBA-GEIGY Corp.

27. Which of the following functions is not mediated from the sympathetic nervous system (SNS)?

A. Vasomotor
B. Sudomotor
C. Pilomotor
D. Trophic
E. All of the above are mediated from the SNS

Chapter 4 Neuroanatomy and Sensory Re-education

The sympathetic nervous system mediates vasomotor (skin color and skin temperature), sudomotor (sweat), pilomotor (gooseflesh), and trophic (skin texture, soft-tissue atrophy, nail changes, hair growth, and rate of healing) functions. After nerve injury, early sympathetic changes include rosy, warm, and dry skin without gooseflesh. Trophic changes include soft, smooth skin texture with hair falling out or becoming longer and finer. Late changes after sympathetic nerve injury include mottling or cyanosis and cool skin with no pilomotor function. The skin is nonelastic, the patient develops curved (talon-like) nails, and hair continues to fall out and become longer and finer.

To treat sympathetic dysfunction, the therapist must return moisture to the skin with daily soaking and oil massage, inspect the patient daily for pressure areas, and use tools or splints that assist in injury prevention.

Answer: **E**
Malick and Kasch, pp. 19, 26

28. Your patient injured her hand on the volar aspect of the palm at the metacarpal head on the radial side of the index finger, 6 inches from her fingertip. She is experiencing sensory loss. How long will it take for her feeling to return after digital nerve repair?

A. 3 weeks
B. 3 months
C. 6 months
D. 12 months
E. You have no way of knowing unless the hand surgeon performs diagnostic testing.

The rate of nerve regeneration is inversely proportional to the distance from the cell body. A Tinel's sign is one way to measure a regenerating axon. When Wallerian degeneration occurs, rates of regeneration vary according to body part; e.g., in the upper arm, regeneration occurs at 8.5 mm/day, whereas 1 to 1.5 mm/day (1 inch/month) has been reported and accepted in the forearm and hand. In this case study, your patient injured herself roughly 6 inches from her fingertip. Nerve regeneration would be expected in approximately 6 months because the distance to the fingertip is roughly 6 inches.

Of interest, the traditional concept that regenerating axons take 3 weeks to cross the suture line and another 3 weeks to establish function once the distal end of the axon reaches its target end organ is now viewed as incorrect by some authors.

Answer: **C**
Hunter, p. 618
Dellon, pp. 38-43

29. A 52-year-old man is referred to you for sensory re-education. Your examination reveals that he cannot perceive 256 Hertz (Hz), but is able to perceive 30 Hz. He exhibits difficulty with localization and touch recognition. Which treatment modality would help with early sensory re-education?

A. Have your patient identify a variety of objects placed in a bag.
B. Occlude your patient's vision and have him identify various coins.
C. Stroke an eraser end across the targeted area.
D. All of the above are excellent tools for early sensory re-education.

Early sensory re-education may begin when 30 Hertz and moving touch are perceived. Your goal in early re-education is to correct false localization and have the patient learn to distinguish constant from moving touch. Early re-education can be accomplished by stroking or pressing an object (e.g., an eraser end of a pencil or a cotton-ball) to the targeted area. This is completed first with the patient's eyes opened, allowing the patient to observe the process. Next, the patient's eyes are closed and the patient is told to concentrate on the stimulus. Afterward, your patient should open his eyes to observe the stimulus. It is helpful to have the patient verbalize to himself the location of perceived movement or pressure when his eyes are opened and closed. A patient will perceive stroking first, followed by constant-touch and pressure.

Dellon invented the terms early and late sensory re-education in 1970. Answers *A* and *B* are performed in late-phase re-education, which is re-education of object identification. It is pointless to attempt object recognition before all sensory submodalities have regenerated to the fingertip. Keep in mind that some authors divide sensory re-education into protective and discriminative rather than early and late phases. For details regarding these categorizations, refer to Hunter, Mackin, and Callahan, pages 704 through 712.

Answer: **C**
Dellon, pp. 20, 246-295

30. If the posterior cord of the brachial plexus were injured, paralysis would be expected in which of the following muscles?

A. Latissimus dorsi
B. Deltoid
C. Extensor carpi radialis longus/extensor carpi radialis brevis
D. Coracobrachialis
E. A and D are correct
F. A, B, and C are correct

The posterior cord receives contribution from all three trunks in the brachial plexus. The posterior cord gives rise to five nerves: (1) the upper subscapular nerve, which supplies the subscapular muscle; (2) the lower subscapular nerve, which supplies the teres major and a branch of the subscapularis; (3) the thoracodorsal nerve, which supplies the latissimus dorsi; (4) the axillary nerve, which supplies the deltoid muscle and teres minor; and (5) the radial nerve, which supplies the extensors of the elbow, wrist, and digits. The coracobrachialis muscle is innervated by the musculocutaneous nerve, which is part of the lateral cord (see Fig. 4-7).

Answer: **F**
Malick, Kasch, pp. 6-9
Hunter, Mackin, Callahan, pp. 888-891,1875

31. A 32-year-old man sustained a brachial plexus injury. He cannot control shoulder abduction or forward elevation. He can extend his elbow, but cannot actively flex his elbow. He is experiencing sensory loss involving the thumb and index fingers. The middle finger sensation is intact. Which nerve roots are damaged?

A. C5 and C6
B. C5, C6, and C7
C. C6, C7, and C8
D. C7 and C8

The brachial plexus anatomy is formed by the anterior primary rami of C5, C6, C7, C8, and T1, and their terminal outflow of the peripheral nerves. Injury to the brachial plexus involves commonly observed patterns. In this case study, the lesion involves the C5 and C6 roots. The paralysis of the deltoid and lateral rotators of the humerus and elbow flexors indicates this particular level of injury. In addition, the sensory loss of the thumb and index fingers is the result of C5 and C6 root damage; the middle finger (C7) is spared (see Fig. 4-7).

Answer: **A**
Hunter, Mackin, Callahan, p. 636

32. After a nerve repair at the wrist, when can "final" evaluation of nerve recovery be assessed?

A. 6 months
B. 2 years
C. 4 to 5 years
D. The nerve is in perpetual recovery

After a nerve suture or nerve graft at the wrist, nerve regeneration to the fingertips occurs by 1 year. After another year of sensory re-education, final assessment can be performed at 2 years following surgical nerve repair.

Answer: **B**
Dellon, pp. 38-43

33. When evaluating the upper limb in a patient with a brachial plexus injury, care should be taken during examination of the shoulder joint. To prevent stress on the roots of the brachial plexus, which maximal shoulder abduction should be allowed?

A. 25°
B. 45°
C. 60°
D. 90°

In brachial plexus injuries, the therapist should be careful not to increase tension on the brachial plexus roots. Coronal abduction, and especially coronal abduction combined with lateral rotation, may cause tension on the brachial plexus roots if the arm is abducted above 90°. Because the rotator cuff often is paralyzed, which may result in humeral subluxation and abduction,

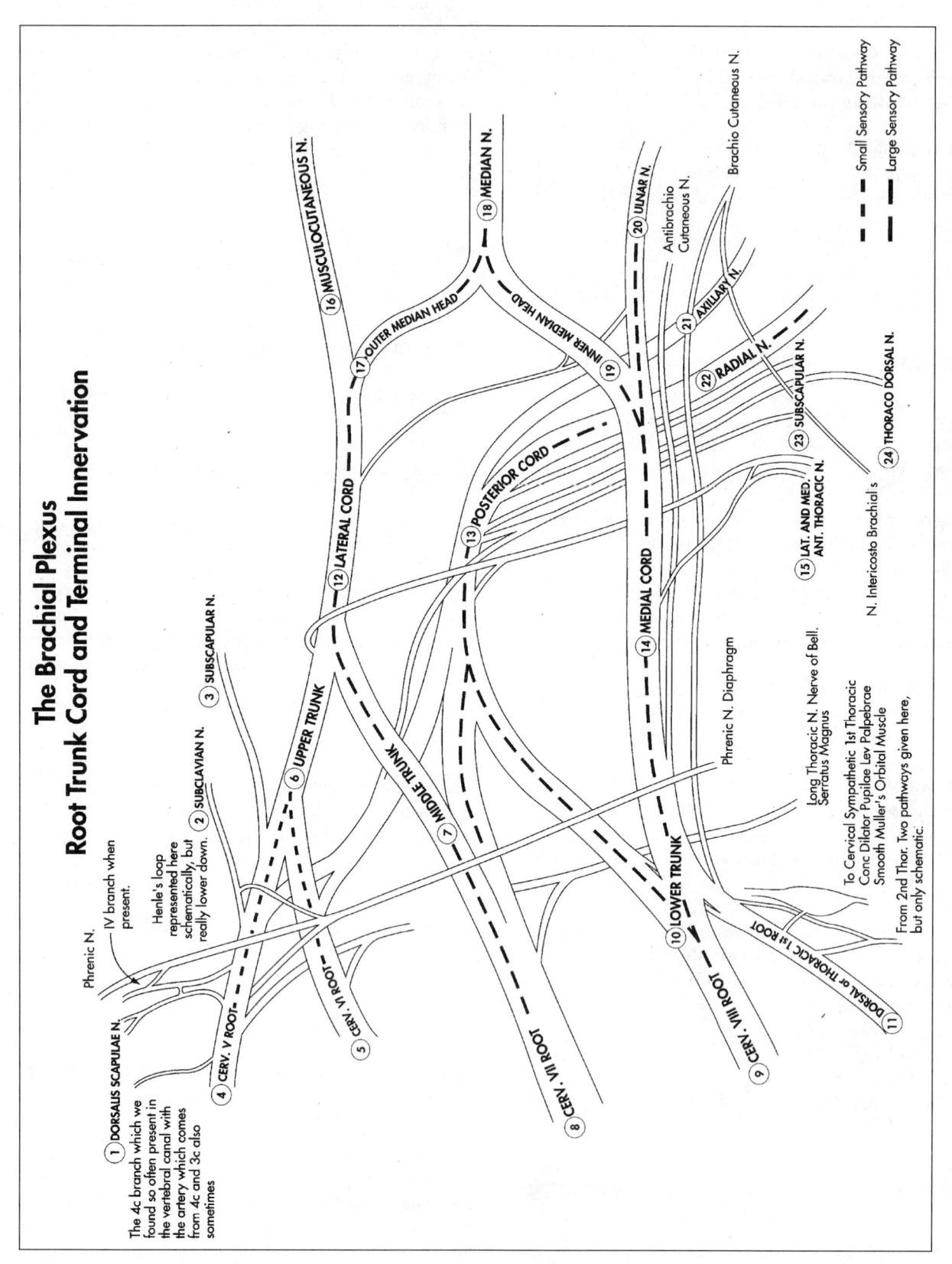

48 CHAPTER 4 Neuroanatomy and Sensory Re-education

Fig. 4-7 ■ The Stevens diagram of the brachial plexus. (Modified from Stevens JH with assistance from Kerr AT: *Brachial plexus paralysis*. In Codman EA, editor: *The shoulder*, Malabar, Fla, 1934, Robert E. Krieger, with permission.)

shoulder motion beyond 90° puts additional stress on the capsule and should be avoided.

Answer: **D**
Hunter, Mackin, Callahan, p. 648

34. **The goals of therapy during treatment of a patient experiencing brachial plexus injuries include:**

A. Protecting the limb from additional trauma
B. Preventing contractures
C. Monitoring sensory recovery
D. Addressing psychological issues
E. All of the above

A brachial plexus injury is a devastating, complex event that requires a team approach to treatment. Both psychological distress and physical involvement affect the functional outcome. The healthcare team should help with psychological issues involving functional loss, depression, or difficulty dealing with the loss. In addition, the goals of therapy are to protect the limb from additional trauma, prevent contractures, and monitor sensory and motor recovery.

Answer: **E**
Hunter, Mackin, Callahan, pp. 647-655

35. **The median nerve usually enters the forearm:**

A. Between the two heads of the supinator
B. Between the two heads of the pronator teres
C. Posterior to the brachial artery
D. Superficial to the lacertus fibrosis

The median nerve enters the forearm between the two heads of the pronator teres, deep to the biceps aponeurosis.

Answer: **B**
Hoppenfeld, deBoer, p. 121

> **CLINICAL GEM:**
> Each major peripheral nerve enters the forearm through a two-headed muscle: the median nerve enters through the pronator teres; the radial nerve through the supinator; and the ulnar nerve through the flexor carpi ulnaris.

36. **The term Klumpke palsy refers to which brachial plexus level of injury?**

A. (C5), C6, C7
B. C6, C7
C. C7, C8
D. (C7), C8, T1

Klumpke palsy is an uncommon lesion in the adult population involving the (C7), C8, and T1 nerve-roots. The shoulder, elbow, and wrist extension are intact. Loss of finger flexion, extension, and intrinsic function of the hand is observed. The sensory loss may be severe and usually involves the little finger, ring finger, and medial aspect of the forearm (see Fig. 4-7).

Answer: **D**
Hunter, Mackin, Callahan, pp. 637, 886

37. **You are treating a patient 4 weeks after distal fingertip amputation. Primary healing has occurred. He describes extreme hypersensitivity and also reports that the fingertip feels as if it is going to "burst open." Which contact particle or texture would be best for this patient during initial treatment?**

A. Burlap texture
B. Velcro hook
C. High-cycle continuous vibration
D. Cotton balls

Desensitization programs should be initiated at the level of vibration texture and contact medium that the patient can tolerate. A patient with extreme hypersensitivity, as described in this situation, would not be able to tolerate Velcro hook, burlap texture, or high-cycle continuous vibration. Initiating treatment with moleskin texture, felt, or cotton would be more appropriate for this patient. This patient probably would benefit from retrograde massage during the early stage of hypersensitivity. The patient also should work on a home program using contact particles and dowel textures to assist with desensitization. Vibration often is more uncomfortable initially but, according to Janet Waylett-Rendall, vibration eventually is preferred over any other desensitization media. Hand-held, battery-operated vibrators can be issued for home use.

Answer: **D**
Hunter, Mackin, Callahan, pp. 698-699
Refer to Fig. 4-8.

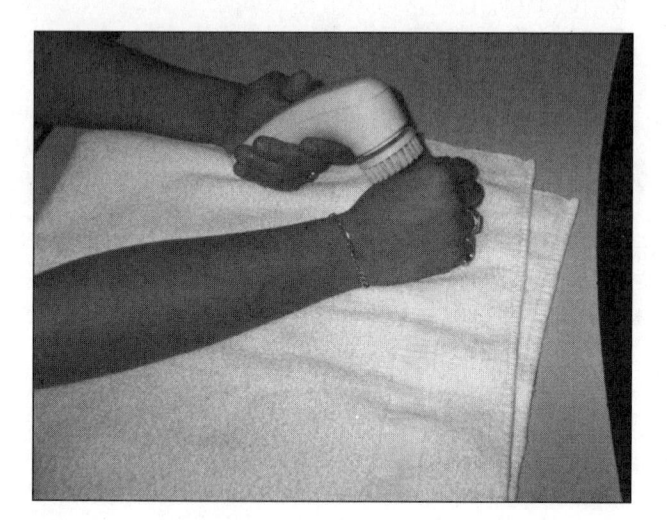

Fig. 4-8

38. A patient who complains of complete loss of sensation in the ring and little finger and along the medial forearm has loss of sensation caused by:

A. C8 nerve-root damage
B. Cubital tunnel compression
C. Guyon canal compression
D. C7 nerve-root damage

Each dorsal root innervates a particular area of skin called a dermatome. This patient has *loss* of sensation from C8 dorsal nerve-root damage. The dermatome for C8 is the ring finger, little finger, and the medial forearm. A relationship exists between dermatomes and areas innervated by peripheral nerves. The ulnar nerve and the antebrachial cutaneous nerve are the peripheral nerves that correspond to the C8 dermatome. Sensory changes associated with cubital tunnel usually are confined to the ulnar aspect of the hand and the ulnar one and a half digits. In nerve compression syndromes, patients rarely have a complete loss of sensation. Alterations of sensitivity result in nerve compression syndromes rather than complete loss (see Fig. 4-6).

Answer: **A**
Tubiana, Thomine, Mackin, p. 318
Kandel, Schwartz, p. 304

CLINICAL GEM:
Form a "6" with your thumb and index fingers by making an "O" and extending the other digits. The "O" in the "6" correlates with the C6 dermatome for the thumb and index fingers (see Fig. 4-9).

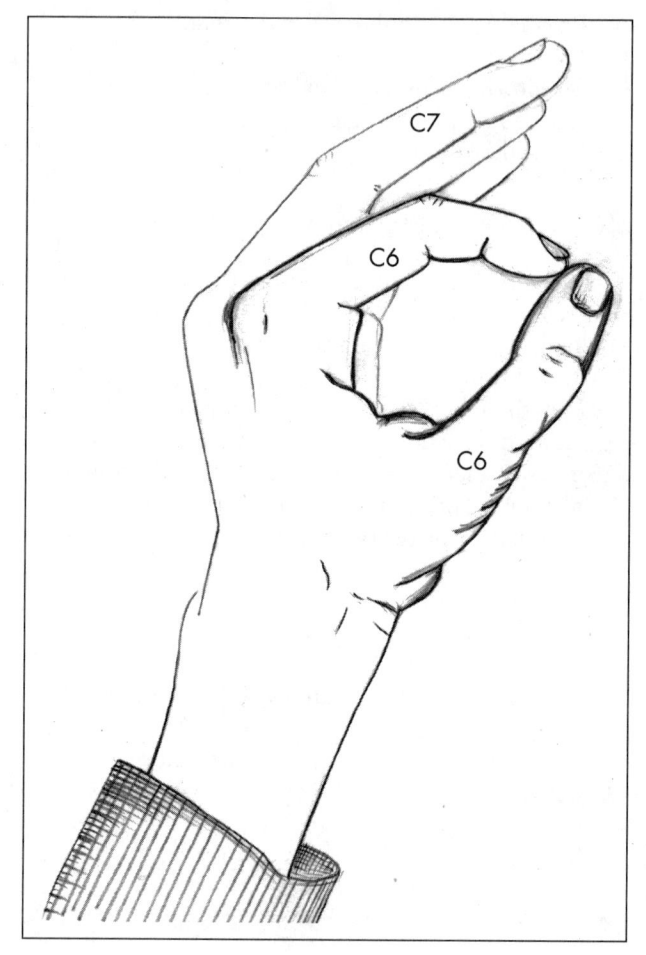

Fig. 4-9

39. Neural gliding to the affected arm is an appropriate treatment for a patient in the irritable phase of thoracic outlet syndrome. True or False?

When a patient is in an irritable state (constant pain that is easily provoked and may take a long time to settle), treatment should revolve around rest, with activities limited to those functions that produce minimal or no discomfort. Between rest periods, the patient must avoid activities and postures that strain or aggravate the tissue. Patients initially may need the support of a sling, pillow, or abduction wedge for the shoulder to reduce pain. When irritability is reduced to a moderate or minimal level, neural gliding exercises may be initiated to the unaffected extremity; examples would include neural gliding on the uninvolved arm or a straight leg raise.

Non-irritable neural restrictions can be treated with nerve gliding techniques. The upper limb tensioning techniques, as proposed by Butler, restore neural motion in patients who are in a non-irritable state. Nerve gliding must begin without development of tension in the involved extremity, especially in patients who previously were highly irritable. Patients can be progressed to increased neural tension and postural ergonomic instructions in preparation to return to activities. Next, strengthening conditioning should ensue for return to full activity.

Answer: **False**
Hunter, Mackin, Callahan, pp. 946-947
Butler, pp. 104-105

40. Which sympathetic function is displayed in Figure 4-10?

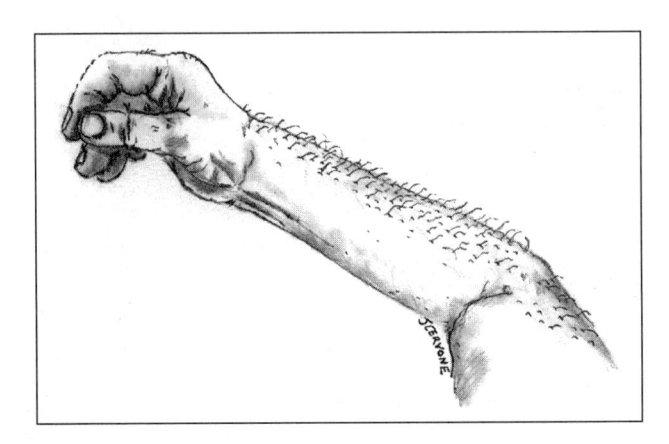

Fig. 4-10

A. Trophic
B. Sudomotor
C. Vasomotor
D. Pilomotor

This figure shows pilomotor function or the "gooseflesh" response of the skin in the upper extremity.

Answer: **D**
Malick, Kasch, p. 19

41. Which obstetric palsy most often affects the C5 and C6 nerve roots?

A. Erb's palsy
B. Duval's palsy
C. Seddon's palsy
D. Klumpke's palsy

Obstetric palsy traction injuries are caused by fetal malposition, cephalopelvic disproportion, or the use of forceps.

Erb's palsy is an upper brachial plexus palsy most often affecting the C5 and C6 nerve roots. It includes paralysis of the supraspinatus, infraspinatus, deltoid, biceps, brachialis, and brachioradialis muscles.

Lower brachial plexus injury, known as Klumpke's or Dejerine Klumpke type, involves the C8 and T1 nerve roots. This injury results in paralysis of the flexors and extensors of the forearm, with sparing of the brachioradialis, supinator, pronator teres, extensor carpi radialis longus, and extensor carpi radialis brevis muscles. The hand intrinsic muscles and part of the triceps are paralyzed. Sensory loss with this injury is severe.

Answer: **A**
Green, p. 1510
Hunter, Mackin, Callahan, p. 886

Chapter 5
Wrist

Topics to be reviewed in random order are:

- Evaluation and treatment of the distal radioulnar joint
- Carpal bone instability, fractures, and management
- Wrist tumors
- Volar intercalated segment instability pattern
- Dorsal intercalated segment instability pattern
- Forearm bone fractures
- Kienböck's disease
- Triangular fibrocartilage complex pathology; evaluation and treatment
- Provocative testing techniques

1. The major stabilizer of the distal radioulnar joint is the:

A. Pronator quadratus muscle
B. Extensor retinaculum
C. Geometric shape of the sigmoid notch
D. Volar radial ulnar ligament
E. Triangular fibrocartilage complex (TFC)

Although all the structures listed contribute to distal radioulnar stability, the triangular fibrocartilage complex has the greatest effect on its stability.

Answer: **E**
Lichtman, p. 224
Refer to Fig. 5-1.

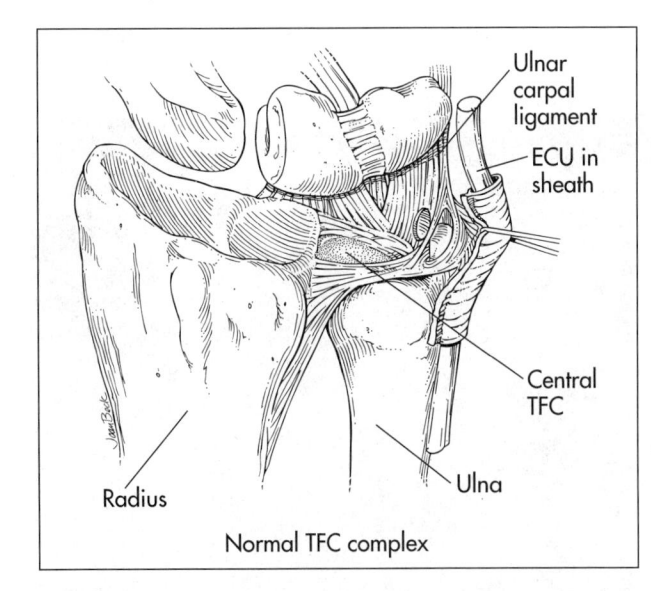

Fig. 5-1 ■ From Cooney WP, Linscheid RL, Dobyns JH: *The wrist: diagnosis and operative treatment,* St. Louis, 1998, Mosby-Year Book.

2. A hand surgeon shows you a posteroanterior radiograph in which there is no visible joint between the lunate and the triquetrum. The patient has no surgical scar and no history of trauma. This condition is:

A. Less frequently seen compared with a similar condition involving the capitate and hamate
B. Associated with restricted wrist motion

53

C. Caused by an incomplete separation of the embryological carpal cartilage
D. Rarely seen in people of African descent
E. Usually associated with more serious congenital anomalies

This patient has a lunotriquetral coalition. A coalition refers to an incomplete separation of the embryological cartilage anlage. One large bone appears without an articulation between two bones. When only two bones are involved, the condition usually is not associated with other congenital anomalies. A lunotriquetral coalition usually is an incidental finding; it does not affect range of motion and typically has no symptoms. However, the referenced article cites one symptomatic case.

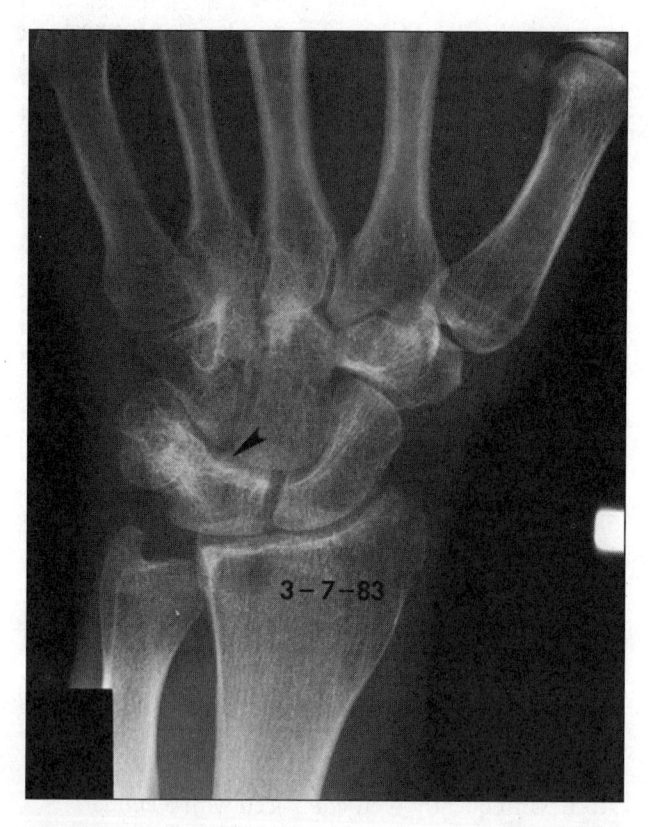

Answer: **C**
Simmons, Mckenzie, pp. 190-193
Refer to Fig. 5-2.

Fig. 5-2 ■ From Cooney WP, Linscheid RL, Dobyns JH: *The wrist: diagnosis and operative treatment,* St. Louis, 1998, Mosby-Year Book.

3. **What is the most commonly fractured carpal bone?**

A. Trapezium
B. Capitate
C. Hamate
D. Scaphoid
E. Lunate

The most commonly fractured carpal bone is the scaphoid. This fracture is common in young adult males. Reports have indicated that these fractures account for 60% to 70% of all carpal injuries. Other carpal fractures include: trapezium (1% to 5% of all carpal injuries); capitate (1% to 2%); hamate (2% to 4%); pisiform (1% to 3%); triquetrum (3% to 4%); trapezoid (less than 1%); and lunate (2% to 7%).

Answer: **D**
Prosser, Herbert, p. 139

> **CLINICAL GEM:**
> The proximal pole of the scaphoid is poorly vascularized; therefore, it is notorious for delayed healing. Fortunately, only about 10% of scaphoid fractures are through this proximal pole; 80% are through the waist, and the remainder are at the tuberosity or distal pole.
> Cooney, Linscheid, Dobyns, p. 395

4. **What percentage of force is transmitted across the radiocarpal joint when loading the wrist in the neutral position?**

A. 80
B. 60
C. 40
D. 20

Eighty percent of force is transmitted at the radiocarpal joint and the remaining 20% is transmitted across the ulnocarpal joint. With pronation, the ulnocarpal force transmission increases up to 37% and with ulnar deviation, the ulnocarpal force increases to 28%.

Answer: **A**
Berger, p. 92

5. Which ligament is known as a ligament of Testut?

A. Deltoid ligament
B. Radioscapholunate ligament
C. Radioscaphocapitate ligament
D. Radiotriquetral ligament
E. Ulnar lunate ligament

The radioscapholunate ligament is also known as the ligament of Testut. This ligament has been described as a remnant of vascular ingrowth to the carpus. The ligament of Testut perhaps is more appropriately classified as a mesocapsule rather than a ligament. It is part of the extrinsic ligamentous system. Extrinsic ligaments are extracapsular and pass from the radius or metacarpals to the carpal bones; intrinsic ligaments are intracapsular and originate from and insert on adjacent carpal bones. The intrinsic ligaments are thicker and stronger volarly than they are dorsally.

Answer: **B**
Bednar, Osterman, pp. 10,11
Cooney, Linscheid, Dobyns, p. 82

6. Which of the following carpal bones acts as a sesamoid bone?

A. Trapezium
B. Trapezoid
C. Pisiform
D. Hamate
E. Scaphoid

The pisiform is considered a carpal bone but functions as a sesamoid bone, onto which the flexor carpi ulnaris tendon inserts. The definition of a sesamoid bone is an oval nodule of bone or fibrocartilage embedded in a tendon or joint capsule. The patella is the largest sesamoid bone. The pisiform is a rounded carpal bone that lies over the triquetrum. Although anatomically the pisiform is located in the proximal carpal row, it does not participate in either the radiocarpal or midcarpal joints. It is a sesamoid bone whose sole function appears to be to increase the moment arm of the flexor carpi ulnaris muscle as its tendon courses over the pisiform. The flexor carpi ulnaris inserts into the pisiform with prolongations to the hamate and the fifth metacarpal.

Answer: **C**
Cooney, Linscheid, Dobyns, p. 66
Taber's

> **CLINICAL GEM:**
> The pisiform is the only carpal bone with a tendon insertion from a forearm muscle.

7. What is the normal radial inclination and palmar tilt in the wrist?

A. Radial inclination of 33° and palmar tilt of 20°
B. Radial inclination of 22° and palmar tilt of 12°
C. Radial inclination of 13° and palmar tilt of 21°
D. Radial inclination of 10° and palmar tilt of 10°

Typically the radial inclination is 22° to 23° (Fig. 5-3, *A*) and the palmar tilt is 11° to 12° (Fig. 5-3, *B*). With a loss of normal palmar tilt, dorsal angulation can occur, the wrist may appear deformed, and range-of-motion deficits are noted. Loss of radial inclination has been correlated with decreased grip strength and range of motion. If the anatomy is not restored, the functional use of the arm may be limited or painful.

Answer: **B**
Laseter, Carter, pp. 117-118
Cooney, Linscheid, Dobyns, pp. 328, 570

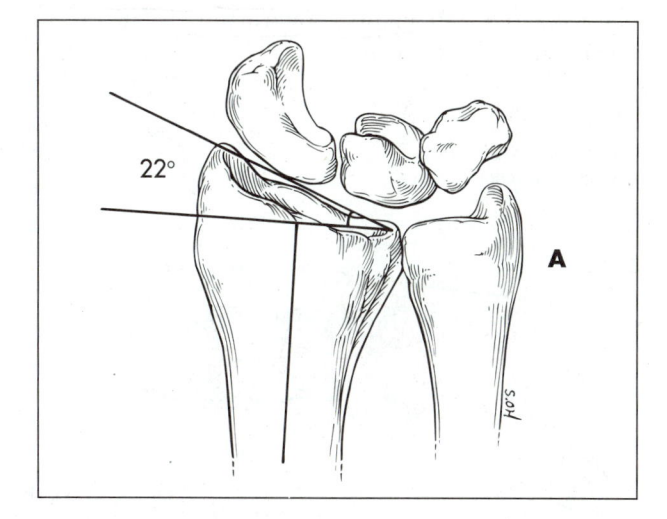

Fig. 5-3 ■ **A,** From Cooney WP, Linscheid RL, Dobyns JH: *The wrist: diagnosis and operative treatment,* St. Louis, 1998, Mosby-Year Book.

Continued

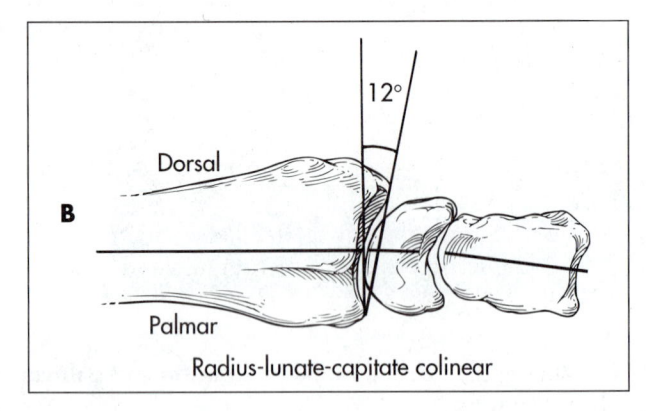

Fig. 5-3, cont'd ■ **B,** From Cooney WP, Linscheid RL, Dobyns JH: *The wrist: diagnosis and operative treatment,* St. Louis, 1998, Mosby-Year Book.

8. Which fracture describes a distal radius fracture with dorsal displacement?

   A. Colles'
   B. Smith's
   C. Palmar Barton's
   D. All of the above present with a dorsal displacement.

A Colles' fracture (Fig. 5-4) is a distal radius fracture with dorsal displacement. A Smith's fracture, also known as a reverse Colles', presents with palmar angulation of the distal radius. A Barton's fracture is a fracture-dislocation in which the rim of the distal radius is displaced dorsally or palmarly along with the hand and carpus. A Barton's fracture is different from both Colles' and Smith's fractures because the **dislocation** is the most obvious radiographic abnormality; a fracture of the radius is noted secondarily.

Answer: **A**
Laseter, Carter, p. 114
Cooney, Linscheid, Dobyns, p. 315

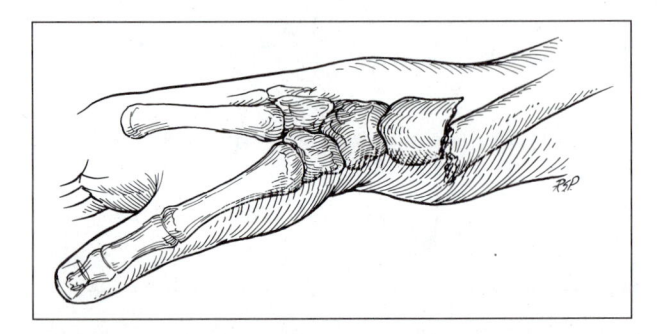

Fig. 5-4 ■ From Malone TR, McPoil TG, Nitz AJ: *Orthopedic and sports physical therapy,* ed 3, St. Louis, 1997, Mosby-Year Book.

9. One of the most important objectives of distal radius fracture rehabilitation is the restoration of:

   A. Digit extension
   B. Digit flexion
   C. Supination
   D. Isolated wrist extension

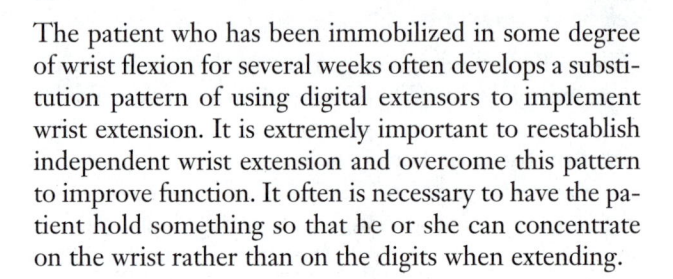

The patient who has been immobilized in some degree of wrist flexion for several weeks often develops a substitution pattern of using digital extensors to implement wrist extension. It is extremely important to reestablish independent wrist extension and overcome this pattern to improve function. It often is necessary to have the patient hold something so that he or she can concentrate on the wrist rather than on the digits when extending.

Answer: **D**
Laseter, Carter, pp. 112-124

10. The most common tumor in the wrist is the:

    A. Dorsal wrist ganglion
    B. Lipoma
    C. Giant cell tumor
    D. Hemangioma
    E. Fibrosarcoma

The word tumor can be misleading. It should be recalled that "tumor" is generic and refers to swelling or enlargement; it does not necessarily imply a solid growth. Commonly seen dorsal wrist ganglions arise from the scapholunate interosseous ligament. Transilluminescence with a pen light over the ganglion can quickly allay the fear of a solid tumor. Malignant tumors (sarcomas) in the wrist and hand are very rare. Giant cell tumors frequently are seen in the fingers. Lipomas occasionally are seen in the wrist.

Answer: **A**
Dorland's Medical Dictionary
Nelson, Sawmiller, Phalen, pp. 1459-1464

11. You are asked to evaluate a 60-year-old patient with a Colles' fracture. In the typical distal radial fracture, treated by traction and percutaneous pinning, you would most likely identify a loss of which motion 6 months after the fracture?

A. Volar flexion
B. Dorsiflexion
C. Flexion lags of the index and long fingers
D. Radial deviation
E. Ulnar deviation

The typical Colles' fracture displaces the articular surface dorsally. Often this can result in as much as 30° to 40° of dorsal articular tilt. Most fractures treated with traction and pinning restore the articular tilt to neutral. It is difficult to restore the 10° to 15° of volar articular tilt seen on the lateral view. Because the articular tilt is neutral, the wrist most likely lacks complete volar flexion but dorsiflexion actually may increase compared with the unaffected extremity. Flexion lags of digits can be seen and commonly are associated with "fracture disease"; they usually are not a result of pinning technique.

Answer: **A**
Rayhack, pp. 287-300

> **CLINICAL GEM:**
> "Fracture disease" is a constellation of symptoms caused by prolonged immobilization. It can lead to a vicious pain cycle, unresolved edema, muscle atrophy, and osteoporosis. It is not a necessary part of fracture management and can be avoided or prevented with early digital motion and edema management.

12. A scapholunate dissociation produces a volar intercalated segment instability. True or False?

A scapholunate dissociation results in a dorsal intercalated segment instability (DISI) (Fig. 5-5, *B*), whereas a lunotriquetral dissociation results in a volar intercalated segment instability (VISI) (Fig. 5-5, *C*). A normal wrist is depicted in Figure 5-5, *A*. DISI and VISI are both determined in reference to which ligament (either the scapholunate ligament or lunotriquetral ligament) is disrupted around the lunate. In a VISI deformity, the lunate and triquetrum ligaments are separated, resulting in a volar rotation of the lunate with extension of the triquetrum. In a scapholunate dissociation, the scaphoid is disrupted from the lunate, producing a dorsally rotated lunate. An untreated DISI can result in a scaphoid-lunate advance collapse wrist.

Answer: **False**
Bednar, Osterman, p. 12
Hunter, Mackin, Callahan, p. 329

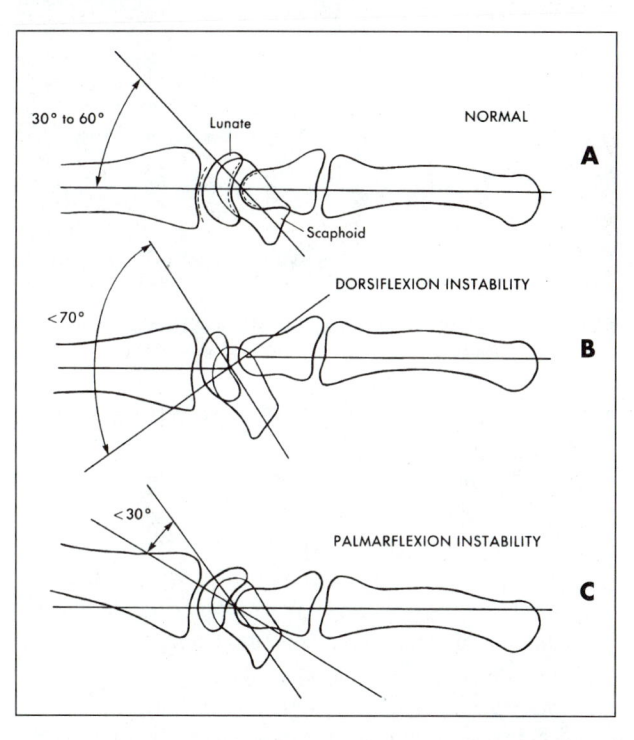

Fig. 5-5 ■ **A,** Normal wrist with the lunate properly aligned. **B,** Dorsal intercalated segment instability pattern. The lunate is dorsally rotated (or looking up in extension). **C,** Volar intercalated segment instability pattern. The lunate is volarly rotated (or looking down in flexion). (From Hunter JM, Mackin EJ, Callahan AD: *Rehabilitation of the hand: surgery and therapy,* ed 4, St. Louis, 1995, Mosby-Year Book.)

> **CLINICAL GEM:**
> A scaphoid-lunate gap has been called the "Terry Thomas" sign. This refers to a British actor with a wide gap between his front teeth (Fig. 5-6).

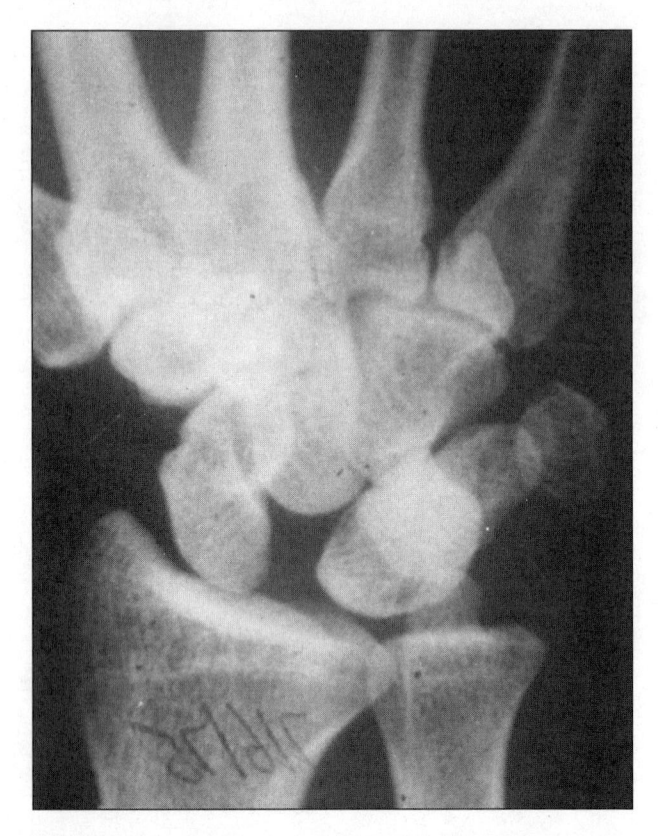

Fig. 5-6 ■ From Hunter JM, Mackin EJ, Callahan AD: *Rehabilitation of the hand: surgery and therapy,* ed 4, St. Louis, 1995, Mosby-Year Book.

CLINICAL GEM:
Another important term to be familiar with is carpal instability dissociative, which is an instability between the carpal bones or through the carpal bones in the same carpal row (proximal or distal). This occurs as a result of intrinsic ligament damage, most frequently of the scapholunate or lunotriquetral ligaments.

A carpal instability nondissociative (CIND) is a fairly uncommon form of wrist pathology involving instability **between** the carpal rows rather than within a single carpal row. CIND often is seen in individuals with ligament laxity and frequently is referred to as a midcarpal instability.

13. A fracture of the radial head combined with distal radioulnar joint dislocation is classified as a (an):

A. Colles' fracture
B. Essex-Lopresti fracture dislocation
C. Barton's fracture dislocation
D. Piano-key fracture
E. Chauffeur fracture

A radial head fracture combined with a distal radioulnar joint dislocation is termed an Essex-Lopresti fracture dislocation. The interosseous membrane tears in this injury result in proximal migration of the radius. An ulnar plus variance of 2 to 3 mm often develops in patients after this injury; however, this becomes symptomatic enough to warrant treatment in only a minority of the cases. Radial head replacements with Silicone prostheses may be of temporary help in stabilizing the radius, but angulation, fragmentation, capitellar erosion, and particulate synovitis frequently are seen as adverse reactions. An ulna resection is a better choice, but persistent radial migration can occur along with other problems. Ulnar head resection is a last resort.

Answer: **B**
Cooney, Linscheid, Dobyns, pp. 851-852

14. Kienböck's disease is related to:

A. Negative ulnar variance
B. Positive ulnar variance
C. Negative radial variance
D. Positive radial variance

Abnormal distribution of the load on the lunate is believed to be a major factor in the development of Kienböck's disease. Anatomic variables reported to increase stress on the lunate include a negative ulnar variance, as well as the shape of the lunate.

There are several ways to measure ulnar variance. Refer to Figure 5-7 for techniques for measuring ulnar variance.

Answer: **A**
Cooney, Linscheid, Dobyns, pp. 201, 220

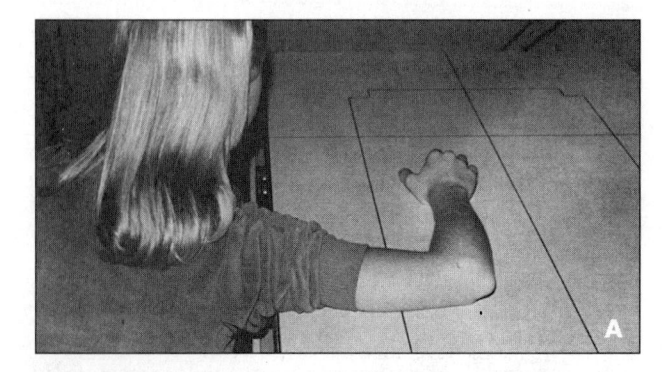

Fig. 5-7 ■ **A**, Standard positioning for wrist radiographs to measure ulna variance. The shoulder is abducted, the elbow is flexed 90°, and the wrist is placed in neutral forearm pronation-supination.

Continued

15. You are treating a patient with undiagnosed wrist pain. The patient reports pain in the wrist, weakness, and diminished motion. Radiographs reveal an ulnar minus variance. What might the diagnosis be for this patient?

A. Preiser's disease
B. Kienböck's disease
C. Madelung's deformity
D. None of the above

In 1910, Kienböck described a condition that was characterized by pain, stiffness, and swelling in the wrist. Kienböck's disease tends to occur in young active adults in the third or fourth decades of life. It usually occurs in the dominant extremity, but can occur bilaterally. The ulnar minus variance noted in 1928 by Hulten is observed in only 23% of radiographs of normal wrists but is present in 78% of patients with Kienböck's disease. The etiology of the disease remains controversial. Some authors have proposed that the ulnar minus variance subjects the lunate to a greater compression or shear stress. This compression or shear stress has been coined the "nutcracker effect."

Answer: **B**
Almquist, p. 141
Refer to Fig. 5-8.

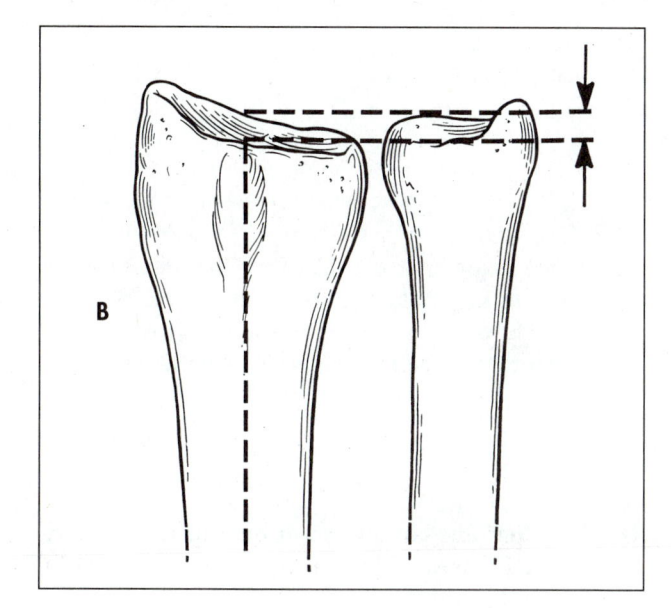

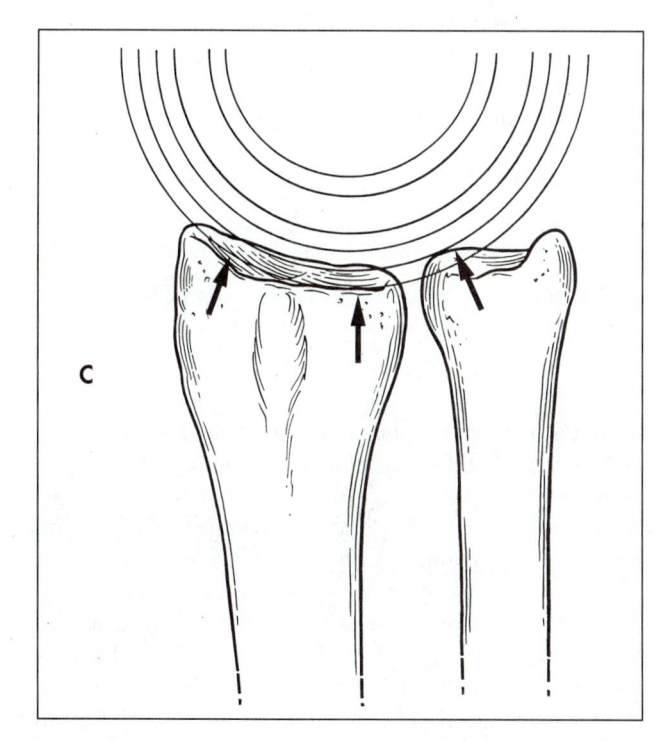

Fig. 5-7, cont'd ■ **B,** Articular surface method. A line from the articular surface of the lunate fossa of the distal radius is drawn toward the ulna. This line should be perpendicular to the longitudinal axis of radius. **C,** Concentric semicircle method. A semicircular template is aligned closely to the contour of the articular surface of the distal radius. The ulnar head is outlined (*right arrow*) and compared with the distal radius articular surface lines (*arrows on the left*). In this case, 2.6 mm of positive ulna variance is measured. (From Cooney WP, Linscheid RL, Dobyns JH: *The wrist: diagnosis and operative treatment,* St. Louis, 1998, Mosby-Year Book.)

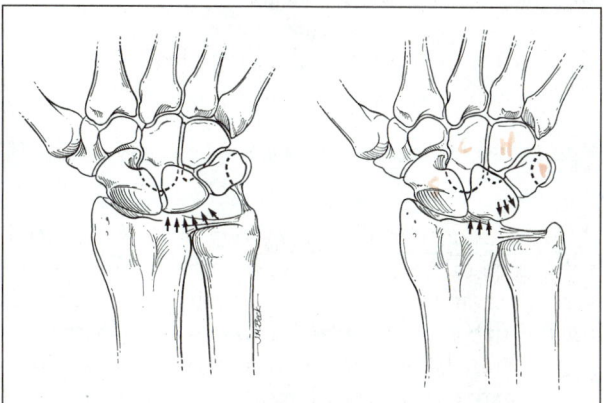

Fig. 5-8 ■ The lunate in a normal wrist is almost completely supported by the distal radius (*left*). In Kienböck's disease, the lunate is not as well covered by the radius and thus is more susceptible to uneven compression (*right*). (From Cooney WP, Linscheid RL, Dobyns JH: *The wrist: diagnosis and operative treatment,* St. Louis, 1998, Mosby-Year Book.)

16. All of the following are possible treatment options for patients with Kienböck's disease who have a 3-mm negative ulnar variance, except:

A. Scaphoid, trapezium, trapezoid arthrodesis
B. Radial shortening
C. Ulnar lengthening
D. Lunotriquetral fusion
E. Capitate shortening

The goal of leveling procedures used to treat Kienböck's disease is to decrease the biomechanical pressure on the lunate. Lunotriquetral fusion would not be effective in decreasing the lunate load. Capitate shortening has been advocated as a treatment option, but some physicians doubt its ability to decrease biomechanical load. The other three procedures do appear to decrease lunate biomechanical load.

Answer: **D**
Coe, Trumble, pp. 417-429

17. Weight-lifters and gymnasts tend to repetitively hyperextend and forcefully load their wrists. A specific nerve injury in these individuals can cause development of perineural fibrosis and pain, without sensory changes. Which nerve is associated with this phenomenon?

A. Palmar cutaneous nerve
B. Radial sensory nerve
C. Posterior interosseous nerve
D. Deep branch of the ulnar nerve
E. Superficial dorsal branch of the ulnar nerve

The posterior (dorsal) interosseous nerve is the terminal branch of the radial nerve. It has no cutaneous sensory innervation. This nerve is located on the floor in the fourth compartment and is accompanied by the posterior branch of the anterior interosseous artery. Irritation of the posterior interosseous nerve often is associated with dorsal wrist ganglia. Less well known is its irritation by repetitive, forceful hyperextension, which causes perineural fibrosis (abnormal scarring around a nerve).

Answer: **C**
Aulicino, pp. 455-466

> **CLINICAL GEM:**
> The posterior interosseous nerve does not have sensory innervation, but does provide proprioceptive innervation to the wrist joint. Therefore, this nerve can cause a painful wrist.

18. Your patient complains of pain in the lunotriquetral (LT) area. The patient reports a painful clicking and point tenderness. Which of the following tests is helpful to assess the LT ligament?

A. Watson's shift test
B. Ballottement test
C. Piano-key test
D. All of the above are appropriate tests

When a patient complains of pain in the lunotriquetral (LT) area, a helpful test is the ballottement test, as described by Reagan (Fig. 5-9, *A*). The lunate is stabilized firmly with the thumb and index finger of one hand while the pisotriquetral unit is rocked with the other hand. A positive test results in pain, crepitus, and laxity. A modification of this test is the "shear" test, as described by Kleinman (Fig. 5-9, *B*). To perform this test, the patient rests the elbow on the table with the forearm in neutral rotation. The examiner's contralateral thumb is placed over the dorsal aspect of the lunate just beyond the medial edge of the distal radius. With the lunate stabilized, the examiner uses his or her opposite thumb to load the pisotriquetral joint from a palmar to dorsal plane, creating a shearing force at the LT joint and causing pain. Although these are good tests, they are less specific at determining LT involvement than we would like. These tests can produce a false positive because of other pathologies.

Answer: **B.**
Green, pp. 894-896
Cooney, Linscheid, Dobyns, pp. 531-533

19. You are treating a patient who fell on his outstretched hand several months ago. The patient presents with pain and tenderness dorsally over the mid-wrist region. You perform a Watson's test and it is positive. Which injury might you suspect?

A. Triangular fibrocartilage complex tear
B. Lunate-triquetrum (L-T) tear
C. Scaphoid-lunate (S-L) tear
D. Distal radius fracture

The Watson's test is used to assess S-L ligament competence. To perform this test, the wrist is placed in ulnar deviation and the examiner's thumb is placed on the scaphoid tuberosity. As the wrist is brought into radial deviation, the normal flexion of the scaphoid is blocked by the examiner's thumb. If there is an instability, a dorsal subluxation of the scaphoid occurs. A click or snap is noted as the scaphoid reduces back to the wrist when the pressure is released from the tuberosity. This diagnosis is further confirmed with a clenched fist radiograph to assess the size of the gap between the scaphoid and the lunate (see Fig. 5-6).

Answer: **C**
Wright, Michlovitz, p. 150
Cooney, Linscheid, Dobyns, pp. 256-258
Refer to Fig. 5-10.

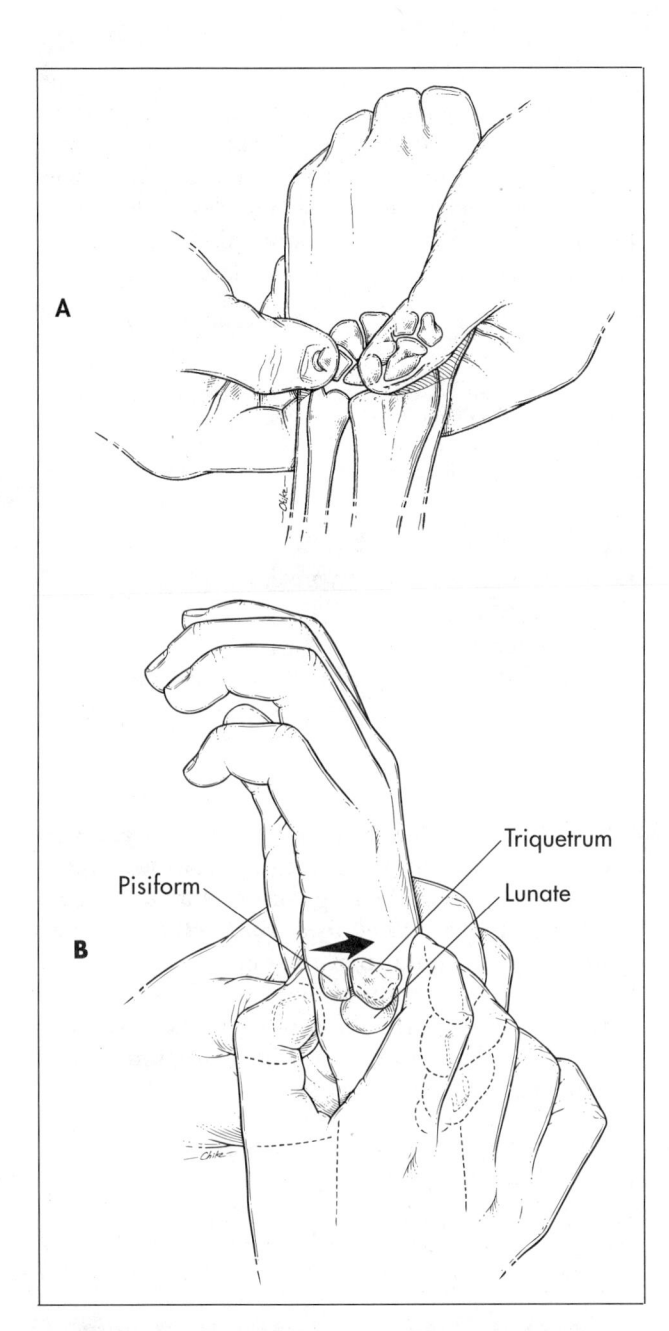

Fig. 5-9 ■ Lunotriquetral stress test. **A,** Ballottement test. The purpose of the test is to rock or "ballotte" the lunate against the triquetrum to demonstrate pain related to instability, cartilage loss, or local synovitis. Both hands are used to grasp the lunate and triquetrum and to stress up and down the lunotriquetral interval. **B,** Lunotriquetral shear test. The purpose of the test is to place a dorsal shear force by lifting the pisiform and triquetrum dorsally on the fixed lunate. The examiner's hands support the lunate dorsally (examiner's contralateral thumb) while the opposite hand (ipsilateral thumb) directly loads the pisotriquetral joint from a palmar to dorsal direction. (From Cooney WP, Linscheid RL, Dobyns JH: *The wrist: diagnosis and operative treatment,* St. Louis, 1998, Mosby-Year Book.)

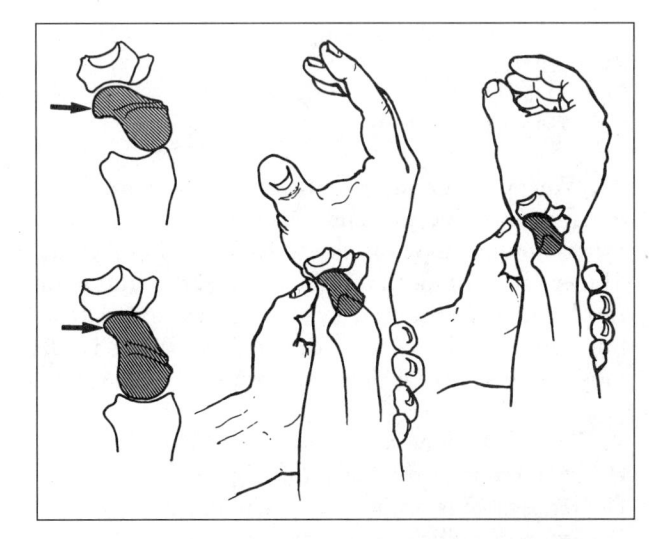

Fig. 5-10 ■ Scaphoid displacement test is performed by pushing upward on the scaphoid tuberosity while the hand is in ulnar deviation. This tends to cause the scaphoid to ride out of the radial fossa over the dorsal rim, at times producing a painful snap. The test might be positive in loose-jointed individuals and requires clinical and radiologic correlation. (From Cooney WP, Linscheid RL, Dobyns JH: *The wrist: diagnosis and operative treatment,* St. Louis, 1998, Mosby-Year Book.)

20. **A patient with an acute onset of wrist pain has a soft-tissue opacity on a lateral carpal radiograph. The patient is treated with indomethacin and the pain quickly resolves. A follow-up radiograph 2 weeks later demonstrates nearly complete disappearance of the amorphous, well-circumscribed opacity. The most likely diagnosis is:**

A. Scaphoid lunate advance collapse with osteoarthritis
B. Gout
C. Acute calcium soft-tissue deposition
D. Rheumatoid arthritis
E. Pseudogout

This remarkable acute onset of symptoms and equally remarkable resolution with indomethacin and rest is infrequently seen but can occur with acute calcium soft-tissue deposition. Opacities are visualized as fluffy, soft-tissue calcium deposits that can disappear on radiographs in as little as 2 weeks.

Pseudogout would show linear calcification in the triangular fibrocartilage complex that would not resolve in 2 weeks. Calcifications seen with rheumatoid arthritis or gout also would not disappear on radiographs in 2 weeks. Osteophytes are common in degenerative joint disease but they would not be seen in the soft tissues as fluffy, opaque deposits.

Answer: **C**
Milford, p. 377
Carroll, pp. 422-426

21. **You are treating a patient with a 6-week-old distal radius fracture and the patient reports that "something snapped in my wrist when I moved it." Finger range of motion is normal and the thumb interphalangeal joint can be actively extended to 0° but cannot achieve hyperextension. What is the most likely cause of these symptoms?**

A. Breakup of adhesions of the radial carpal joint
B. Incongruity at the radial carpal joint
C. Tenosynovitis of the flexor carpi radialis
D. Extensor pollicis longus rupture

The extensor pollicis longus may rupture following a distal radius fracture. A roughened surface and possibly some slight dorsal articular tilting predisposes rupture of the extensor pollicis longus. Vascularity is probably compromised and the tendon attenuates and ultimately ruptures. The thumb interphalangeal joint often can extend to zero using the intrinsic muscles of the thumb, but hyperextension will be lacking. Also lacking will be the ulnar border of the snuffbox during the physical examination.

Answer: **D**
Engkvist, Lundburg, pp. 76-86
Tubiana, Thomine, Mackin, p. 312
Hunter, Mackin, Callahan, pp. 60, 551

> **CLINICAL GEM:**
> With an extensor pollicis longus rupture, the patient is unable to lift his or her thumb off of the table. This motion is termed retroposition.

22. **A patient with a diagnosis of wrist sprain is referred to you from a general physician for evaluation and treatment. During your evaluation, the patient reveals that he fell from the back of a moving vehicle last week but that the emergency room radiographs were negative. He currently is wearing a Futuro® wrist splint. The patient has exquisite tenderness in the snuffbox during palpation. Which injury might this patient have?**

A. Triangular fibrocartilage complex tear
B. Scaphoid fracture
C. Lunate-triquetral tear
D. Colles' fracture

Often early radiographs are reported negative with scaphoid fractures but this patient's extreme tenderness should alert you to a possible fracture. When the patient is seen immediately after injury, the fracture may not be readily apparent. Negative initial films should be followed up after 2 weeks of cast immobilization with a second radiograph. This allows osteoporosis adjacent to the fracture to develop and provides radiographic evidence of the fracture.

Answer: **B**
Cooney, Linscheid, Dobyns, p. 393

23. You are treating a patient who has obvious signs of ulnar abutment after distal radius fracture. The patient has pain with extremes of rotation and ulnar deviation, which are aggravating his discomfort. At times, the patient complains of a clicking sensation, activity-related swelling, and decreased strength and motion. Radiographs reveal an ulnar plus variance of 2.6 mm. Surgery will be performed. What is the surgical treatment of choice according to Cooney, Linscheid, and Dobyns when there is minimal distal radioulnar joint involvement?

A. Bower's hemiresection
B. Darrach procedure
C. Suave-Kapandji procedure
D. Ulnar resection (shortening)

Each of the procedures mentioned has potential benefit through relieving stress on the ulnar side of the wrist by effectively unloading the ulna. However, each may result in residual symptoms that may bother the patient. According to Cooney, Linscheid, and Dobyns, the ulnar resection (shortening) is the procedure of choice for most cases of ulnar abutment. The ulnar shortening has the advantage of maintaining the articular surfaces of the ulnocarpal joint and the distal radioulnar joint. Another benefit of ulnar shortening is tightening of the ulnocarpal ligaments and the triangular fibrocartilage complex, providing a stabilizing effect for patients with ligament laxity or injury. Postoperatively, the extremity is immobilized in a Muenster-type cast for 6 weeks to control forearm rotation. This is followed by use of a removable, custom-made splint until complete union is obtained.

Answer: **D**
Cooney, Linscheid, Dobyns, pp. 776-782

> **CLINICAL GEM:**
> - The Suave-Kapandji procedure can lead to instability at the site of pseudoarthrosis (Fig. 5-11, *A*).
> - Bower's hemiresection may result in residual impingement at the sigmoid notch (Fig. 5-11, *B*).
> - Darrach resection may result in residual weakness and instability (Fig. 5-11, *C*).

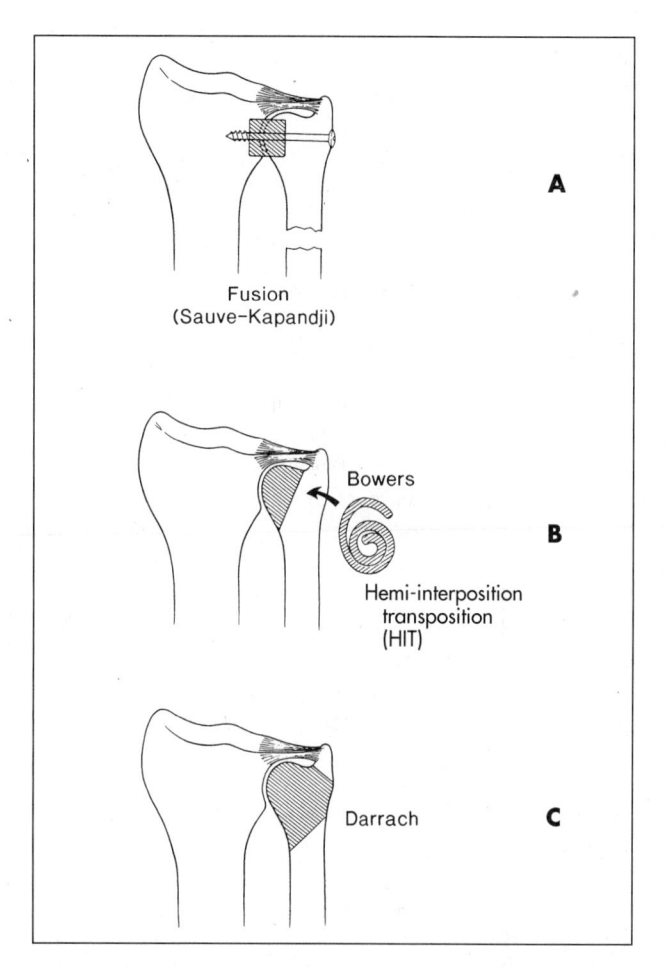

Fig. 5-11 ■ From Cooney WP, Linscheid RL, Dobyns JH: *The wrist: diagnosis and operative treatment,* St. Louis, 1998, Mosby-Year Book.

24. Fusion of the scaphoid, trapezium, trapezoid joint, also termed the triscaphe joint, is a useful procedure for all of the following, except:

A. Carpal instability
B. Kienböck's disease
C. Triscaphe arthritis
D. Radioscaphoid arthritis

A fusion of the scaphoid, trapezium, trapezoid (STT) joint is best used as a treatment for triscaphe arthritis, carpal instabilities, and Kienböck's disease. An STT fusion would not be used for a patient with radioscaphoid arthritis. In fact, one of the long-term side effects of an STT fusion is radiocarpal arthritis. This often is caused by a failure to achieve scaphoid realignment during fusion. The creation of a four-bone fusion using the capitate, hamate, lunate, and triquetrum with a scaphoid excision is one possible procedure for radioscaphoid arthritis.

Answer: **D**
Leibozic, pp. 616, 617

25. A peripheral tear of the triangular fibrocartilage complex almost always occurs secondary to direct force. True or False?

A peripheral tear of the triangular fibrocartilage complex (TFCC) almost always occurs secondary to direct force. It often is associated with distal radius fractures. The patient complains of ulnar-sided wrist pain and weakness. Central tears of the TFCC occur traumatically or from deterioration.

With a TFCC tear, the patient often complains of pain with resisted forearm rotation and sometimes reports a painful click. The central one third of the TFCC is a cartilaginous weightbearing area that does not have or require a vascular supply. Central tears are treated with surgical débridement and peripheral tears most often are treated with surgical repair (see Fig. 5-1).

Answer: **True**
Cooney, Linscheid, Dobyns, pp. 720-723

> **CLINICAL GEM:**
> Clinical assessment of the central triangular fibrocartilage complex (TFCC) can be performed with a TFCC load test in which the examiner ulnarly deviates the patient's wrist and moves the proximal carpal row in a volar/dorsal direction, with gentle manual compression over the TFCC. With a TFCC tear, patients typically have pain with forearm pronation, ulnar deviation, and gripping.

26. After a triangular fibrocartilage complex peripheral tear is treated with surgical repair, when are passive supination and pronation allowed for a patient with limited range?

A. After 2 weeks
B. After 4 weeks
C. After 6 weeks
D. After 10 weeks

After a peripheral repair of the triangular fibrocartilage complex, the patient is immobilized for 1 week in a long-arm cast. This is followed by use of a long-arm Muenster-style splint or Sugar Tong splint until weeks 2 to 4. Supination and pronation are restricted during this time to limit stress on the repair. During weeks 4 to 6, the patient is in a short-arm splint and he or she can begin elbow range of motion. From week 6 through week 10, active range of motion is begun, avoiding extremes of motion—especially supination and pronation—to avoid stress on the repair. At week 10, no restrictions apply. Gentle passive range of motion is initiated if limitations are noted for supination and pronation. Strengthening also is initiated at this time.

Answer: **D**
Skirven

27. You are treating a patient with a distal radius fracture. He complains of pain with ulnar deviation of the wrist and with gripping when the forearm is pronated. He is unable to open jars or use a screwdriver without difficulty. Loading the wrist also is painful for him. This patient might be exhibiting symptoms of:

A. Posterior interosseous neuritis
B. Scaphoid impingement
C. Ulnar impaction syndrome
D. Scaphoid-trapezial arthritis
E. None of the above

Ulnar impaction syndrome frequently occurs after malreduction of distal radius fractures, premature closure of the radial physis, or Madelung's deformity. Ulnar impaction syndrome is a common cause of dorsal ulnar wrist pain; it causes the patient pain with ulnar deviation and loading of the wrist. When the forearm is in pronation, the radius migrates proximally in relation to the ulna, increasing the ulnocarpal abutment. Diagnosis is made by testing forearm pronation-supination with the wrist in ulnar deviation, as well as by compression of the ulnar side of the wrist against the distal ulna with the forearm pronated. Diagnostic procedures to confirm ulnocarpal impingement include a bone scan, an arthrogram, and arthroscopy, after routine and stress radiographs have been taken.

Answer: **C**
Cooney, Linscheid, Dobyns, pp. 244-245

28. Which of the following tools is used primarily to diagnose ligament injuries of the wrist?

A. Tomography
B. Arthrography
C. Ultrasonography
D. Computed tomography scan

Wrist arthrography is used primarily to evaluate the integrity of the wrist ligaments and the triangular fibrocartilage complex. In a normal wrist, injection of contrast material through arthrography does not have leakage from one joint to another. If there is a crossing of the contrast material from one interval to another, it is consistent with a ligament injury.

Ultrasonography can be helpful in evaluation of the painful wrist, especially if a ganglion cyst is present. Ultrasound also is helpful in evaluating the tendons, as well as the tendon sheaths. Computed tomography (CT) is helpful in evaluating possible distal radioulnar joint disruption; it is more accurate than radiographs, especially when the patient is in pain or when cast immobilization makes positioning difficult. CT scans also are helpful in detecting subtle fractures, evaluating the healing fracture, and identifying occult tumors, bone lesions, scaphoid fractures, and Kienböck's disease. Tomography is used for evaluating position alignment and articular involvement of fractures.

One tool not yet mentioned is magnetic resonance imaging (MRI). MRI is useful when assessing a patient with possible osteonecrosis, soft-tissue masses, and neural compression in the carpal tunnel. The primary benefit of MRI for the wrist involves the assessment of avascular changes that may be present in the scaphoid, lunate, or capitate bones.

Answer: **B**
Cooney, Linscheid, Dobyns, pp 272-278

29. A radial styloid fracture is classified as a:

A. Smith's fracture
B. Barton's fracture
C. Colles' fracture
D. Chauffeur fracture
E. None of the above

A Chauffeur fracture is one in which the radial styloid is fractured off the radius. This fracture usually can be treated with closed reduction and percutaneous pin fixation. However, if the fracture is displaced more than 3 mm, there may be an associated scapholunate dissociation; in this case open reduction with repair of the ligament and anatomic reduction of the distal radial styloid is performed.

Answer: **D**
Cooney, Linscheid, Dobyns, p. 352
Refer to Fig. 5-12.

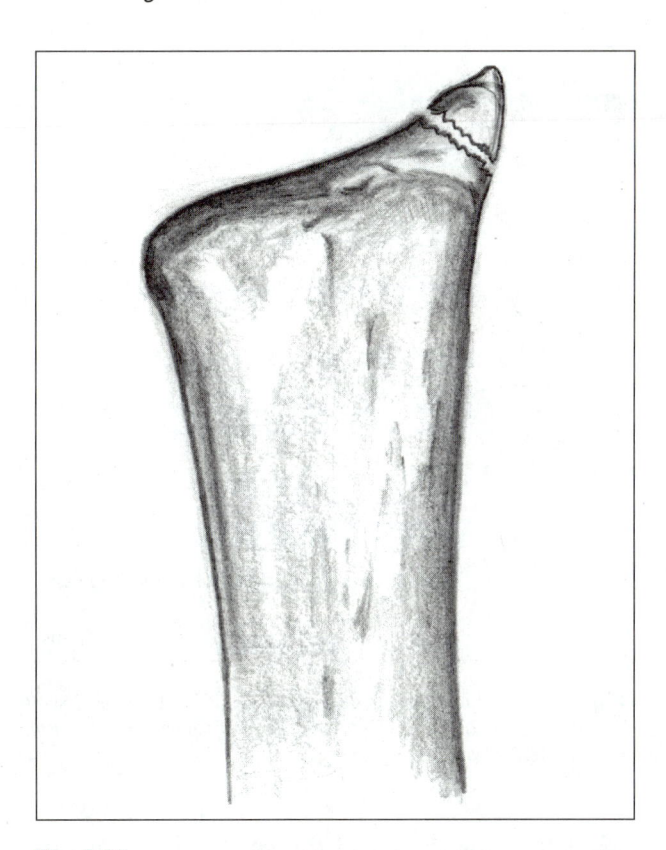

Fig. 5-12

30. In ulnar deviation of the wrist, the proximal carpal row extends. True or False?

In wrist ulnar deviation, the proximal carpal row extends, glides volarly, and translates radially. The distal carpal row in ulnar deviation flexes, glides dorsally, and translates ulnarly. The reverse occurs in radial deviation.

Answer: **True**
Cooney, Linscheid, Dobyns, p. 528

CHAPTER 5 Wrist

31. Complete palmar dislocation of the lunate occurs in the end stages of perilunate dislocation. True or False?

A lunate dislocation is merely the end phase of a perilunate dislocation in which the lunate is spit out volarly, often into the carpal canal. This is considered the most severe form of a perilunate instability—a grade four carpal injury. Clinically, most lunate dislocations are thought to be caused by wrist dorsiflexion injuries as a result of a fall on the outstretched hand.

Answer: **True**
Cooney, Linscheid, Dobyns, pp. 696-697
Refer to Fig. 5-13.

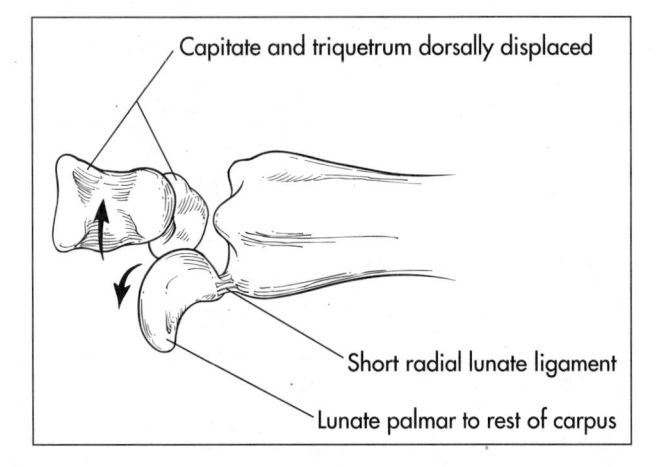

Fig. 5-13 ■ Complete palmar dislocation of the lunate. (From Cooney WP, Linscheid RL, Dobyns JH: *The wrist: diagnosis and operative treatment,* St. Louis, 1998, Mosby-Year Book.)

32. Ulnar translation of the carpus is not associated with:

A. Severe carpal (wrist) trauma
B. Rheumatoid arthritis
C. Psoriatic arthritis
D. Preiser's disease

Ulnar translocation frequently occurs after attenuation of ligament support caused by rheumatoid or psoriatic arthritis. On a rare occasion, ulnar translation of the carpus may be seen after severe wrist trauma. The diagnosis is made with radiographs showing abnormal translation of the lunate in an ulnar direction. In a traumatic, rheumatoid, or psoriatic condition, a radiolunate fusion is the best choice for a successful outcome. There is no place for nonsurgical treatment. Preiser's disease is an avascular necrosis of the scaphoid and is not associated with ulnar translation of the carpus.

Answer: **D**
Taleisnik, pp. 305-307

33. You have been asked to fabricate a low temperature thermoplastic ulnar gutter splint for a patient with a triquetral avulsion fracture. Where would this patient be most tender and swollen?

A. Volarly over the pisiform
B. Over the triangular fibrocartilage
C. Laterally over the ulnar collateral ligament attachment
D. On the ulnar side of the dorsum of the carpus over the dorsal triquetral body
E. Over the space of Poirier

This unusually tender injury presents with pain and swelling directly over the dorsal triquetral body on the ulnar side of the dorsum of the carpus. A lateral or oblique radiograph typically shows small avulsion fracture fragments. Symptoms commonly subside within 3 to 4 weeks of ulnar gutter splinting. Persistence of pain beyond 6 weeks suggests that a more serious intraligamentous injury may be present. The space of Poirier is described in Chapter 1, question 20 (see Fig. 1-10).

Answer: **D**
Taleisnik, pp. 149-151

34. What is considered a functional wrist range of motion for performing most activities of daily living?

A. 5° of flexion, 30° extension, 10° radial deviation, and 15° ulnar deviation
B. 40° of flexion and extension and 40° of composite radial and ulnar deviation
C. A and B
D. None of the above are considered functional

Studies have revealed a range of numbers for functional wrist range of motion. Palmer indicates that 5° of flexion, 30° of extension, 10° of radial deviation, and 15° of ulnar deviation is needed for functional use. More recently, Ryu and the Mayo Clinic Group found that 40° of wrist flexion, 40° of wrist extension, and 40° of composite radial and ulnar deviation is needed for functional range of motion. Most important to remember is that a person can be functional with less than normal wrist range of motion. Our goal is to maximize range of motion in a painfree range.

Answer: **C**
Ryu, Mayo Clinic Group
Skirven
Weidrich

35. A patient is referred to you for evaluation and treatment with a diagnosis of wrist sprain. During your evaluation, the patient reveals normal range of motion and 50% strength, with tenderness in the triangular fibrocartilage complex region. Your initial treatment should include the following:

A. Splinting the wrist at 0° extension and activity modification
B. A strengthening program
C. Referral for surgical intervention
D. Ultrasound and hot packs for pain management; no splint

This patient may have a triangular fibrocartilage complex (TFCC) tear. Initial treatment for a TFCC injury is conservative treatment. Treatment involves splinting with 0° of wrist extension, antiinflammatory medication, and activity modification. After a trial of 3 to 6 months of conservative measures, surgical intervention may be considered. Before surgical intervention, further diagnostic studies are helpful to confirm the diagnosis of TFCC tear.

Answer: **A**
Jaffe, Chidgery, LaStayo, pp. 129-135

36. A lunotriquetral fusion results in approximately what percentage of flexion loss?

A. 80
B. 55
C. 27
D. 12

Fusions crossing the radiocarpal joint (e.g., scaphoradiolunate fusion) lose approximately 55% of flexion/extension. Fusions crossing the intercarpal row (e.g., scaphotrapeziotrapezoid fusion) lose approximately 27% of flexion/extension. However, fusions within a single carpal row (e.g., lunotriquetral fusion) lose approximately 12% of flexion/extension.

Answer: **D**
Meyerdierks, Werner, p. 528

37. When performing pronation and supination, the ulna rotates around the radius. True or False?

Pronation-supination is a complex movement. It combines rotation of the radius around the ulna with horizontal and axial translation. The actual movement of the radius on the ulna in pronation-supination is a combination of rolling and sliding. When the arm is pronated, the radius crosses the ulna. In this pronated position, the radius proximally migrates in relation to the ulna, leading to a more positive ulnar variance.

Answer: **False**
Cooney, Linscheid, Dobyns, p. 222

Chapter 6
Shoulder

Topics to be reviewed in random order are:

- Shoulder anatomy
- Evaluations
- Provocative tests
- Rotator cuff pathology
- Impingement syndrome pathology
- Thoracic outlet syndrome pathology and treatment
- Bankart and Superior labrum anterior to posterior lesions: Evaluation and treatment
- Acromioclavicular joint pathology and treatment
- Shoulder fracture pathology
- Frozen shoulder pathologies
- Therapy for specific diagnoses

1. When this muscle is paralyzed or weakened, the scapula "wings":

A. Subscapularis
B. Serratus anterior
C. Rhomboid major
D. Serratus posterior

During normal scapulohumeral rhythm, the serratus anterior holds the scapula in place as it slides over the rib cage. Winging of the scapula occurs when the serratus anterior muscle becomes weak from an injury to the long thoracic nerve. The muscle originates from ribs one through nine and inserts along the medial border of the scapula.

Answer: **B**
Norris, p. 277
Rockwood, Matsen, pp. 56-57
Greenfield, Syen, pp. 201-207
Refer to Fig. 6-1.

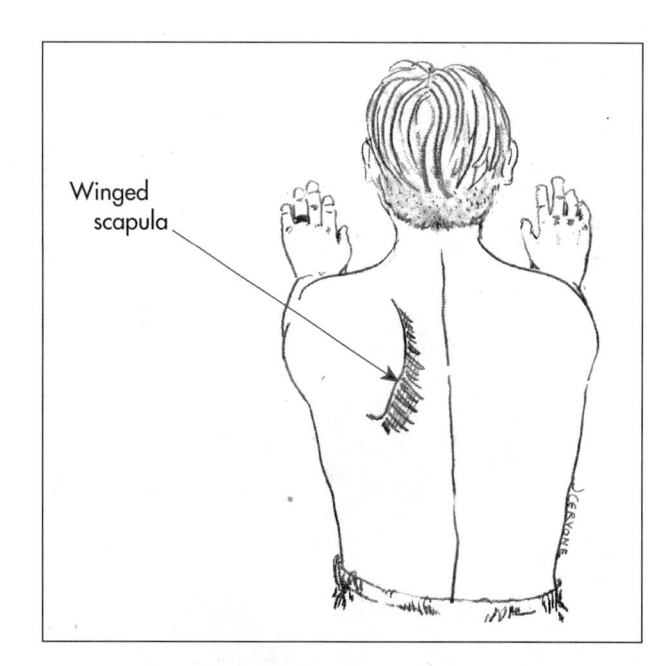

Fig. 6-1 ■ While performing a push up "winging" of the scapula is evident.

2. **Two prime retractors of the scapula are the rhomboid major and the rhomboid minor. Name the nerve that innervates these muscles.**

A. Thoracodorsal nerve
B. Long thoracic nerve
C. Subscapular nerve
D. Dorsal subscapular nerve

The dorsal scapular nerve is derived from C4 and C5 nerve roots and innervates the rhomboid major, rhomboid minor, and levator scapulae.

Answer: **D**
Magee, p. 104

3. **The nerve most commonly injured in fractures around the shoulder is the _____ nerve.**

A. Musculocutaneous
B. Radial
C. Axillary
D. Suprascapular

The axillary nerve exits the axilla from the brachial plexus and wraps around the posterior aspect of the surgical neck of the humerus, innervating the deltoid and teres minor muscles. This nerve is susceptible to trauma from fractures to the proximal humerus.

Answer: **C**
Donatelli, p. 202
Basti et al, pp. 111-112
Refer to Fig. 6-2.

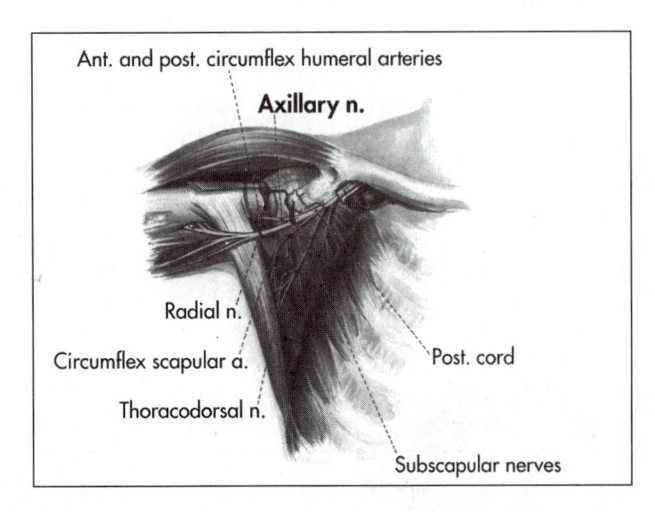

Fig. 6-2 ■ From Hunter JM, Mackin EJ, Callahan AD: *Rehabilitation of the hand: surgery and therapy*, ed 4, St. Louis, 1995, Mosby-Year Book.

4. **The coracoclavicular ligament is the only non-contractile structure suspending the scapula from the clavicle. True or False?**

The coracoclavicular ligament is the only noncontractile structure suspending the scapula from the clavicle. The major support of the acromioclavicular joint is the coracoclavicular ligament. It is comprised of two parts, the conoid and the trapezoid ligaments, and it connects the clavicle and coronoid process. The two parts are oriented differently and resist different forces placed on the scapula and clavicle.

Answer: **True**
Pratt, pp. 66-67
Refer to Fig. 6-3.

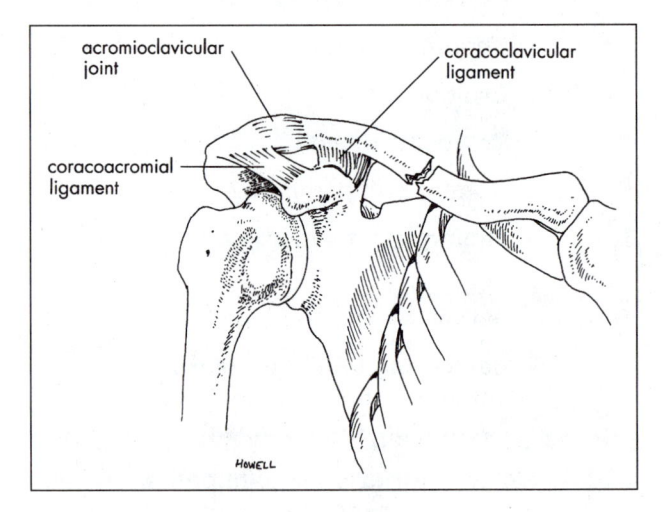

Fig. 6-3 ■ From Hawkins RJ, Bell RH, Lippitt SB: *Atlas of shoulder surgery*, St. Louis, 1996, Mosby-Year Book.

5. **A primary extensor of the shoulder is the:**

A. Teres minor
B. Long head of the triceps
C. Latissimus dorsi
D. Trapezius

Primary extensors of the shoulder include the posterior portion of the deltoid, the teres major, and the latissimus dorsi. The teres minor and the long head of the triceps are secondary extensors.

Answer: **C**
Hoppenfeld, p. 26

6. The three structures that make up the coracoacromial arch are the acromion, the coracoacromial ligament, and the coracoid process. True or False?

The coracoacromial arch comprises the acromion, the coracoacromial ligament, and the coracoid process. The arch is anatomically above the rotator cuff. The compression of the rotator cuff, especially the supraspinatus tendon, is believed to lead to rotator cuff degeneration and possibly even biceps tendon rupture. This is because of supraspinatus compression between the humeral head below and the coracoacromial arch above (see Fig. 6-3).

Answer: **True**
Flatow, pp. 20-21

7. In normal shoulder biomechanics, both the deltoid and the rotator cuff allow elevation of the humerus to occur. True or False?

Elevation of the shoulder occurs because of the combined actions of the rotator cuff muscles and the deltoid muscle acting as a "force-couple." As abduction occurs, the action of the deltoid causes the humerus to move into the glenoid fossa. At the end range of motion, the deltoid causes the head of the humerus to translate downward out of the glenoid cavity. This action is counteracted by the group of muscles known as the rotator cuff. The rotator cuff acts to stabilize the humerus in the glenoid fossa.

Answer: **True**
Loth, Wadsworth, p. 395

8. Match each muscle to the correct innervation:

Muscle

1. Coracobrachialis
2. Subscapularis
3. Levator scapulae
4. Subclavius
5. Latissimus dorsi

Innervation

A. Subscapular nerve
B. Thoracodorsal nerve
C. Musculocutaneous nerve
D. Fifth and sixth cervical nerves
E. Dorsal scapular nerve

Answers: **1. C; 2. A; 3. E; 4. D; 5. B**
Sieg, Adams, pp. 27, 30, 34, 36

9. When shoulder abduction is measured in the sitting position, the fulcrum of the goniometer is placed over the lateral aspect of the glenohumeral joint. True or False?

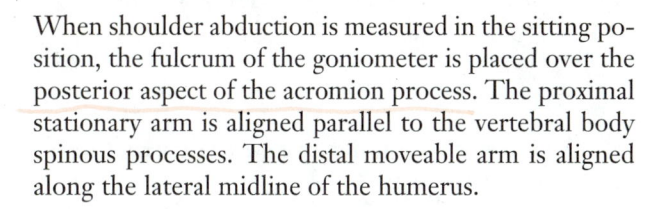

When shoulder abduction is measured in the sitting position, the fulcrum of the goniometer is placed over the posterior aspect of the acromion process. The proximal stationary arm is aligned parallel to the vertebral body spinous processes. The distal moveable arm is aligned along the lateral midline of the humerus.

Answer: **False**
Norkin, White, p. 61

10. Which of the following muscles comprise the rotator cuff?

A. Supraspinatus, teres minor, teres major, infraspinatus
B. Teres minor, subscapularis, posterior deltoid, infraspinatus
C. Supraspinatus, infraspinatus, teres minor, subscapularis
D. Supraspinatus, teres major, infraspinatus, subscapularis

The four muscles in answer C originate on the scapula and become tendons that fuse with the capsule of the shoulder, forming a musculotendinous cuff, which is termed the rotator cuff.

Answer: **C**
DeLee, Drey, p. 467
Refer to Fig. 6-4.

72 CHAPTER 6 Shoulder

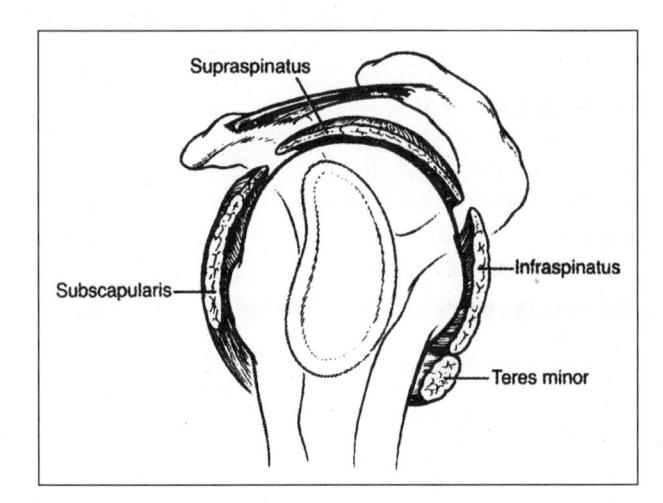

Fig. 6-4 ■ From Rockwood CA Jr, Matsen FA: *The shoulder,* Philadelphia, 1990, WB Saunders.

> **CLINICAL GEM:**
> One way to remember the muscles of the rotator cuff is to recall that **SITS** stands for **S**upraspinatus, **I**nfraspinatus, **T**eres minor, and **S**ubscapularis.

11. Match each shoulder test to the correct interpretation of the test:

Shoulder Test

1. Apprehension test (Crank Test)
2. Hawkins-Kennedy impingement test
3. Lippman test
4. Drop-Arm test

Test Interpretation

A. Rotator cuff tear
B. Bicipital tendinitis
C. Anterior instability
D. Supraspinatus tendinitis

Answers: **1. C; 2. D; 3. B; 4. A**
Magee, p. 118

12. Rotator cuff pathology almost always occurs with a supraspinatus component. True or False?

Because of the rotator cuff's insertion on the greater tuberosity of the humerus, the supraspinatus has a "critical zone" that is prone to calcium deposits and potential rupture. There is constant pressure from the head of the humerus and impingement against the coracoacromial arch during normal joint movements (see Fig.1-7).

Answer: **True**
Marks, Warner, Irrgang, pp. 91-93

13. What combination of nerves would have to be damaged in order to inhibit abduction of the shoulder?

A. Musculocutaneous and upper and lower subscapularis
B. Axillary and suprascapular
C. Suprascapular and long thoracic
D. Axillary and upper and lower subscapular

The suprascapular nerve supplies the supraspinatus muscle, which is responsible for abduction initiation. The axillary nerve innervates the deltoid, whose middle portion is a primary abductor. Injuries to both of these nerves will inhibit abduction of the shoulder.

Answer: **B**
Hoppenfeld, p. 27
Pratt, p. 73

14. Which of the following actions occur when the infraspinatus, subscapularis, and teres minor all contract at the same time?

A. Internal shoulder rotation
B. Shoulder flexion
C. External shoulder rotation
D. Depression of the humeral head in the glenoid fossa

The rotator cuff functions to approximate the humeral head to the glenoid cavity. The supraspinatus assists the deltoid in abduction, and the subscapularis, infraspinatus, and teres minor depress the humeral head during elevation of the arm.

Answer: **D**
Marks, Warner, Irrgang, p. 90

15. Of the three types of acromion shapes, which two are most often associated with rotator cuff tears?

A. Types one and two
B. Types one and three
C. Types two and three
D. None of the above

There are three types of acromion shapes: type one is flat and has been found in approximately 17% of the population (Fig. 6-5, *A*); type two is curved and has been found in approximately 43% of the population (Fig. 6-5, *B*); and type three is hooked and is believed to be found in approximately 39% of the population (Fig. 6-5, *C*). Types two and three are more often associated with rotator cuff tears because the impingement caused by the anterior curving or hooking leads to degeneration and tearing of the rotator cuff.

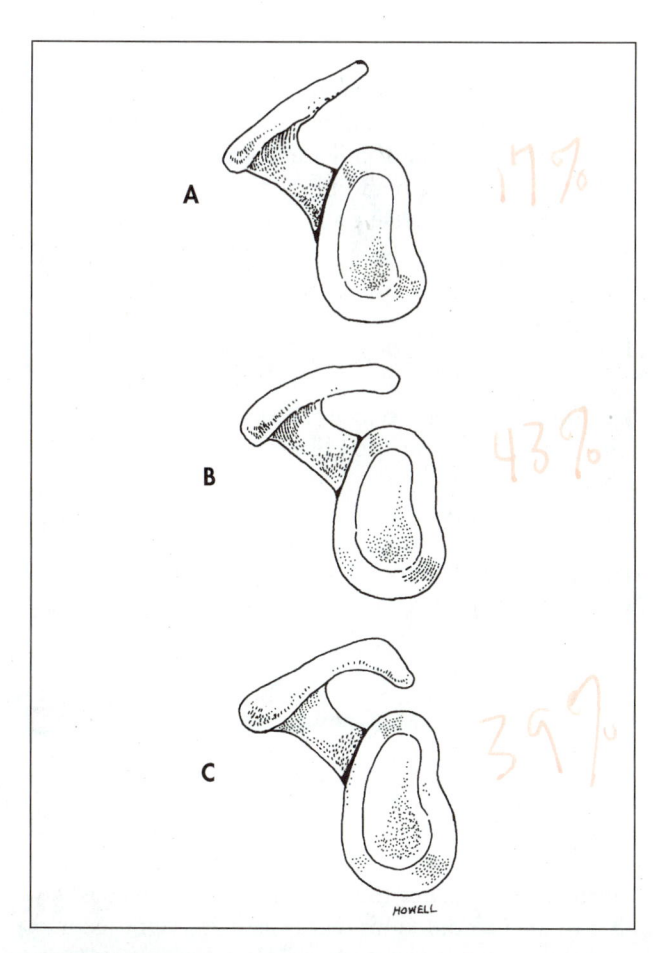

Answer: **C**
Flatow, p. 21

Fig. 6-5 A to C ■ From Hawkins RJ, Bell RH, Lippitt SB: *Atlas of shoulder surgery*, St. Louis, 1996, Mosby-Year Book.

16. A positive clunk test would indicate:

A. Rotator cuff tear
B. Labral tear
C. Impingement
D. Frozen shoulder

The clunk test is performed by rotating (internally and externally) the flexed shoulder with the elbow extended. A feeling of a clunk in the joint is believed to indicate that a labral fragment has been caught in the glenohumeral joint.

Answer: **B**
Flatow, p. 45

17. Generally speaking, postsurgical shoulder rehabilitation can be divided into the following three phases. True or False?

Phase I: Passive or assisted exercises to maintain or gain motion.
Phase II: Active range of motion.
Phase III: Resistive exercises to gain strength.

Progression among phases is a balancing act dependent upon tissue healing status; therefore timing among phases is critical. For example, if strict immobilization is required in Phase I, to promote tissue healing, active motion (Phase II) frequently is delayed for 6 to 8 weeks, depending on the rate of healing of violated tissues. Resistive exercise (Phase III) is initiated several weeks after Phase II begins.

Answer: **True**
Hawkins, Bell, Lippitt, pp. 309-310

18. Impingement syndrome at the shoulder may be caused by:

A. Decreased suboccipital space
B. Weakness in rotator cuff
C. Weakness of deltoid musculature
D. A and B
E. A and C

When abduction of the shoulder occurs, the tuberosity approximates the acromion and several structures may become pinched between the tuberosity and the coracoclavicular ligament. If there is repeated trauma, edema results, increasing soft tissue volume and decreasing the subacromial space. Weakness of the rotator cuff can cause instability when the deltoid overpowers the cuff muscles, allowing the humeral head to "ride up" during deltoid contraction and resulting in impingement (see Fig. 1-7).

Answer: **B**
Norris, p. 282

19. Rehabilitation of a patient with shoulder impingement should focus primarily on which of the following?

A. Rotator cuff strengthening
B. Scapular rotator strengthening
C. Pectoralis strengthening
D. A and B

In the rehabilitation of a patient with a shoulder impingement problem, it is important to strengthen both the rotator cuff and the scapular rotators. Strengthening the rotator cuff allows for depression of the humeral head into the glenoid fossa and prevents excessive superior movement of the humeral head in shoulder elevation, thus helping to prevent impingement. Strengthening the scapular rotators ensures that the scapula will follow the humerus in shoulder elevation, thus providing proper scapulohumeral rhythm. If the scapulothoracic muscles are weak, abnormal posture of the scapulae exists. This can cause disruption of the normal scapulohumeral rhythm that occurs with arm elevation, leading to impingement of the rotator cuff as it passes under the coracoacromial arch. Strengthening of the pectoralis muscles is contraindicated because it can increase impingement; however, stretching of the pectoralis is beneficial in the treatment of impingement syndrome.

Answer: **D**
Brotzman, pp. 93-94

20. Postural correction exercises, including scapular strengthening, pectoral stretching, and external rotation of the shoulder, can be useful in reducing stage-one impingement of the rotator cuff tendons. True or False?

In 1972, when Neer first introduced the concept of rotator cuff impingement, he believed that the majority of rotator cuff lesions were a result of mechanical impingement of the rotator cuff tendons. This impingement is beneath the anterior inferior portions of the acromion, particularly when the shoulder is placed in forward elevation and internal rotation. Therefore, if postural correction exercises are used, including scapular strengthening, pectoral stretching, and external rotation of the shoulder, the impingement will lessen.

Answer: **True**
Pettrone, p. 143

21. After arthroscopic surgery for subacromial decompression (ASAD), range-of-motion exercises should be delayed for 2 to 4 weeks and resistive exercises should not be attempted for 8 weeks. True or False?

After arthroscopic surgery for subacromial decompression, passive range-of-motion exercises are initiated immediately after surgery and are progressed to active exercise as soon as pain and motion will allow—typically in 4 to 5 days. Resistive exercises may be added at 3 to 4 weeks.

Answer: **False**
Hawkins, Bell, Lippitt, p. 284

22. The term for a tear of the superior labrum and biceps tendon from the glenoid is:

A. Bankart lesion
B. Superior labrum anterior to posterior lesion
C. Labral tear
D. Rotator cuff tear

The term SLAP lesion denotes a tear of the **S**uperior **L**abrum **A**nterior to **P**osterior. This area of the labrum also attaches the long head of the biceps tendon to the glenoid. This tear usually is diagnosed with magnetic resonance imaging (MRI), arthrography, or arthroscopy.

Answer: **B**
Sneider and Karzel, p. 49

23. After a superior labrum anterior to posterior lesion repair, which motion of the shoulder should be delayed?

A. Shoulder flexion beyond 90°
B. Internal rotation beyond 30°
C. External rotation beyond neutral
D. Shoulder extension
E. C and D

After sling immobilization for the first week, the patient can begin gentle active range of motion with restrictions. The patient should avoid external rotation of the shoulder beyond a neutral position and extension of the arm behind the body with the elbow extended for an additional 4 weeks to prevent stresses to the repaired structures. Patients generally are restricted from activities that place a significant stress on the biceps tendon until 3 to 4 months after surgery.

Answer: **E**
Pettrone, p. 124

24. A Bankart lesion usually results from:

A. An acromiohumeral impingement
B. A direct blow to the shoulder
C. An anterior dislocation of the shoulder
D. A posterior dislocation of the shoulder

An anterior dislocation of the shoulder usually results in an avulsion of the attachment of the anterior inferior glenohumeral ligament to the glenoid labrum from the anterior glenoid neck. It is believed that the anterior inferior glenohumeral ligament is the key static stabilizer of any anterior dislocation of the shoulder.

Answer: **C**
Sneider, Karzel, p. 57

25. After a Bankart lesion repair of the shoulder, the earliest recommended time to begin external rotation beyond 0° is 3 weeks. True or False?

After a Bankart repair, it is recommended that patients begin external rotation beyond 0° at 6 weeks. Gentle Codman exercises begin at approximately 2 weeks, with a gradual progression of range-of-motion exercises. Gentle strengthening exercise is initiated at 6 weeks.

Answer: **False**
Sneider, Karzel, p. 57

> **CLINICAL GEM:**
> Remember: protocol varies depending on the surgeon's preference and the tension on the repair site.

26. What is the preferred medical term for a "frozen shoulder" that is not related to any other shoulder problem?

A. Secondary adhesive capsulitis
B. Rotator cuff arthropathy
C. Degenerative arthritis of the glenohumeral joint
D. Primary adhesive capsulitis

Because "frozen shoulder" is a general term for loss of shoulder motion, the use of a more specific term is preferred. Most clinicians refer to idiopathic loss of shoulder motion as a primary adhesive capsulitis. Certain disease processes are believed to predispose an individual to this condition, including cardiovascular disease, neurologic conditions, and especially diabetes mellitus. The exact cause of the disease is unknown, but possibilities include immunologic, inflammatory, biochemical, and endocrine problems. Secondary frozen shoulder occurs in patients who develop decreased shoulder range of motion after trauma.

Answer: **D**
Warner, p. 130

27. The capsular pattern for the shoulder is: internal rotation (IR) is more limited than abduction (ABD), which is more limited than external rotation (ER) (IR > ABD > ER). True or False?

When a joint is injured, a limitation of movement occurs in characteristic proportions. The patterns vary from joint to joint. In the shoulder, the capsular pattern: is external rotation is more limited than abduction, which is more limited than internal rotation (ER > ABD > IR).

Answer: **False**
Cyriax, p. 54

28. When treating adhesive capsulitis of the shoulder with ultrasound, the sound head should be directed toward the anterosuperior portion of the capsule. True or False?

Most adhesions occur in the anteroinferior portions of the capsule. This should be the area of focus with mobilizations, modalities, and stretching. When ultrasound is performed, the arm is abducted and externally rotated and the sound head is directed toward the anteroinferior portion of the capsule.

Answer: **False**
Saunders, p. 161
Michlovitz, p. 203

29. Occupational or physical therapy treatment for primary frozen shoulder would appropriately include all of the following, except:

A. Heat and ultrasound
B. Transcutaneous electrical nerve stimulation or interferential electrical stimulation
C. Massage
D. Aggressive passive stretching
E. Active range-of-motion exercises

Therapy should include the use of modalities such as heat, ultrasound, and massage of trigger-points to increase soft-tissue extensibility. The use of nonsteroidal antiinflammatory agents or subacromial space injection enhances therapy tolerance. This is followed by *gentle* passive and active range-of-motion exercises. Aggressive passive stretching should be avoided. If significant improvement is not attained after 6 months, manipulation of the shoulder under anesthesia usually is considered.

Answer: **D**
Pettrone, p. 223

30. Injury to the acromioclavicular joint typically is caused by landing on the acromion during a fall or by a blow to the lateral shoulder. True or False?

Inferior and sometimes posterior forces to the shoulder stress the acromioclavicular ligament and the coracoclavicular ligament. If the force is excessive, these ligaments are disrupted sequentially. Rockwood describes six grades/types of injury. For a detailed description of these six grades, refer to Hunter, Mackin, and Callahan.

Answer: **True**
Pettrone, p. 167
Hunter, Mackin, Callahan, p. 1652
Refer to Fig. 6-6.

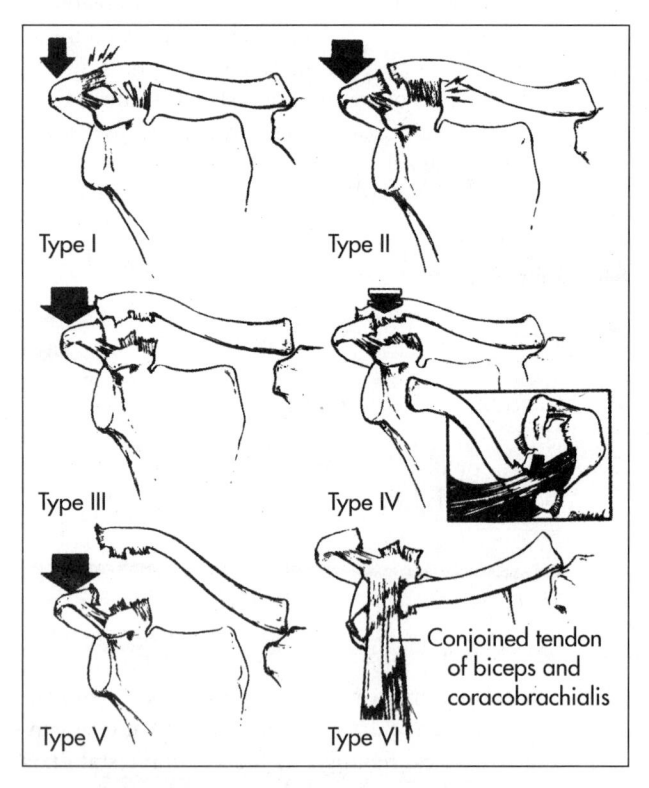

Fig. 6-6 ■ The six types of acromioclavicular disruptions. (From Rockwood CA Jr, Williams GR, Young DC: *Injuries to the acromioclavicular joint.* In Rockwood CA Jr, Green DP, Bucholz RW, editors: *Rockwood and Green's fractures in adults,* ed 3, Philadelphia, 1991, JB Lippincott.)

31. After a type-two acromioclavicular injury (e.g., acromioclavicular joint subluxed, acromioclavicular ligament disrupted), active range of motion should be initiated when acute pain subsides. Which of the following shoulder motions usually is not limited?

A. Flexion
B. Abduction
C. Elevation
D. Internal rotation

Shoulder abduction, forward flexion, and elevation often are limited because of injury to the trapezius and deltoid. Internal rotation usually is not limited.

Answer: **D**
Pettrone, p. 171

> **CLINICAL GEM:**
> Acromioclavicular injury types one through three, as described by Rockwood, usually can be treated conservatively, but types four through six may require surgical reconstruction.

32. A 50-year-old patient presents to an orthopedic surgeon with a 6-month history of severe shoulder pain without any history of injury. The range of motion of the shoulder is diminished by approximately 50% and testing is positive for impingement. The patient also exhibits a positive drop-arm test. The patient refuses any injections or medicines. What should the surgeon do next?

A. Order immediate occupational/physical therapy
B. Instruct the patient in a home exercise program
C. Order an arthrogram
D. Order a magnetic resonance imaging

The best choice for this patient would be to order a magnetic resonance imaging for evaluation of the rotator cuff. Evaluation of the cuff would be essential before deciding on further treatment. Occupational or physical therapy would likely aggravate the pain at this stage, and therefore would not be indicated. A home exercise program most likely would be ineffective because this would aggravate the pain. Because the patient refuses injection, an arthrogram would not be possible.

Answer: **D**
Flatow, pp. 43-45

33. The patient in question 32 had a magnetic resonance imaging that showed a greater than 50% partial tear of the articular surface of the supraspinatus tendon and anterior acromiohumeral impingement. The patient refuses injection, medication, or therapy and wants something done operatively. The surgeon most likely would:

A. Abandon this patient because the patient obviously is uncooperative
B. Perform arthroscopy and débride the tear only
C. Perform arthroscopy with acromioplasty and a mini open repair
D. Insist that the patient attend occupational or physical therapy

The most appropriate treatment for a greater than 50% partial tear of the rotator cuff would be: first, confirm the presence of the partial tear with arthroscopy; second, perform an arthroscopic acromioplasty; and third, perform a mini open repair of the partial thickness tear. It has been found that arthroscopy and débridement alone for these types of tears is not as effective.

Answer: **C**
Flatow, pp. 79-82

34. The same patient in questions 32 and 33 is seen in the doctor's office three days after surgery. The patient is doing well and the wounds are healing with no evidence of infection. Pain is controlled with analgesics. What should be done next?

A. Occupational/physical therapy with active range of motion should be ordered
B. Patient should be kept completely immobilized for 6 weeks
C. Occupational/physical therapy with passive range of motion only should be ordered
D. Patient should receive massage therapy

During the postoperative period after mini open repair, the patient should be on a passive range-of-motion program for the first 3 to 6 weeks. If the deltoid was detached and reattached, active range of motion is prohibited for 6 weeks. If the patient has undergone arthroscopic débridement only, gentle active motion may begin immediately. Specific protocols vary depending on surgeon preference and facility guidelines.

Answer: **C**
Flatow, p. 80

35. Immediately after shoulder surgery, it is best to assign the patient a complex home exercise program that is performed once a day. True or False?

When appropriate in the early days after surgery, it is best to instruct the patient in a short, simple exercise program that is performed frequently. A session should be limited to 10 to 15 minutes and performed 5 to 6 times a day. As healing progresses, the length of the sessions should be expanded and their frequency should be decreased. After discharge from formal therapy, the patient should be reminded to continue stretching and strengthening once a day.

Answer: **False**
Hawkins, Bell, Lippitt, p. 310

36. A patient presents to the orthopedic surgeon's office with a minimally displaced proximal humeral fracture through the surgical neck. She is quite stoic and does not want any pain medication. What should be done next?

A. The arm and shoulder should be immobilized in a sling for approximately 6 weeks.
B. The arm and shoulder should be immobilized in a sling for approximately 3 weeks.
C. The arm and shoulder should be immobilized in a sling for approximately 7 to 10 days.
D. An open reduction internal fixation should be performed.

Approximately 80% of proximal humeral fractures are slightly displaced. However, most of these fractures are stable. Thus, better results have been seen with early motion—typically as early as 7 to 10 days after injury. When displacement is excessive, various forms of open reduction internal fixation may be considered.

Answer: **C**
Frymoyer, p. 285
Refer to Fig. 6-7.

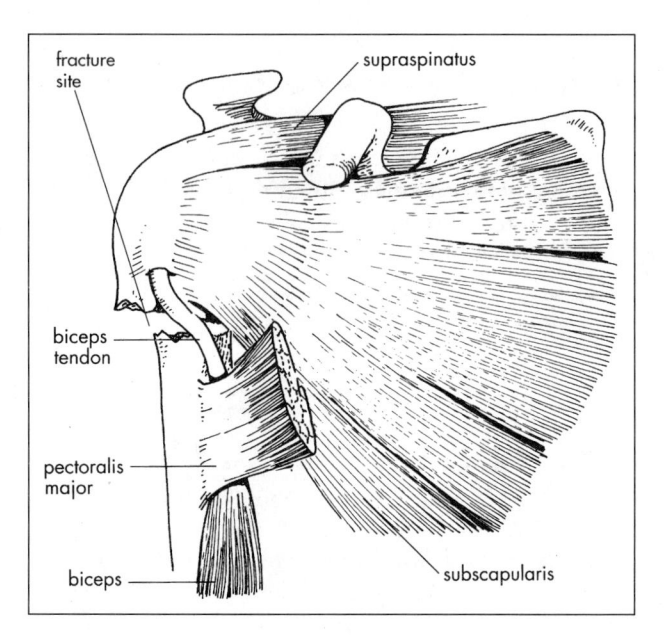

Fig. 6-7 ■ From Hawkins RJ, Bell RH, Lippitt SB: *Atlas of shoulder surgery,* St. Louis, 1996, Mosby-Year Book.

37. Codman's exercises frequently are used as postoperative or postfracture exercises for almost all shoulder pathologies. These exercises are appropriate because:

A. Strengthening of the pectoral girdle occurs without shoulder motion during this exercise.
B. Achieving joint approximation through weightbearing on the extremity occurs rather than muscle contraction.
C. They assist in reduction of the distal postoperative edema while protecting the shoulder joint.
D. Shoulder motion is gained passively, using gravity and body position rather than muscle contraction.

Codman's exercises are performed by having the patient bend at the waist, allowing the arm to dangle away from the body. In this position, gravity alone can achieve up to 90° of shoulder flexion without any muscle contraction. The patient also can use body motion to swing the arm gently clockwise, counterclockwise, forward and back, and side to side. These exercises can be performed with or without a sling to maintain elbow flexion and are easily progressed to an active exercise with minimal use of the shoulder musculature.

Answer: **D**
Pettrone, p. 214
Refer to Fig. 6-8.

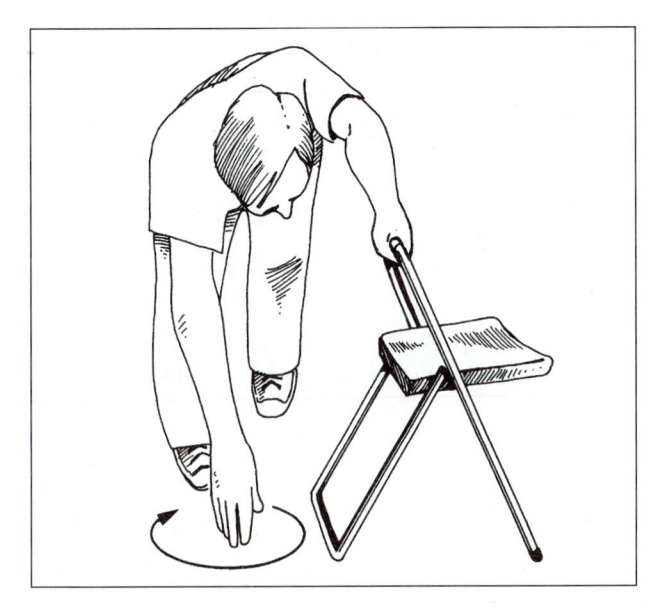

Fig. 6-8 ■ From Hawkins RJ, Bell RH, Lippitt SB: *Atlas of shoulder surgery,* St. Louis, 1996, Mosby-Year Book.

38. Nonoperative treatment for multidirectional instability of the shoulder after acute injury should include:

A. A prolonged period of immobilization (4 to 6 weeks)
B. Codman's exercises with weights after the acute phase
C. Weighted exercise to create an inferior traction force on the shoulder after the acute phase
D. Rotator cuff strengthening after the acute phase

After acute dislocation resulting in multidirectional instability, an arm sling is worn for a few days to decrease pain. Traction on the shoulder should be avoided. A rehabilitation program that emphasizes rotator cuff and periscapular muscle strengthening is employed after acute pain decreases. Traumatic dislocations respond less favorably to therapy than atraumatic dislocations.

Answer: **D**
Pettrone, p. 132

39. Osteoarthritis of the glenohumeral joint can be identified by sharp, intermittent pain—frequently when the joint is at rest. True or False?

Osteoarthritis of the glenohumeral joint causes a non-localizing "toothache"-like pain that is aggravated by motion and that may result in muscle atrophy and contractures. Crepitation is noted with motion. Treatment consists of gentle therapy and pain-relieving measures.

Answer: **False**
Pettrone, p. 240

> **CLINICAL GEM:**
> Crepitation is a clicking or crackling sound heard during the movement of certain joints; it is caused by irregularities in the articulating surfaces.

40. After a biceps tenodesis procedure, passive range-of-motion exercises are started on the second postoperative day for both the shoulder and the elbow. True or False?

Biceps pathology is encountered during rotator cuff repair and proximal humeral fractures; occasionally it is caused by acute tears, or rarely, by attritional deterioration. Biceps tenodesis is the fixation of the long biceps tendon in the bicipital groove of the humerus. Passive range-of-motion exercises are started on the second postoperative day for the elbow and shoulder. The patient is taught to perform progressive elbow extension as pain allows. Full extension may not be achieved for 5 to 6 weeks. The patient is cautioned against active elbow flexion to protect the tenodesis. Active exercise is started for the elbow and shoulder at 2 to 3 weeks, with strengthening at 4 to 6 weeks. Heavy resistance should be avoided for 2 to 3 months.

Answer: **True**
Hawkins, Bell, Lippitt, p. 144

41. A 72-year-old woman is seen by an orthopedic surgeon. Her primary complaint is severe pain and a loss of motion in her shoulder during the past 6 months. She was referred to the orthopedic doctor by her primary care physician after 3 months of nonoperative treatment, including occupational/physical therapy, antiinflammatory medications, and steroid injections. Radiographs confirm a superior subluxation of the humeral head with some degenerative changes. The magnetic resonance imaging shows a large retracted rotator cuff tear. The patient wants her shoulder to work as well as possible. What is the best option for the surgeon?

A. Explain to the patient that she is too old for surgery
B. Order more occupational/physical therapy
C. Schedule the patient for arthroscopic débridement with no attempt at repair of the tear
D. Schedule the patient for arthroscopy with possible open repair

Rotator cuff tears have been classified as: small, which is less than 1 cm in diameter; medium, which is 1 to 3 cm; large, which is 3 to 5 cm; and massive, which is greater than 5 cm. Many studies have shown that débridement provides satisfactory results for the short term. Long-term studies, however, indicate that for all types of tears a patient is best served by operative repair of the tear.

Answer: **D**
Flatow, pp. 117-124

42. Which of the following test(s) identify(ies) thoracic outlet syndrome:

A. Halstead maneuver
B. Speeds test
C. Adson maneuver
D. B and C
E. A and C

The Adson maneuver is a common test for identifying thoracic outlet syndrome. The radial pulse is monitored while the head is rotated toward the involved shoulder. The patient extends his or her head and the shoulder is placed in extension and external rotation as the patient takes a deep breath and holds it. If the radial pulse decreases or disappears, the test is positive. In some individuals it may be necessary to rotate the head to the opposite side to have an effect on the radial pulse. Therefore, both positions must be tested.

The Halstead maneuver is performed by locating the radial pulse and applying a downward traction on the arm while the patient hyperextends the neck and rotates his or her head to the opposite side. A diminished or absent pulse indicates a positive test for thoracic outlet syndrome.

The two tests just described help determine neurovascular compression within the thoracic outlet; however, they specifically address vascular compression.

Compression at the thoracic outlet can involve the subclavian artery, the subclavian vein, or the brachial plexus.

Answer: **E**
DeLee, Drey, p. 796
Magee, p. 122

CLINICAL GEM:
Thoracic outlet syndrome presents with vascular and/or neurological symptoms. Controversy surrounds the actual percentage for each category; however, it is accepted that neurological presentation is more common.

43. Which of the following is not a suitable treatment technique for thoracic outlet syndrome?

A. Strengthening the trapezius, rhomboids, and levator scapulae
B. Strengthening the pectoralis major, pectoralis minor, and subscapularis
C. Postural reeducation
D. Biofeedback

Conservative treatment for thoracic outlet syndrome (TOS) consists of modifying aggravating factors (e.g., avoiding overhead activities). Important aspects of rehabilitation for a patient with TOS include strengthening the shoulder girdle and postural reeducation. The muscles to be strengthened include the trapezius, the rhomboids, and the levator scapulae. Other treatments include antiinflammatory medications, ultrasound, transcutaneous electrical nerve stimulation, and biofeedback. Strengthening the pectoralis major, the pectoralis minor, and the subscapularis would cause increased impingement; therefore, it is best to stretch these structures.

Answer: **B**
Oates, Daley, pp. 711-712

> **CLINICAL GEM:**
> If a patient has an arterial obstruction, he or she will report symptoms of coolness, cold sensitivity, numbness in the hand, and exertional fatigue. These symptoms indicate compression at the pectoralis minor loop. If a patient has a venous obstruction, he or she will report symptoms of cyanotic discoloration, arm edema, finger stiffness, and a feeling of heaviness. These symptoms indicate a compression at the first rib.

Chapter 7

Flaps/Grafts/Thermal Conditions

Topics to be reviewed in random order are:

- Burn classifications
- Keloid/hypertrophic scarring
- Splinting the burned hand
- Exercising the burned hand
- Grafting of burns
- Pressure treatment for burns
- Flap coverage techniques
- Skin graft coverage techniques
- Rehabilitation for flaps and grafts
- Raynaud's disease/phenomenon
- Splinting for flaps and grafts
- Edema management techniques

1. Which of the following should be avoided when treating a patient with edema?

A. Home exercise program
B. Pneumatic compression device
C. Whirlpool
D. All of the above should be avoided

The use of a whirlpool should be avoided because it requires the arm to be placed in a dependent position, which leads to increased edema.

Answer: **C**
Vasudevan, Melvin, pp. 520-523

2. Which is the most effective and accessible method for preventing and reducing edema?

A. Jobst pressure garments
B. Retrograde massage
C. Elevation
D. Coban wrap

All of the above are used to manage edema. Elevation is the most effective and accessible method for preventing and reducing edema because it requires no assistance.

Answer: **C**
Vasudevan, Melvin, pp. 520-523

3. Edema is synonymous with oedema. True or False?

Oedema is the spelling used in Great Britain. The terms are synonymous.

Answer: **True**
Taber's

83

CHAPTER 7 Flaps/Grafts/Thermal Conditions

4. Raynaud's disease occurs with a causative disease. True or False?

Raynaud's disease (idiopathic Raynaud's phenomenon) occurs without a specific causative disease. It occurs most often in young women and presents bilaterally, with an absence of primary disease. Raynaud's syndrome or secondary Raynaud's phenomenon, in contrast, is associated with disease. Some of the causes of Raynaud's phenomenon may include connective tissue disorders (rheumatoid arthritis or scleroderma), arterio-occlusive disorders, and late sequelae to cold injury. Recently, vibratory trauma to the digits from power tools has been associated with Raynaud's phenomenon.

Answer: **False**
Hunter, Mackin, Callahan, pp. 972-973

5. The first color response in patients with Raynaud's phenomena is:

A. Cyanosis
B. Erythema
C. Pallor
D. No color changes occur with Raynaud's phenomena

Color changes related to Raynaud's phenomena occur in a "triple-response" pattern. The first color change is ischemic pallor, which is followed by cyanotic coloring; as blood flow returns, a reactive erythema is noted.

Answer: **C**
Hunter, Mackin, Callahan, p. 962

6. A good choice for treatment of Raynaud's phenomena is thermal biofeedback. True or False?

Thermal biofeedback is an excellent modality for pain relief and for learning rewarming techniques for patients experiencing Raynaud's phenomena.

Answer: **True**
Hunter, Mackin, Callahan, p. 1567

CLINICAL GEM:
The use of a Neoprene glove is helpful with vascular or cold injuries. These can be purchased at diving and water skiing shops. Because the gloves are thin, they allow for hand motion while maintaining heat to keep joints pliable and increase perspiration, which aids edema reduction.

7. What is the mildest type of cold injury?

A. Chilblains
B. Frostbite
C. Immersion injuries
D. All of the above are mild types of injuries

Chilblains are the mildest form of cold injury. They occur when individuals are exposed repeatedly to the cold with limited protection. Acute forms often are resolved within a week, but the condition can become chronic.

Immersion injuries occur from exposing an extremity to wet cold at a temperature above freezing. Common sequelae from immersion injuries are Raynaud's phenomena, hyperhidrosis, muscle wasting, and cold sensitivity. Frostbite results from a crystallization of tissue water and occurs with exposure to temperatures below freezing. (Tissue freezes at approximately −2° C; the body's normal core temperature is 37° C or 98.6° F.)

Answer: **A**
Hunter, Mackin, Callahan, pp. 1295-1296

8. The Hunting reaction is a protective reaction to cold exposure. True or False?

The Hunting reaction is a cyclic vasodilation and constriction that occurs with exposure to water or air at about 0° C (32° F). However, if an individual experiences prolonged cold exposure, the protective Hunting reaction will be overcome and the tissues will freeze.

Answer: **True**
Hunter, Mackin, Callahan, p. 1296

9. Rewarming treatment after frostbite should be performed slowly. True or False?

Only a few years ago physicians advocated rewarming the extremity slowly, first with cold water baths or by allowing the extremity to thaw at room temperature. More recently, evidence has shown that rapid rewarming at 40° to 44° C (104° to 112° F) is the most important step in salvaging the tissue and function of a frostbitten limb. Rewarming usually occurs within 30 minutes.

Answer: **False**
Green, p. 2034

10. All of the following should be used in the management of a patient with acute frostbite except:

A. Whirlpool b.i.d.
B. Range-of-motion exercises
C. Static and/or dynamic splints as needed
D. Always remove blisters

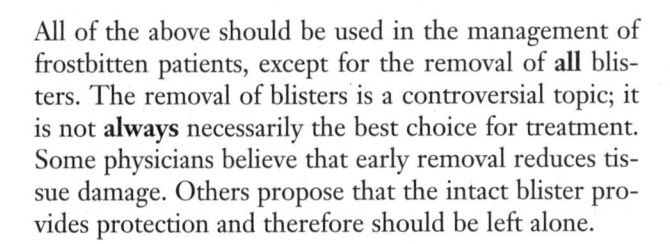

All of the above should be used in the management of frostbitten patients, except for the removal of **all** blisters. The removal of blisters is a controversial topic; it is not **always** necessarily the best choice for treatment. Some physicians believe that early removal reduces tissue damage. Others propose that the intact blister provides protection and therefore should be left alone.

Answer: **D**
Hunter, Mackin, Callahan, p. 1299

11. The American Burn Association classifies a hand burn as a major injury. True or False?

The American Burn Association has established criteria for defining major burns that require hospitalization or care in a burn center. A burn to the hand is included among the definitions of a major burn. After a burn injury, mobility of the hand must be preserved, function must be restored, and soft-tissue coverage must be stable and soft. A failure to achieve these objectives can result in the individual not returning to work or functional independence. Burn center personnel have experience in treating critical hand burns and can assist patients in achieving good, functional outcomes.

Answer: **True**
Herndon, p. 506
Richards, Staley, pp. 114-115

12. According to the "rule of nines," the hand constitutes which percentage of total body surface area?

A. 1
B. 3
C. 5
D. 7

During evaluation of a burn wound, an estimate of the size of the wound is made. This helps assess the severity of the injury and determine the patient's prognosis. Knowing the size of the wound also helps establish treatment protocols for fluid resuscitation, nutritional support, and surgery. Burn size is estimated by calculating the total body surface area (TBSA) covered by the wound. Only partial- and full-thickness wounds are used in estimation. The percentage of TBSA covered by a burn is most often determined with a diagram that divides the body into 11 segments, with each one representing 9% TBSA. With this method, called the "rule of nines," a hand is calculated to be approximately 3% of an individual's TBSA. Therefore, a circumferential burn to the hand would be classified as a 3% burn.

Answer: **B**
Richards, Staley, pp. 109-110
Herndon, p. 35
Refer to Fig. 7-1.

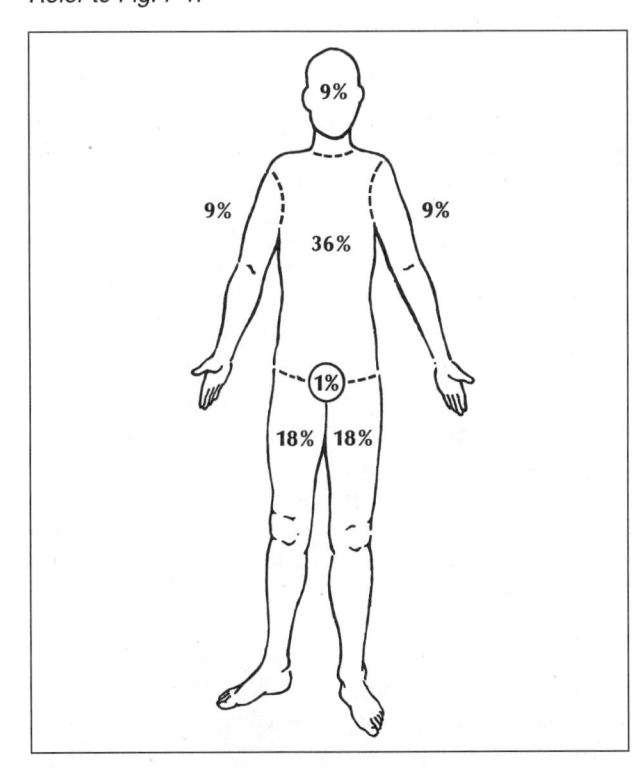

Fig. 7-1 ■ Rule of nines. (From Pedretti LW: *Occupational therapy: practice skills for physical dysfunction,* ed 4, St. Louis, 1996, Mosby-Year Book.)

86 CHAPTER 7 Flaps/Grafts/Thermal Conditions

13. Full-thickness (third-degree) burns are quite painful. True or False?

Full-thickness (third-degree) burns destroy the full thickness of the skin, which may include the muscle, tendon, and bone. These burns often are pain-free and insensitive to pinprick because of the loss of nerve endings in the skin. However, most third-degree burns are surrounded by second-degree burns, which are very painful.

Answer: **False**
Hopkins, Smith, pp. 571-572

14. A patient in the clinic presents with an erythematous and blistering burn on his right thumb. How would you classify this burn?

A. Superficial (first-degree)
B. Superficial partial-thickness (second-degree)
C. Deep partial-thickness (second-degree)
D. Full-thickness (third-degree)

Historically, burns have been classified as first-, second-, or third-degree. Currently the terms superficial, partial-thickness, and full-thickness are commonly used.

Superficial (first-degree) burns are confined to the epidermis. These burns are characterized by erythema and blanching under pressure. There is some pain and edema but no blistering. An easy way to remember this burn is to think of a sunburn. These burns heal within 3 to 7 days.

Second-degree burns are known as partial-thickness burns. Partial-thickness burns are classified as either superficial partial-thickness, or deep partial-thickness. Superficial partial-thickness burns involve the epidermis and part of the papillary dermis. These burns characteristically are more painful and present with blisters and subcutaneous edema. **The patient in this question falls into this classification.** These burns typically heal in 7 to 21 days. Deep partial-thickness burns involve the epidermis, papillary, and reticular layers of the dermis and sometimes the fat domes of the subcutaneous layers. Healing time is 21 to 35 days for these burns as long as the wound is free from infection. These burns may develop hypertrophic scars.

Full-thickness (third-degree) burns destroy the full thickness of the skin. The skin varies from a dry, leathery appearance to charred skin, depending on burn severity. Full-thickness burns can be subcategorized as minor, moderate, or severe. The patient may experience minimal to no pain because nerve endings have been burned. Most large areas will require grafting. If these areas are left to heal on their own, they may take many months. Hypertrophic scarring can be severe.

Answer: **B**
Hopkins, Smith, pp. 571-572
Richards, Staley, pp. 110-112

15. A keloid scar has distinct characteristics that distinguish it from a hypertrophic scar. True or False?

Controversy regarding the difference between a keloid scar and a hypertrophic scar has continued for almost 200 years. The keloid was first described in 1802. Hypertrophic scars were defined in 1847. Since then, their differences have been questioned. Historically, a keloid has been characterized as a scar that extends beyond the boundaries of the original wound. This definition continues to be used by some authors. However, some studies suggest that there is little difference between these two types of scars and that a keloid may be an extreme variant of a hypertrophic scar. Further research is needed to solve this complex issue.

Answer: **False**
Richards, Staley, pp. 381-382
Herndon, pp. 388-389
Hunter, Mackin, Callahan, p. 1269

16. How long does a hypertrophic scar take to fully mature?

A. 4 to 6 months
B. 6 months
C. 1 year
D. 2 years

During the first 6 to 12 weeks of wound healing, biomechanical and cellular changes accelerate and hypertrophic scars begin to appear. Collagen synthesis is active during this healing phase. Attempts to alter the scar are most effective between the sixth and twelfth weeks. A scar becomes fully mature approximately 2 years after injury.

Answer: **D**
Richards, Staley, pp. 383-385
Hunter, Mackin, Callahan, p. 1273

17. The application of superficial heat can be beneficial in the treatment of a burned hand after wound closure. True or False?

Therapeutic heat can increase blood flow, reduce pain caused by passive stretching, and decrease muscle spasms. When connective tissue is heated and stretched simultaneously, its ability to lengthen increases. Heating the burn wound after wound closure can help temporarily elongate scar tissue. Moist hot packs, fluidotherapy, or paraffin can be used to decrease hand stiffness and increase the extensibility of tissues. It is important to remember that applying heat before wound closure is contraindicated because it may increase edema or cause hemorrhaging.

Answer: **True**
Richards, Staley, pp. 420-421, 568

18. When can exercises be safely initiated after a burn injury?

A. First 48 hours
B. 4 to 5 days
C. 7 to 10 days
D. 2 to 3 days

Edema formation, which is the body's initial response to a burn injury, occurs within the first 24 to 48 hours. Exercise programs for burn injury must be initiated as soon as possible (in the first 48 hours) after injury. Exercises are designed to help reduce edema, increase circulation, and assist with wound healing. Burn scar contraction begins to develop in the first 4 days after injury. A tightness in tendons, sheaths, and muscles occurs between 5 and 21 days after injury. Exercises are progressed to address strength deficits and functional loss and to provide resistance against the contracting scar.

Answer: **A**
Hunter, Mackin, Callahan, p. 1271
Herndon, p. 453
Richards, Staley, pp. 324-329

19. All of the following are factors that influence the development of scar tissue. Which one is most important in predicting hypertrophic scar development?

A. Race
B. Burn depth
C. Age
D. Length of time for wound closure

All of the above factors affect hypertrophic scar development.

AGE: Most hypertrophic scars develop in individuals 30 years of age and younger, perhaps because this age group has a higher incidence of trauma and a higher rate of collagen synthesis when compared with older individuals.

RACE: Darker pigmented races (Black and Asian) have a higher incidence of hypertrophic scar development when compared with Caucasians. One study found that black populations have twice the incidence of hypertrophic scar development compared with Caucasians.

BURN DEPTH: Hypertrophic scars develop from deep wounds that involve the reticular dermis. The reticular dermis is a deep plane in which collagen fibers are thicker and numerous elastic fibers form undulating (up-and-down) patterns. These wounds take longer than 3 weeks to heal, contributing to scar hypertrophy.

LENGTH OF TIME FOR WOUND CLOSURE: Hypertrophic scars develop from wounds that take longer than 3 weeks to close. If a wound is open for an excessive amount of time, greater amounts of collagen are deposited, making the length of time for wound closure **the most important factor** in predicting hypertrophic scarring. Collagen deposition results in the formation of thick, rigid scar tissue. Seventy-eight percent of wounds that take longer than 21 days to close develop hypertrophic scars.

Answer: **D**
Richards, Staley, pp. 385-387
Hunter, Mackin, Callahan, pp. 1268-1271

88 CHAPTER 7 Flaps/Grafts/Thermal Conditions

20. A patient in the clinic presents with a dorsal hand burn. In which position should she be splinted?

A. Wrist neutral, metacarpophalangeal joints at 90° flexion, and interphalangeal joints flexed
B. Wrist neutral, metacarpophalangeal joints at 45° flexion, and interphalangeal joints at 30° flexion
C. Wrist at 15° extension, metacarpophalangeal joints at 60° flexion, and interphalangeal joints extended
D. Wrist at 30° extension, metacarpophalangeal joints extended, and interphalangeal joints extended

Because of edema and wound tightness, the unsupported hand will position itself in a claw deformity of wrist flexion, metacarpophalangeal joint hyperextension, and interphalangeal flexion. To prevent this deformity, the wrist should be placed in slight extension, with metacarpophalangeal joints at 60° to 70° of flexion and interphalangeal joints in full extension. If the thumb is involved, it should be splinted in abduction, with the interphalangeal joint slightly flexed. Splinting the hand in this position helps preserve the extensor mechanism and assists in preventing collateral ligament tightness.

Answer: **C**
Hunter, Mackin, Callahan, p. 1273
Richards, Staley, p. 283
Herndon, p. 446
Refer to Fig. 7-2.

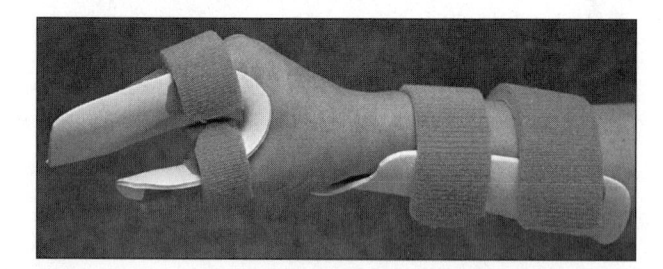

Fig. 7-2 ■ A resting hand splint. The hand is in an antideformity (intrinsic plus) position. (From Coppard BM, Lohman H: *Introduction to splinting: a critical-thinking and problem-solving approach*, St. Louis, 1996, Mosby-Year Book.)

21. A 21-year-old woman is referred to therapy with a hand burn, she has limited motion; you choose joint mobilization to increase finger flexion. When can you begin joint mobilization techniques after a burn injury?

A. During the acute phase
B. After reduction of edema
C. During the scar maturation phase
D. After wound closure

A burn scar must have good tensile strength to tolerate the friction that occurs during joint mobilization. Therefore, joint mobilization should not be performed until the scar maturation phase; complications may occur if this technique is used earlier.

Answer: **C**
Richards, Staley, p. 336

22. During burn reconstruction, tenolysis is a successful surgical procedure for releasing tendon adhesions in the hand. True or False?

In deep burn wounds, scar tissue encircles the tendon and forms along the full length of the wound. Skin quality often is poor; therefore, tenolysis rarely is successful in releasing adhesions in the burned hand.

Answer: **False**
Herndon, p. 512

23. A 7-year-old boy sustained an amputation of the tip of his nondominant ring finger. The resulting wound measures 1 cm in diameter. No bone is exposed at the base of the wound. Which of the following would be the most appropriate form of management?

A. Healing by secondary intention
B. Full-thickness skin graft from the groin
C. Cross-finger flap
D. Thenar flap
E. Atasoy V-Y advancement flap

Healing by secondary intention is the most appropriate management of this injury. It provides good, functional results with few complications at a low cost. The primary disadvantage is an extended period of healing. Although skin grafting would require a shorter period of healing, additional procedures would be necessary and the overall cost would be higher. In addition, there is no evidence that skin grafting results in improved function. Grafting is more appropriate for volar oblique amputations.

A flap should be considered if pulp loss is greater than 1.5 cm in diameter and bone remains intact. Local flaps, such as the V-Y advancement flap, usually provide good sensibility but are difficult to mobilize when more than 1 cm of tissue is required.

Cross-finger flaps and thenar flaps are excellent for reconstruction of the volar fingertip but are not necessary for small, uncomplicated injuries. Although the cross-finger flap causes less flexion contracture of the proximal interphalangeal joint, the thenar flap provides more tissue bulk and is consistently more successful in reconstructing large injuries.

Answer: **A**
Yaremchuk, p. 125

24. When nerves, blood vessels, and tendons are not injured and a healthy recipient bed is present, which of the following is the most appropriate form of reconstruction of the dorsal hand:

A. Skin graft
B. Cross-finger flap
C. V-Y advancement flap
D. Free flap

Treatment alternatives for soft-tissue coverage of the hand should be considered logically. Options range from simple (primary closure or skin grafts) to complex (flap or free-tissue transfer). The simplest method that will preserve form and function should be used. In this example, a skin graft would be the best choice because of its simplicity in the presence of a healthy recipient bed.

Answer: **A**
American Society for Surgery of the Hand, pp. 281, 287

25. The part of a flap that provides the blood supply is termed the "pedicle." True or False?

A flap is skin with varying amounts of underlying tissue that is used to cover a defect. A flap receives its blood supply from a source other than the tissue in which it is placed. The part of the flap that provides the blood supply is termed the "pedicle." All flaps have pedicles of varying types.

Answer: **True**
Green, p. 1741

26. The most common cause of skin graft failure is:

A. Excessive pressure on a fresh graft
B. Infection
C. Hematoma
D. Movement of the grafted area

A hematoma is a mass of clotted blood caused by a break in a blood vessel. The clot resides in the undersurface of the graft, isolated from the endothelial buds of the recipient bed, preventing revascularization and causing skin graft failure. Infection is the second most common cause of graft loss and is minimized by proper preparation of the wound bed. The other causes listed also can lead to graft failure and must be prevented.

Answer: **C**
Orenstein, pp. 1-30

27. The most appropriate coverage for a burn wound involving the entire dorsum of the hand is:

A. Full-thickness skin graft
B. Split-thickness skin graft
C. Primary closure
D. Latissimus dorsi myocutaneous free flap

In this example, a split-thickness skin graft (Fig. 7-3) is the best and simplest solution. The graft can be harvested with minimal donor site morbidity and yields an excellent functional result. A full-thickness skin graft would not be large enough to reconstruct this defect without grafting the donor area. Primary closure is not possible in this large defect. A latissimus dorsi myocutaneous free flap carries a significant donor site morbidity, and its thickness would not be needed in this case.

Answer: **B**
Orenstein, pp. 1-30

CHAPTER 7 Flaps/Grafts/Thermal Conditions

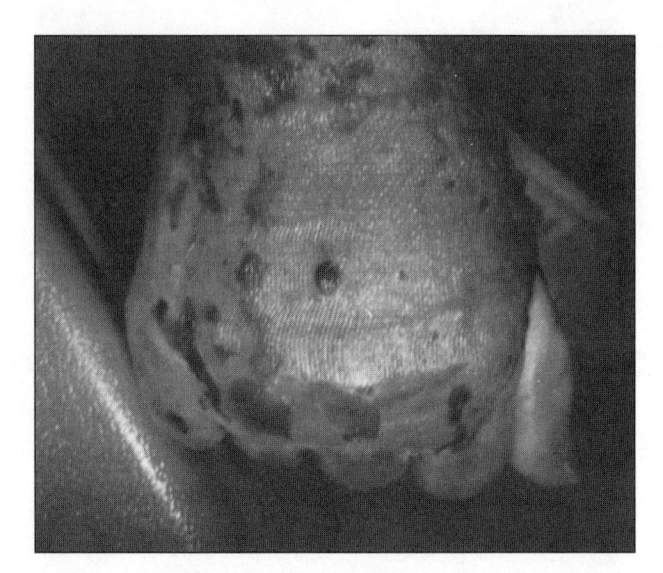

Fig. 7-3 ■ From Hunter JM, Mackin EJ, Callahan AD: *Rehabilitation of the hand: surgery and therapy*, ed 4, St. Louis, 1995, Mosby-Year Book.

28. Splinting helps to minimize contractures after skin grafting. True or False?

Splinting is essential to minimize the risk of joint contractures after skin grafts. Most surgeons use splinting in the immediate postoperative period. Early mobilization and joint range of motion also are used once the graft has demonstrated good adherence.

Answer: **True**
American Society for Surgery of the Hand, pp. 281-287

29. Primary treatment objectives in fingertip amputations include all of the following, except:

A. Closing the wound
B. Maximizing sensory return
C. Preserving length
D. Maintaining joint function
E. Maintaining cosmetic appearance

Ten percent of all accidents seen in emergency facilities in the United States involve hand and fingertip amputations. The first four choices are primary treatment objectives; cosmetic appearance is of secondary concern.

Answer: **E**
Orenstein, pp. 1-30

30. Match each graft with the appropriate definition.

Graft

1. Autograft
2. Isograft
3. Allograft
4. Xenograft (heterograft)

Definition

A. Graft tissue is transferred from a member of one species to a member of another species
B. Transplant tissue is transferred between two genetically dissimilar members of the same species
C. A graft is transferred between people who are identical in histocompatibility antigens (e.g., identical twins)
D. A graft is taken from a donor site and placed in a different site in the same person

Answers: **1. D; 2. C; 3. B; 4. A**
Rockwood, Green, p. 159
Taber's

31. After skin grafting to a burn wound on the dorsum of the hand, a patient is likely to have some degree of sensory loss. True or False?

A limited number of studies have addressed sensory loss after thermal injury. There has been documentation of permanent sensory deficits in dorsal hand burns involving the dermis layer, regardless of skin grafting. Closure of the wound with skin grafting does not improve sensation. Clinicians should anticipate some degree of permanent impairment of light touch and temperature.

Answer: **True**
Richards, Staley, pp. 540-541

32. How soon after skin grafting can pressure therapy be applied?

A. 1 to 2 weeks
B. 2 to 4 weeks
C. 4 to 6 weeks
D. 6 to 8 weeks

Pressure therapy ranges from interim pressure techniques, including co-wraps, Isotoner gloves, and pressure bandages (Fig. 7-4, *A*) to commercially made custom-fitting pressure garments (Fig. 7-4, *B*). Wounds must be able to tolerate minimal sheering force before pressure therapy can begin at 1 to 2 weeks. The purpose of early pressure is not only to inhibit scar contracture and hypertrophy but also to inhibit vascular and lymphatic pooling and decrease hypersensitivity of the skin. When applying commercially fit gloves, wounds should be no larger than the size of a quarter, with minimal edema and adherent grafts.

Answer: **A**
Richards, Staley, p. 393
Herndon, p. 449
Hunter, Mackin, Callahan, pp.282, 1281, 1282

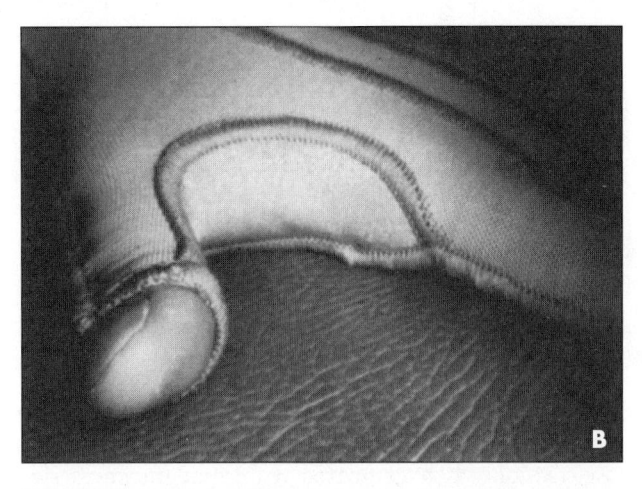

Fig. 7-4, cont'd ■ **B**, Bio-Concepts glove. (From Hunter JM, Mackin EJ, Callahan AD: *Rehabilitation of the hand: surgery and therapy*, ed 4, St. Louis, 1995, Mosby-Year Book.)

CLINICAL GEM:
Although it is possible to apply a commercially fit garment to a burned extremity 1 to 2 weeks after the burn, patients frequently are unable to tolerate these garments until a later date because of skin sensitivity and decreased tolerance to pressure.

33. Which of the following is the optimum capillary pressure for the reduction of hypertrophic scar?

A. 5 mmHg
B. 10 mmHg
C. 25 mmHg
D. 45 mmHg

Many studies currently are examining the amount of pressure needed to alter scar maturation. Studies have shown that the application of compression with pressures greater than 15 mmHg has a positive influence on scars; however, pressures greater than 40 mmHg can macerate a scar. Twenty-five mmHg is thought to be necessary to reduce blood flow to collagenous tissue; this amount of pressure results in a smoother, flatter, and more pliable scar.

Answer: **C**
Richards, Staley, pp. 393-394
Hunter, Mackin, Callahan, p. 1282

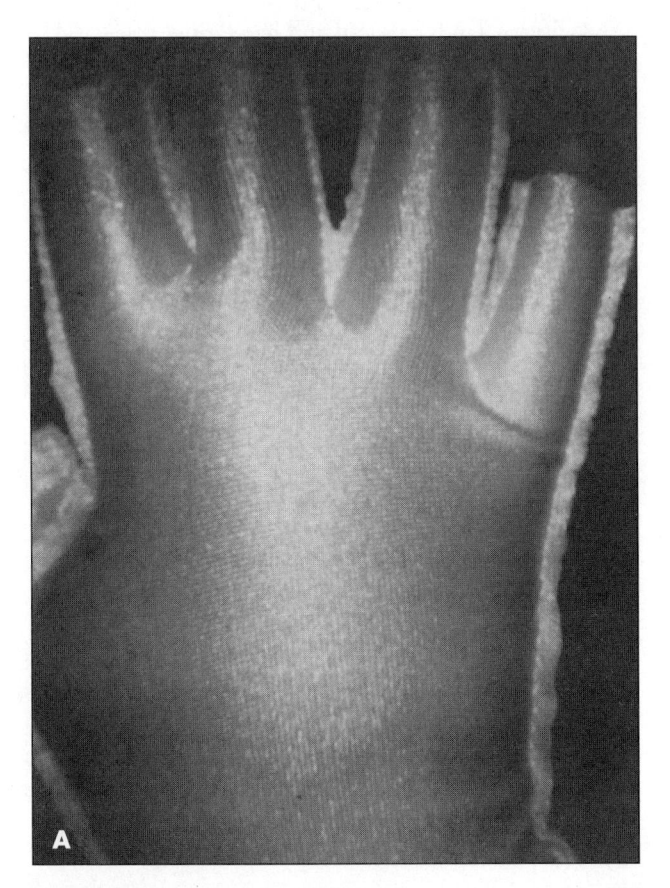

Fig. 7-4 ■ **A**, Interim pressure glove.

Continued

92 CHAPTER 7 Flaps/Grafts/Thermal Conditions

34. What is the optimal wound technique closure for a deep palmar wound?

A. Full-thickness skin graft
B. Meshed split-thickness skin graft
C. Split-thickness skin graft
D. Primary closure

Full-thickness skin grafts (FTSG) (Fig. 7-5) placed on palmar burns are reported to be more durable, with less contraction when compared with split-thickness skin grafts. FTSGs require less therapy and a shorter wearing time of pressure garments.

Answer: **A**
Hunter, Mackin, Callahan, p. 1278
Richards, Staley, p. 195

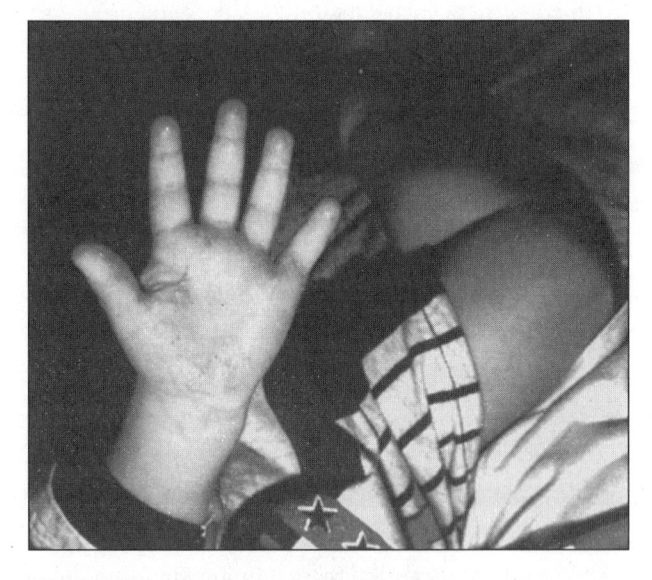

Fig. 7-5 ■ Full-thickness skin graft on the palm of a pediatric patient who was treated for a contact burn. The patient required minimal therapy. (From Hunter JM, Mackin EJ, Callahan AD: *Rehabilitation of the hand: surgery and therapy*, ed 4, St. Louis, 1995, Mosby-Year Book.)

35. Full-thickness skin grafts contract more postoperatively than split-thickness skin grafts. True or False?

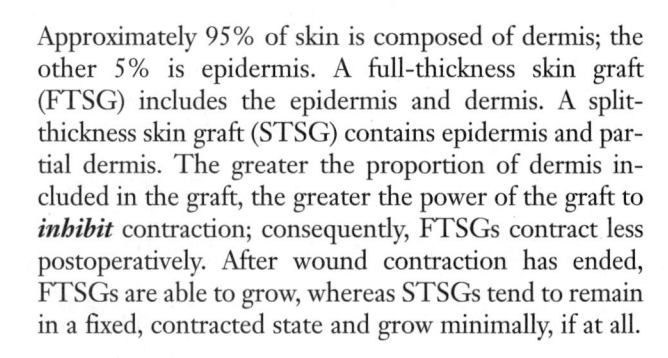

Approximately 95% of skin is composed of dermis; the other 5% is epidermis. A full-thickness skin graft (FTSG) includes the epidermis and dermis. A split-thickness skin graft (STSG) contains epidermis and partial dermis. The greater the proportion of dermis included in the graft, the greater the power of the graft to *inhibit* contraction; consequently, FTSGs contract less postoperatively. After wound contraction has ended, FTSGs are able to grow, whereas STSGs tend to remain in a fixed, contracted state and grow minimally, if at all.

Answer: **False**
Orenstein, pp. 1-30

36. The cross-finger flap is used primarily to cover digital defects. True or False?

Crouier first described the cross-finger flap for fingertip reconstruction in 1951. It brings durable cover to exposed bone, joint, and/or flexor tendons when local advancement flaps do not suffice. Blood supply of the cross-finger flap is random and based upon the subdermal plexus of an adjacent digit. The dorsum of the proximal or middle phalanx of the long finger is the most common source of flap tissue.

Answer: **True**
Smith, Aston, p. 868
Orenstein, pp. 1-30
Refer to Fig. 7-6.

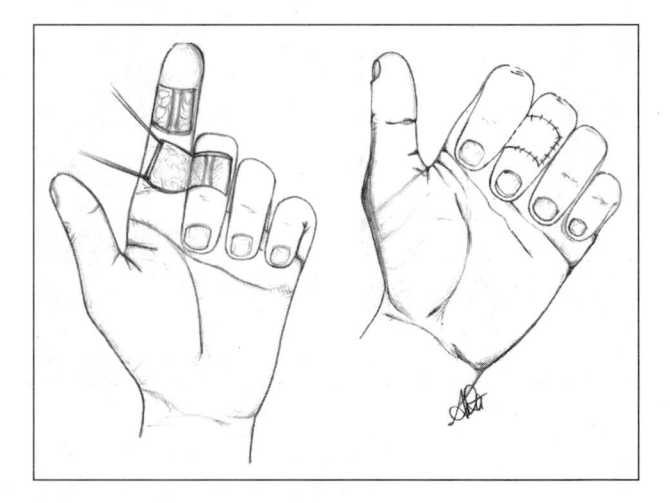

Fig. 7-6

37. Which of the following is an example of a random pattern flap?

A. Groin flap
B. Thoracoabdominal flap
C. Scapular flap
D. Temporoparietal flap

Flaps can be classified into axial and random types, as well as by method of transfer, destination, geometry, and tissue composition. The thoracoabdominal flap is an example of a random pattern flap. Choices A, C, and D are axial-pattern flaps. Axial-pattern flaps are single-pedicle flaps that receive their blood flow from a single, constant vessel, whereas random pattern flaps receive their blood supply from many vessels of the subdermal or subcutaneous plexus.

Answer: **B**
Hodges, pp. 1-30
Green, pp. 1741-1742

38. A 45-year-old woman has loss of skin and subcutaneous tissue of the volar aspect of the distal third of the dominant thumb; the distal phalanx is exposed. Which of the following procedures would be best for soft-tissue coverage of this crush injury?

A. Dressing changes and healing by secondary intention
B. Full-thickness groin skin graft
C. Split-thickness hypothenar skin graft
D. Index cross-finger flap
E. Volar advancement flap

The most appropriate management for this thumb defect is coverage with a double neurovascular thumb volar advancement flap, which was first proposed by Moberg to treat amputations of the thumb that occurred distal to the interphalangeal joint. This volar advancement flap provides stable sensate coverage of the wound, using adjacent tissue that is similar in color and texture. Coverage can be augmented by temporarily flexing the interphalangeal joint, by creating an island flap using V-Y advancement, or by skin grafting of the proximal defect.

Dressing changes and healing by secondary intention are appropriate only for injuries of 1 cm or less. Full-thickness groin skin grafts result in diminished sensory recovery and poor match of color and texture. Split-thickness skin grafts applied directly to exposed bone provide inadequate coverage and little padding. The index cross-finger flap is inappropriate and would unnecessarily traumatize an adjacent digit, further impairing hand function.

Answer: **E**
Yaremchuk, p. 143
Refer to Fig. 7-7.

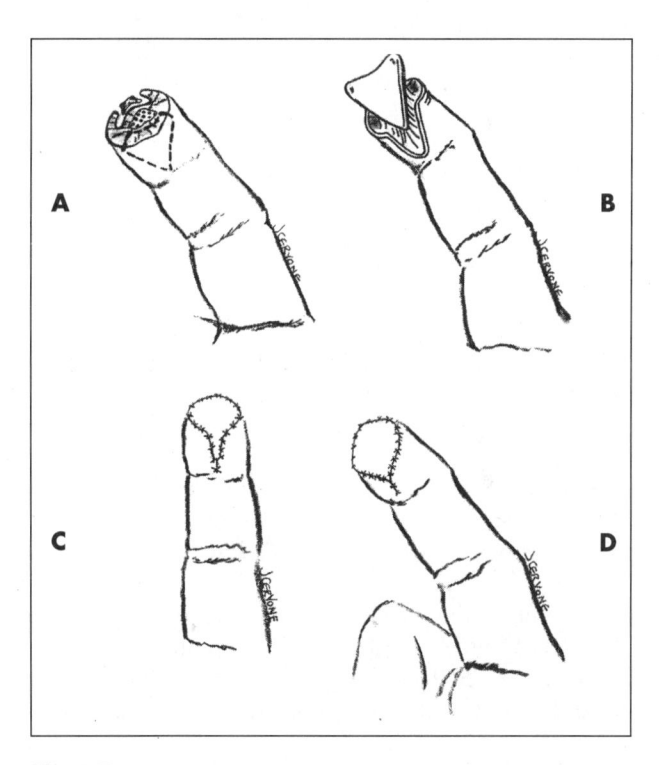

Fig. 7-7 ■ **A**, Plan. **B**, Advancement. **C**, *Inset.* **D**, *Inset;* oblique view.

39. Full-thickness or deep partial-thickness burns of the hand can benefit from early excision and grafting. True or False?

Most authors advocate early excision and grafting after the extent of a burn is known. This reduces edema formation and permits early joint motion. The hand should be splinted with the metacarpophalangeal joints flexed and the interphalangeal joints extended. The use of STSGs or FTSGs helps to minimize joint contracture. Early aggressive occupational therapy can help obtain optimal function.

Answer: **True**
Smith, Aston, pp. 857-887
Orenstein, pp. 1-30

40. All of the following are true statements about thenar flaps, except:

A. They are most commonly used for coverage of the distal phalanx of the index or long finger.
B. A proximal interphalangeal joint flexion contracture can occur as a result of flap design and positioning.
C. A thick flap is raised in the subcutaneous tissue plane near the volar metacarpophalangeal crease.
D. This flap can be surgically performed in a single stage.

Choices A, B, and C are correct. This flap can be proximally, distally, or laterally based, overlying the metacarpophalangeal joint crease. The flap is inset and the finger is protected with a splint. The pedicle is transected during the second surgical stage, usually 14 days after insetting. A proximal interphalangeal joint contracture can occur, especially in older individuals. Some surgeons use this flap only in younger patients.

Answer: **D**
Smith, Aston, pp. 870-873

41. The radial forearm flap can be used for coverage of major dorsal tissue losses of the hand. True or False?

The radial forearm flap is a fasciocutaneous flap based on the radial artery and its nerve and located in the lateral intermuscular septum. The radial artery supplies blood to most of the skin of the forearm. The radial forearm flap may be raised as a distally based island axial flap (Fig. 7-8, *A*) or as a free neurovascular transfer. This flap may be used for complex tissue losses where there is exposed tendon, bone, or joints. The flap is inset (Fig. 7-8, *B*) and the donor site is closed with a skin graft in a one-stage procedure. A bone segment from the radius also can be incorporated when bone is needed for reconstruction.

Answer: **True**
Smith, Aston, pp. 870-880

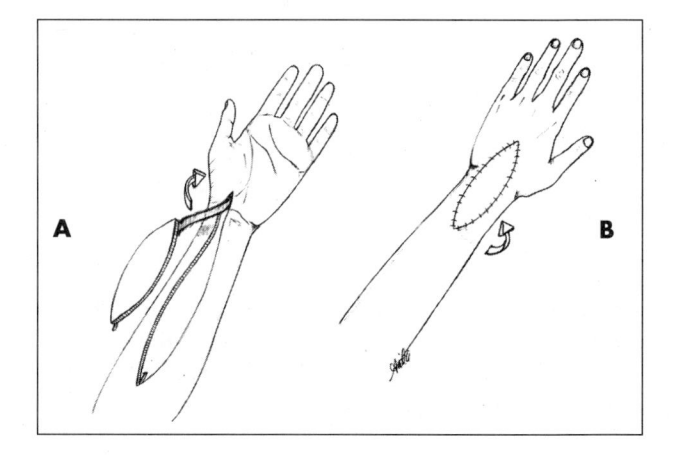

Fig. 7-8

42. The temporoparietal fascia free flap is ideally suited for coverage of hand defects requiring soft-tissue bulk. True or False?

This flap is obtained from the temporoparietal area of the skull, which is located between the subcutaneous tissues and the temporalis muscle fascia. The superficial temporal artery and vein provide the blood supply. The flap is thin and vascular and is an excellent means of palmar reconstruction. The donor scar usually is well hidden. Maximum dimensions of the flap usually do not exceed 13 cm by 9 cm. This flap is used as a free flap transfer and usually is skin-grafted after insetting; it is not appropriate for defects requiring significant tissue bulk.

Answer: **False**
Smith, Aston, pp. 875-883

43. All of the following are true about the groin flap, except:

A. It is an axial-pattern flap based on the superficial circumflex iliac artery.
B. It may be used as a pedicle flap or a free neurovascular transfer.
C. The most common associated complication is infection.
D. It may be used for coverage of complex open wounds of the hand and wrist.

Infection is not the most common complication associated with the groin flap. A primary concern is if the groin flap will "take." Answers A, B, and D are true statements about the groin flap.

The groin flap may be used as a free neurovascular transfer; however, the variable arterial and venous anatomy may limit its use. Other more commonly used free flaps for hand coverage are the radial forearm flap, the lateral arm flap, and the temporoparietal fascia flap. Each of these can provide thin, supple, well-vascularized coverage of difficult wounds.

Answer: **C**
Smith, Aston, pp. 875-878

Chapter 8

Wounds/Infection

Topics to be reviewed in random order are:

- **Stages of wound healing**
- **Key wound healing terms**
- **Wound classifications**
- **Common hand infections**
- **Antibiotic indications**
- **Wound dressings**
- **Therapeutic management of wounds and infections**
- **Fasciotomy**
- **Replantation**
- **Compartment syndrome**

1. **All of the following are terms used for the inflammatory stage of wound healing, except:**

A. Exudative
B. Proliferative
C. Lag
D. Substrate

Exudative, lag, substrate, and inflammatory are all terms for the first stage of wound healing; proliferative, fibroblastic, and reparative are all names for the second stage of wound healing. The first stage of wound healing is a complex arena of cellular activity; this stage begins with injury and usually lasts 3 to 5 days. Stage two lasts until day 21 and is termed proliferative with respect to collagen deposition and connective tissue. An infected wound cannot progress to stage two of wound healing. Stage three (the remodeling stage) generally begins around day 21 and may last for 24 months. This stage focuses on contraction and collagen degradation. It is important to understand that the three stages of wound healing overlap and are influenced by many variables. These variables include, but are not limited to, diet, age, infection, and other medical conditions. All of these factors can alter wound healing time frames.

Answer: **B**
Hunter, Mackin, Callahan, p. 228
McCulloch, Kloth, Feedar, p. 3
Refer to Fig. 8-1.

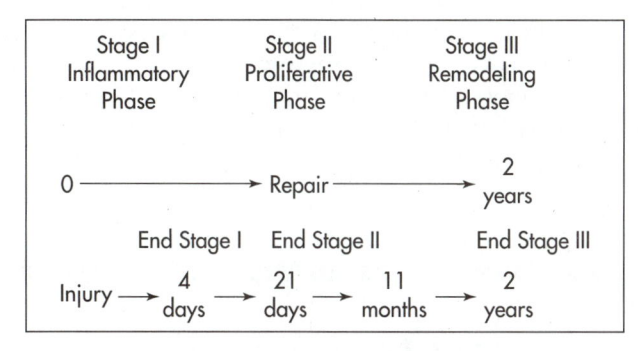

Fig. 8-1 ■ Time frame of wound healing stages.

2. **The inflammatory stage in an untidy wound is completed in how many days?**

A. 2 days
B. 5 days

C. 10 days
D. The length of this stage is indefinite.

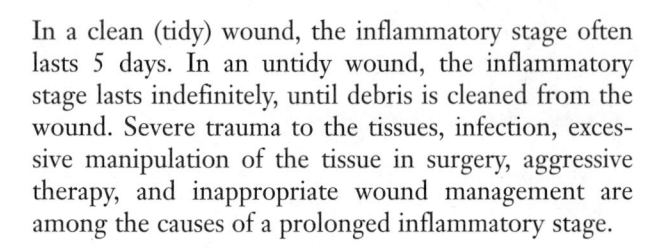

In a clean (tidy) wound, the inflammatory stage often lasts 5 days. In an untidy wound, the inflammatory stage lasts indefinitely, until debris is cleaned from the wound. Severe trauma to the tissues, infection, excessive manipulation of the tissue in surgery, aggressive therapy, and inappropriate wound management are among the causes of a prolonged inflammatory stage.

Answer: **D**
Hunter, Mackin, Callahan, pp. 237-238

3. Match each term with the correct definition:

Term

1. Collagen
2. Chemotaxis
3. Dehiscence
4. Exudate
5. Ground substance

Definition

A. Accumulation of a fluid in a cavity, matter that penetrates through vessel walls into adjoining tissue, or the production of pus or serum
B. A fibrous, insoluble protein found in connective tissues that represents about 30% of total body protein
C. The bursting open of a wound
D. The fluid, semifluid, or solid material that occupies the intercellular space in fibrous connective tissue, cartilage, or bone
E. The movement of additional white blood cells to an area of inflammation in response to the release of chemical mediators by neutrophils, monocytes, and injured tissue

Answers: **1. B; 2. E; 3. C; 4. A; 5. D**
Taber's

4. Most open wounds of the hand require antibiotics. True or False?

Most open wounds do not require antibiotics. Antibiotics should be reserved for wounds in which there is a high risk for infection, such as bite wounds, penetrating wounds, crush injury wounds, highly contaminated wounds, and wounds that have a delay of a few hours before débridement occurs. Because of the widespread use of antibiotics in the past, many bacteria populations currently are now able to resist the medicine; therefore, it is recommended that antimicrobial therapy be delayed until laboratory results are known. One alternative treatment for infection is the use of a hyperbaric chamber.

Answer: **False**
Green, p. 1545
McCulloch, Kloth, Feedar, p. 81

5. An open crush injury is classified as which type of wound?

A. Tidy wound
B. Untidy wound
C. High-level wound
D. Low-level wound

A tidy wound is defined as a clean laceration with minimal tissue injury and contamination; examples include surgical incisions, flaps, and grafts. An untidy wound has a significant amount of soft-tissue injury with a high degree of contamination and an unknown amount of deeper structure viability. Delayed primary closure or secondary wound healing is used for untidy wounds because of the higher degree of contamination associated with them. Answers C and D are incorrect because these categories do not exist.

Answer: **B**
Clark et al, pp. 1-3

6. Collagen synthesis usually begins between 3 and 5 days after an injury. True or False?

Collagen synthesis begins during the second stage of wound healing. This stage typically begins 3 to 5 days after an injury and ends between the fourteenth and twenty-eighth day. Fibroblasts produce collagen molecules that are complex helical structures. It is the collagen molecule that provides the strength and rigidity of scar tissue.

Answer: **True**
Ablove, Howell, p. 166

7. Platelets and macrophages release growth factors essential for tissue repair. True or False?

Both platelets and macrophages release growth factors essential for tissue repair. Platelets most likely are the first cells at an injury site. They attempt to form a balance or a hemostatic environment. Platelets release growth factors that contribute to fibrin deposition, fibroplasia, and angiogenesis. Platelets assist in clot formation, which stops bleeding.

Macrophages are essential regulatory cells in the repair process and they release growth factors essential for tissue repair. The macrophage performs phagocytosis of bacteria, dead cells, foreign bodies, and damaged tissue.

Answer: **True**
McCulloch, Kloth, Feedar, pp. 10, 17-18

8. Match each wound definition with the correct classification. Each classification is used twice.

Definition/Term

1. Serosanguinous drainage
2. Necrotic tissue
3. Surgical débridement
4. Thick, creamy exudate
5. Macrophages attempting to clean exudate
6. Wound may appear clean or pink to bright red, or may be composed of dark red granulation tissue

Classification

A. Red wound
B. Yellow wound
C. Black wound

Answers: **1. A; 2. C; 3. C; 4. B; 5. B; 6. A**
Crossland, ASHT Course
Hunter, Mackin, Callahan, pp. 222-225

9. The maximal strength of healed skin is which percentage of the strength of normal tissue?

A. 30%
B. 50%
C. 75%
D. 100%

At week 3, a normal sutured wound has less than 15% to 25% of its normal strength. Reorganized collagen reaches a maximal strength of 70% to 80% of original tissue.

Answer: **C**
Ablove, Howell, p. 166

10. A keloid is classically thought of as a raised scar within the boundaries of the original wound. True or False?

A keloid scar results from excessive collagen deposition during the healing process. This imbalance occurs when collagen synthesis (production) exceeds collagen lysis (breakdown). Keloids are more common in areas of increased skin tension (e.g., trunk, shoulders, and earlobes). Keloids migrate beyond the boundaries of the wound, whereas hypertrophic scars stay within those boundaries. However, this definition, which distinguishes the keloid from the hypertrophic scar, is not accepted by all authors. Some authors suggest that the only difference between the two is that the keloid is an extreme variant of a hypertrophic scar.

Answer: **False**
McCulloch, Kloth, Feedar, p. 27
Richards, Staley pp. 381-382
Herndon, pp. 388-389

11. Which level of organism is indicative of sepsis?

A. 10 organisms per gram of tissue
B. 10^2 organisms per gram of tissue
C. 10^3 organisms per gram of tissue
D. 10^7 organisms per gram of tissue

Wound sepsis (infection) is determined by bacterial contamination **exceeding** 10^5 organisms per gram of

100 CHAPTER 8 Wounds/Infection

tissue. This level can be determined only by tissue biopsy. It is estimated that 10^3 organisms per gram of tissue normally is present in skin. The U.S. Institute of Surgical Research recommends that wounds with greater than 10^5 organisms per gram of tissue heal by secondary intention to reduce bacterial count.

Answer: **D**
Green, pp. 1545, 1713
McCulloch, Kloth, Feedar, pp. 114, 126

12. Cellulitis involving the fold of soft tissue around the fingernail is which type of infection?

A. Felon
B. Collar button infection
C. Lymphangitis
D. Paronychia

A paronychia (Fig. 8-2) occurs after the introduction of staph (staphylococcus) into a hangnail. This may occur to one side of the nail or it may surround the nail plate. It is the most common infection that occurs in the hand. In the early phase, it can be treated successfully with warm saline soaks, oral antibiotics, and rest. Surgical drainage is indicated for a more extensive lesion. After surgery, the packing is removed at 48 to 72 hours and warm saline soaks are initiated. These are discontinued when the inflammatory reaction ceases.

A felon is a suppurative abscess on the fat pad of the finger that often decompresses spontaneously. Surgical drainage is indicated if a felon is present for more than 48 hours. A collar button infection occurs in the web space through a fissure (break) in the skin and is treated with surgical drainage. Lymphangitis is a serious and rapidly progressing infection that is characterized by fine, red streaks extending from the infection site to the groin or axilla along the pathways of the lymphatics. Fever, chills, myalgia (pain in muscles), and headaches often are reported and prompt medical attention is necessary.

Answer: **D**
Green, pp. 1022-1023
Mosby dictionary
Kasdan, p. 463

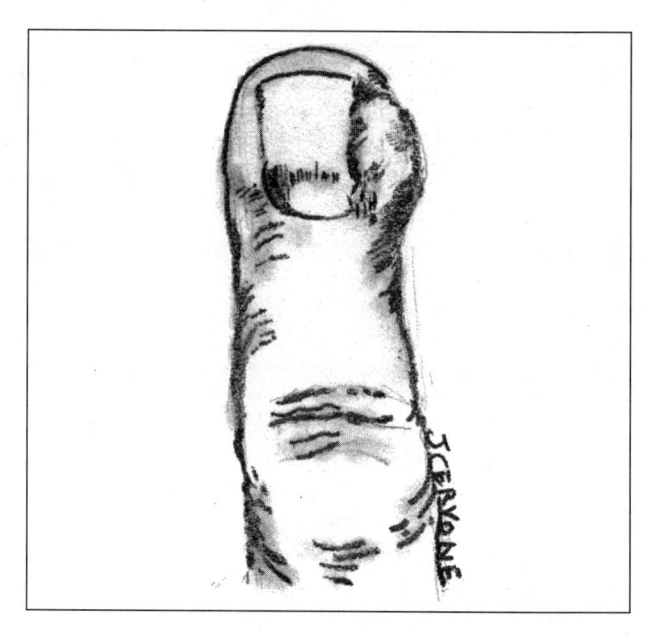

Fig. 8-2

13. Pus always is a sign of infection. True or False?

Pus is not necessarily an indication of active infection. During stage one of wound healing, a complex orchestra of vascular and cellular activities occurs. A neutrophil is a leukocyte that is classified as a polymorphonuclear granulocyte. Neutrophils migrate into a wound through chemotactic attraction immediately after an injury. The survival of neutrophils is short-lived (from 6 hours to several days). Neutrophils are present when a wound is contaminated. Simply put, pus is a large amount of dead, engorged neutrophils at the wound site. If lab results are negative for sepsis, the pus is referred to as "sterile pus;" therefore, pus is not a cardinal sign of infection.

Answer: **False**
McCulloch, Kloth, Feedar, pp. 6-9

14. High-pressure injection injuries may result in amputation. True or False?

High-pressure injection injuries usually are innocuous in appearance; however, these can be devastating injuries that may result in amputation and disfigurement.

These injuries occur when paint, grease, or diesel fuel is accidentally injected into a worker during use of airless spray or grease guns. These injuries may be invasive and require prompt medical attention for optimal results. A visual assessment cannot determine the level of injury; surgical exploration and débridement are necessary.

Answer: **True**
Kasdan, p. 465

15. Which of the following is contraindicated with infection?

A. Antimicrobial therapy
B. Retrograde massage
C. Immobilization
D. Heat

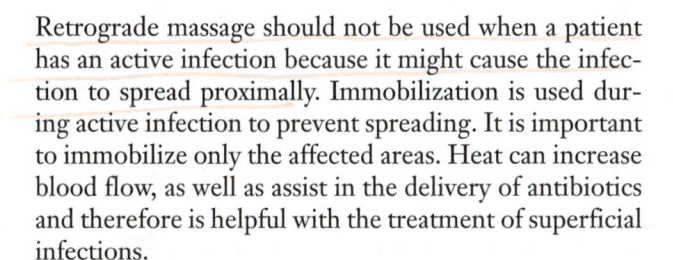

Retrograde massage should not be used when a patient has an active infection because it might cause the infection to spread proximally. Immobilization is used during active infection to prevent spreading. It is important to immobilize only the affected areas. Heat can increase blood flow, as well as assist in the delivery of antibiotics and therefore is helpful with the treatment of superficial infections.

Answer: **B**
Hunter, Mackin, Callahan, p 252

16. Which animal bite is most common?

A. Dog
B. Cat
C. Bird
D. Potbelly pig

Most animal bites are inflicted by dogs. However, bites from cats are associated with more complications.

Answer: **A**
Hunter, Mackin, Callahan, p. 256

17. Your patient, who is a fisherman, presents with an obvious hand infection. Which organism might be present?

A. *Pasteurella multocida*
B. *E. coli*
C. *Neisseria gonorrhoeae*
D. *Mycobacterium marinum*

Mycobacterium marinum is a species of mycobacteria that is found in warm water environments. A person with an open wound may be exposed while working in water or while swimming at the beach or in a lake, river, or pool.

Answer: **D**
Green, p. 1036

18. What is one of the four cardinal signs of Kanavel?

A. Extreme tenderness over the proximal interphalangeal joint
B. Severe pain on attempted passive extension of a digit
C. Isolated swelling at the proximal interphalangeal joint
D. Involved digit postures in full extension

Tenosynovitis of the tendon sheath can be identified by the four cardinal signs of Kanavel, which are: (1) uniform swelling of the digit; (2) digit held in a flexed posture; (3) tenderness over the affected tendon sheath; and (4) severe pain with passive extension/hyperextension of the digit. Flexor tenosynovitis is a serious infection that requires immediate medical attention. The treatment most commonly includes surgical decompression and drainage, along with intravenous antibiotics.

Answer: **B**
Kasdan, p. 467
Refer to Fig. 8-3.

CHAPTER 8 Wounds/Infection

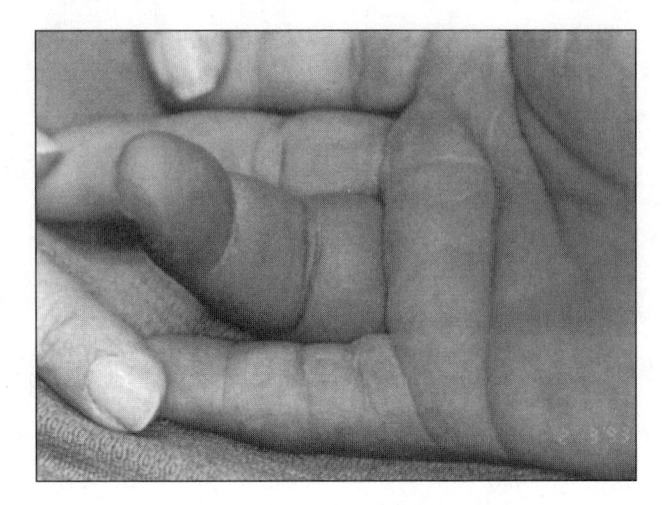

Fig. 8-3 ■ From Hunter JM, Mackin EJ, Callahan AD: *Rehabilitation of the hand: surgery and therapy*, ed 4, St. Louis, 1995, Mosby-Year Book.

19. Which of the following is most compatible with wound healing?

A. Saline
B. Hydrogen peroxide (H_2O_2)
C. Povidone-iodine
D. Chlorhexidine gluconate (Hibiclens)

Of the above answers, saline is the most compatible with wound healing. The only solution that should be placed in a wound is one that can safely be poured into the eye. Many wound specialists condemn the use of antiseptics. Studies have shown that all antiseptic agents are cytotoxic. Hydrogen peroxide has minimal bacterial effect and is often misused along with povidone-iodine and Hibiclens. Some wound therapists currently believe that the pH of saline is too acidic for wounds and recommend lactated Ringer's solution because it is more compatible with the wound environment.

Answer: **A**
Hunter, Mackin, Callahan, pp. 226-228
McCulloch, Kloth, Feedar, p. 145

20. What is the most common source of replant failure?

A. Arterial insufficiency
B. Venous insufficiency
C. Vasospasm
D. None of the above

Three types of vascular compromise may cause replant failure: vasospasm, arterial insufficiency, and venous insufficiency. Vasospasm can occur from manipulation of the replant, often during dressing changes. Conservative measures are employed to relieve vasospasm; these measures include gentle massage, vasodilators, analgesics, warm compresses, and regional anesthetic blocks to assist in restoring circulation to the part. Arterial insufficiency is noted when the digit remains pale. Re-exploration must be immediate to salvage the failing replant. Venous insufficiency is probably the most common cause of replant failure. Congestion is identified by the dusky hue present in the replant. If no adequate veins are available during surgery, the surgeon may try to achieve venous drainage through other means. The nail bed can be removed and heparin soaks can be applied to maintain a constant ooze from the part while venous channels are reestablished. Leaches also have been used under such conditions and have proved helpful in sustaining "the artery-only replant."

Answer: **B**
Hunter, Mackin, Callahan, p. 1084

21. You have a patient with a mild crush injury from a printing press. A minimal amount of serous drainage is observed from the healthy, granulating tissue. Which dressing would you use?

A. Dry, sterile dressing (DSD)
B. Wet-to-dry dressing
C. Adaptic dressing
D. Coban dressing

Your goal is to promote the healing process. Adaptic dressing, classified as an impregnate, allows reepithelialization and prevents adherence of the secondary dressing. You would not choose a dry, sterile dressing alone because it would interrupt the healing process by disturbing the wound bed when removed. In current practice, wet-to-dry dressing has limited use because of the aggressive nature of débridement, which affects both healthy and unhealthy tissue. A wet-to-dry technique is not recommended for wounds with less than 70% necrotic tissue, for wounds with tendon exposures, when it causes bleeding or pain, or when infection is present.

Answer: **C**
Crossland, ASHT Course
McCulloch, Kloth, Feedar, p. 152

22. A 25-year-old male patient is sent to hand therapy for evaluation and treatment after flexor digitorum superficialis/flexor digitorum profundus repair of the ring finger. The patient has minimal drainage from the wound with 2 mm of exposed tendon. Which dressing would you choose?

A. Coban (Elastic wrap)
B. Tegaderm (Semipermeable film)
C. Kaltostat (Calcium alginate dressing)
D. Kerlix (Dry, sterile dressing)

Exposed tendons **must** be protected to prevent desiccation. The best choice is a semipermeable film (SPF) such as Tegaderm, Op-Site, or Bioclusive. These SPFs help regulate the wound environment by preventing dehydration without maceration. SPFs are contraindicated for infected or moderately heavy exuding wounds. Coban and Kerlix are not appropriate because they would not protect the tendons or keep a moist environment. Kaltostat is used for débridement and for moderate-to-heavy exuding wounds.

Answer: **B**
McCulloch, Kloth, Feedar, p. 163

> **CLINICAL GEM:**
> If leakage, nonadherence, or maceration occurs when using semipermeable film, a possible solution is to use a pouch dressing. This is a type of semipermeable film that has the ability to collect exudate. A therapist also may choose to use a more absorbent dressing or change the wearing schedule to allow for more frequent dressing changes.

23. A 24-year-old, right-hand-dominant mill-worker arrives in the emergency room 3 hours after sustaining blunt trauma to his left forearm. The patient's radiographs are normal. The patient complains of severe, progressive pain in the forearm. Physical examination reveals swelling of the proximal one third of the forearm with pain on deep palpation and pain with passive muscle stretches. The hand is warm and pink. Radial and ulnar pulses are normal. Two-point discrimination is normal over all five digits. Which of the following is the most appropriate next step in management?

A. Immobilization and inpatient observation
B. Gallium scan
C. Immediate fasciotomy
D. Immobilization and outpatient observation
E. Technetium scan

Compartment syndrome is a surgical emergency. Muscle that is ischemic for 4 hours is irreparably damaged. The diagnosis of compartment syndrome is made during clinical examination. Compartment pressures of more than 45 mmHg also are diagnostic, but this test is not necessary when the history, signs, and symptoms are consistent. The hallmark of muscle and nerve ischemia is pain. The pain is persistent, progressive, and unrelieved by immobilization. In this patient, the muscle compartments are swollen; distal pulses and distal perfusion are not affected because the radial and ulnar arteries pass adjacent to and between muscle compartments, not through them. In this case, the appropriate next step in management is emergency decompression through fasciotomy.

Answer: **C**
Green, pp. 670-673

24. You are treating a 75-year-old woman who had an olecranon fracture treated with open reduction internal fixation. The hardware was removed at 2 weeks after surgery because of ulnar nerve complications and the patient was immobilized for an additional 4 weeks. When the cast is removed, a yellow wound measuring 2.5 cm wide, 2.0 cm long, and 1.5 cm deep is noted on the elbow. The wound is infected and has moderate amounts of thick, creamy exudate. Which dressing would you choose?

A. Hydrogel dressing (HDG)
B. Calcium alginate dressing (CAD)
C. Hydrocolloid dressing (HCD)
D. Semipermeable film dressing (SPF)

You must choose a dressing that has absorbing properties and is not contraindicated with infection. A calcium alginate dressing (CAD), such as Sorbsan or Kaltostat, can be used with an infected wound and is highly absorbent. CADs are seaweed derived and when used, the CAD converts, through ion exchange, into a gel providing a moist environment that is essential for wound healing. The disadvantages of CADs are cost and the inability to monitor the wound because one cannot see through the dressing; in addition, a secondary dressing is required—at additional cost. The other choices would not be appropriate for this patient because they are contraindicated for infected wounds.

Answer: **B**
McCulloch, Kloth, Feedar, p. 160
Alverez, Rozint, Wiseman, pp. 35-51

25. A patient presents with a bright red to dark red wound. You notice granulating tissue. Which would be the best treatment for this patient?

A. Whirlpool
B. Wet-to-dry dressing
C. Protect the wound; keep it moist
D. Clean the wound of eschar

A red wound is a healthy, healing wound. Your goal is to protect the fragile, budding, granulating tissue by keeping it moist and protected. A whirlpool is contraindicated because it can disturb granulating tissue; the same is true of a wet-to-dry approach (dead matter or necrosed tissue). Eschar is not present in a healthy, red wound.

Answer: **C**
Crossland, ASHT Course
McCulloch, Kloth, Feedar, pp. 138-143

> **CLINICAL GEM:**
> Remind your patients not to overapply ointments for moist wound healing. Overapplying will cause the surrounding healthy tissue to become macerated.

26. You are treating a patient with an external fixation device. You notice a heavy crusted exudate around the pins. How do you provide pin care?

A. Soap and water
B. Hydrogen peroxide
C. Neosporin
D. Hibiclens

Pin care is a very important aspect of hand therapy that is necessary to prevent infection. Hydrogen peroxide would be the best choice in this example; however, once the wound exhibits new granulation tissue, its use is discontinued or it is diluted because of its cytotoxic effects. Hibiclens, another wound cleaner, also is known to have cytotoxic effects. Neosporin is advocated by some; however, it may seal the area, preventing drainage. Soap and water is not as effective as hydrogen peroxide on a crusted wound.

Answer: **B**
Hunter, Mackin, Callahan, p. 226

27. An emergency room doctor calls a hand surgeon to consult about a patient regarding possible replantation. Which of the following individuals is the least likely candidate for replantation?

A. A 68-year-old retiree with an amputated thumb
B. A 9-year-old child with an amputated index finger through the proximal interphalangeal joint
C. A 22-year-old musician with an amputation of the small finger through the metacarpophalangeal joint
D. A 39-year-old laborer with an amputated index finger through the proximal interphalangeal joint

Replantation requires the ability to reliably repair small vessels using microvascular techniques. The best candidates for replants are patients who have sustained sharp lacerations. The time that has elapsed since injury is critical, especially for more proximal injuries in which the ischemic part contains muscle. Contraindications include multiple levels of injury, avulsions, and a prolonged warm ischemic interval. Acceptance criteria for replantation varies from center to center and among surgeons. Most microsurgeons would question the advisability of a single finger replant except under certain circumstances (e.g., thumbs, or in children or patients with special requirements, such as musicians). In the above example, the 39-year-old laborer would be best served by amputation: time off to work is minimized and the index finger is the most expendable because of the seamless integration of the long finger for tasks involving fine grip. Replanted digits often are stiff and in the way, and can be cold-intolerant and painful for prolonged periods.

Answer: **D**
Green, pp. 1085-1102

> **CLINICAL GEM:**
> The maximal warm ischemic time (when the amputated part is not cooled) is 12 hours for digit replantation and 6 hours for proximal replantation (proximal to the carpus).
> The maximal cold ischemic time is 24 hours for digit replantation and 12 hours for proximal amputation.

Chapter 9

Dupuytren's Disease and Tumors

Topics to be reviewed in random order are:

- Surgical and therapeutic techniques
- Complications
- Lipoma
- Carpometacarpal boss
- Ganglion cyst
- Inclusion cyst
- Enchondromas
- Xanthoma
- Hepatic whitlow
- Myositis ossificans

1. Dupuytren's contracture is a type of tumor. True or False?

Dupuytren's contracture also is known as palmar fibromatosis, which is a type of tumor. The word tumor refers to a swelling or enlargement. Dupuytren's contracture affects 1% to 2% of the population and is the most common form of fibromatosis.

Answer: **True**
Conrad, Enneking, p. 12
Taber's

CLINICAL GEM:
Areas affected by fibromatosis, other than the palm, are: (1) dorsum of the penis (Peyronie's disease); (2) plantar fascia (Ledderhose's disease); and (3) knuckle pad (Garrod's nodes).

2. What is the initial manifestation of Dupuytren's disease?

A. Nodule
B. Cord
C. Band
D. Pain

Dupuytren's disease, which typically affects the palmar fascia, appears to be of genetic origin. It is a progressive disease most often seen in people of northern European descent. It typically occurs during the fifth decade in men and during the sixth decade in women and is more common in men. Dupuytren's disease is casually associated with insulin-dependent diabetes mellitus, epilepsy, and chronic alcoholism. The initial presentation is a firm nodule in the palm near the distal palmar crease.

Answer: **A**
McFarlane, pp. 8-13

3. Elevated uric acid indicates:

A. Compartment syndrome
B. Tendon sheath infection

108 CHAPTER 9 Dupuytren's Disease and Tumors

C. Mycobacterium
D. Gout

Gout is caused by an excessive amount of uric acid in blood, tissues, and urine. The uric acid crystallizes in the joints and acts as an abrasive, causing pain and edema. Approximately 90% of patients with gout are male. Uric acid is a byproduct that is caused by a poor diet and/or stress. Gout is common in the great toe.

Answer: **D**
Balch, Balch, p. 191
Taber's

4. What is the most common benign bone tumor?

A. Tophus
B. Lipoma
C. Carpometacarpal boss
D. Enchondroma

A tophus is a gouty deposit. A lipoma is a tumor composed of benign fat cells or lipid cells. A carpometacarpal boss is a rounded eminence on the surface of a bone, which is most often seen at the second and third carpometacarpal joints. An enchondroma, which is a benign growth of cartilage that arises in the metaphysis of a bone, is the most common benign bone tumor.

Answer: **D**
Hunter, Mackin, Callahan, p. 1017

5. Match each disorder to the appropriate definition:

Disorder

1. Bowler thumb
2. Bowen disease
3. Pyogenic granuloma
4. Ganglia
5. Lipoma
6. Wart

Definition

A. Synovial cyst
B. Most common skin tumor
C. Skin lesion; either benign or malignant
D. Vascular tumor protruding through the skin
E. Benign tumor composed of fat
F. Nerve tumor

Answers: **1. F; 2. C; 3. D; 4. A; 5. E; 6. B**
Hunter, Mackin, Callahan, pp. 1027-1031

6. Surgical intervention is indicated for Dupuytren's disease when there is:

A. Metacarpophalangeal joint contracture of 60° and proximal interphalangeal joint contracture of any degree
B. Metacarpophalangeal joint and proximal interphalangeal joint contracture of 40°
C. Metacarpophalangeal joint contracture of 30° and proximal interphalangeal joint contracture of any degree
D. Metacarpophalangeal joint contracture of 50° and proximal interphalangeal joint contracture of 60°

A 30-degree contracture at the metacarpophalangeal joint is a significant disability that justifies surgery; however, metacarpophalangeal joint contractures are correctable no matter how severe or long-standing. In contrast, the proximal interphalangeal joint contracture is not always correctable, and because it is difficult to maintain extension gains, surgery is advisable as soon as proximal interphalangeal joint contractures begin.

Answer: **C**
Green, p. 567

7. After a Dupuytren's contracture is surgically released at the proximal interphalangeal joint, a splint is worn continuously for _____, except during daily hygiene and exercises:

A. 1 week
B. 3 weeks
C. 6 weeks
D. 12 weeks

A splint is indicated after surgical release of the proximal interphalangeal joint in all instances, regardless of the type of surgical correction. Splinting usually is initiated 2 or 3 days postoperatively. However, a splint is not always required after surgical correction of the metacarpophalangeal joint, especially if it was fully corrected. A skilled therapist must assess the situation and make a clinical judgment in collaboration with the referring physician. Various authors propose a variety of splints, including dorsal-based, volar-based, metacarpophalangeal joint flexed at 30° to 40°, and interphalangeal joint in full extension. Positioning the wrist in the splint to minimize tension on the flexor tendons also has been suggested. Some authors propose early dynamic splinting regimens.

During the first 3 weeks after proximal interphalangeal joint surgery, the splint is worn at all times, except during exercises and hygiene. To maintain extension gains, night splinting is continued for 2 or 3 additional months; however, some authors recommend splinting for 6 months or longer.

Answer: **B**
McFarlane, pp. 8-13
Hunter, Mackin, Callahan, p. 990
Green, p. 589

8. What is the most common origin of the wrist ganglion?

A. Scapholunate ligament
B. Flexor tendons
C. Lunotriquetral ligament
D. Extensor tendons

The dorsal wrist ganglion accounts for 60% to 70% of all hand and wrist ganglions. The most frequent site for this cyst is over the scapholunate (S-L) ligament. The dorsal cyst also may arise between extensor tendons or from other carpal joints but frequently has attachments to the S-L ligament. The S-L ligament must be dissected to prevent recurrences.

Answer: **A**
Green, p. 2159

9. When should wrist range of motion begin after a dorsal wrist ganglion is surgically removed?

A. Immediately
B. In 5 days
C. In 14 days
D. In 21 days

Early motion for the wrist is important, especially for flexion, and is initiated at day 5 when the dressing is debulked. Sutures are removed approximately 14 days after surgery and therapy continues until full range of motion is attained.

Answer: **B**
Green, pp. 2160, 2166

> **CLINICAL GEM:**
> A carpometacarpal boss is an osteoarthritic spur that develops at the base of the second and third metacarpal and often is mistaken for a dorsal wrist ganglion. After a carpal boss is removed, the wrist is immobilized for 2 to 3 weeks to allow for healing and to avoid carpometacarpal stress.

10. Which two fingers does Dupuytren's disease typically affect?

A. Thumb and/or index fingers
B. Index and/or middle fingers
C. Index and/or ring fingers
D. Ring and/or little fingers

In approximately one half of patients with Dupuytren's disease, both hands are affected, with the ring and/or little fingers being the digits most commonly involved.

Answer: **D**
Conrad, Enneking, pp. 12, 14
Taber's
Hunter, Mackin, Callahan, pp. 981-982
Refer to Fig. 9-1.

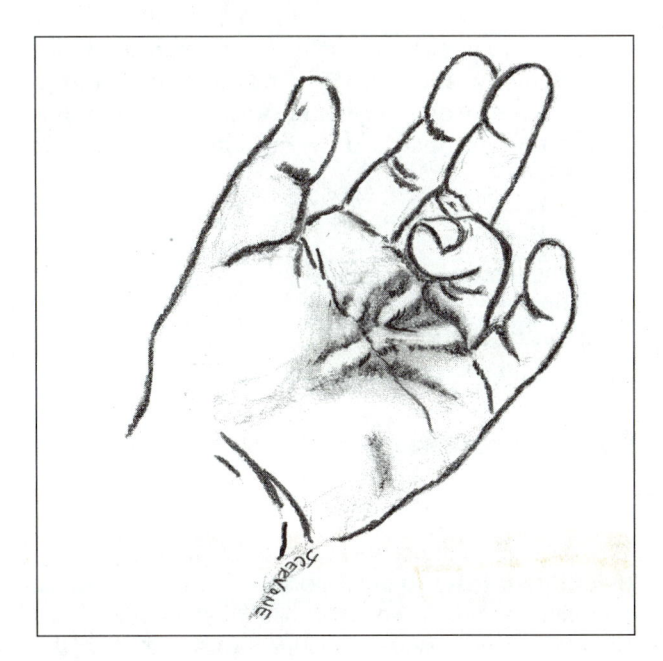

Fig. 9-1

CHAPTER 9 Dupuytren's Disease and Tumors

> **CLINICAL GEM:**
> It is interesting to note that there is a causal link between Dupuytren's disease and trauma to the hand. The disease also is more common among manual laborers.

11. You are treating a patient who has had a dermofasciectomy. When can strengthening exercises begin?

A. Immediately
B. In 2 weeks
C. In 4 weeks
D. In 8 weeks

A dermofasciectomy is a surgical procedure that involves removal of the skin overlying the diseased tissue, as well as the underlying fascia. A full-thickness skin graft (FTSG) is performed for coverage. Typically, strengthening begins 3 to 4 weeks postoperatively for release with primary closures, 4 weeks after skin grafting (dermofasciectomy), and 4 to 6 weeks after open palm technique.

Answer: **C**
Hunter, Mackin, Callahan, pp. 985, 993, 1005

12. A 16-year-old patient presents with a painful soft-tissue swelling in the arm after sustaining a blunt trauma while playing hockey. The patient has a mass that originates in the muscle. The diagnosis might be:

A. Schwannoma
B. Ganglion cyst
C. Fibroma
D. Myositis ossificans

When ossification occurs in a muscle, the term myositis ossificans (MO) is appropriate. This tumor is more prevalent in patients younger than 30 years of age who complain of increasing pain within 3 to 4 weeks after the incident. An erythematous mass develops over the injured area. Surgery is indicated when nerve compression is evident. Treatment involves rest and therapy. Differential diagnoses include malignant tumors. A correct diagnosis is imperative because treatment for a malignant tumor often is radical amputation.

Answer: **D**
Giannakopoulos et al, p. 195
Taber's

13. The most common site for Maffucci's syndrome is in the hand. True or False?

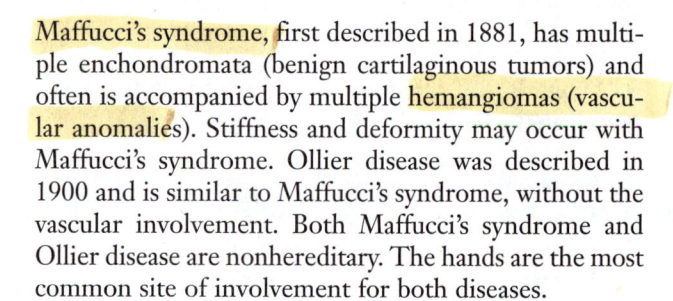

Maffucci's syndrome, first described in 1881, has multiple enchondromata (benign cartilaginous tumors) and often is accompanied by multiple hemangiomas (vascular anomalies). Stiffness and deformity may occur with Maffucci's syndrome. Ollier disease was described in 1900 and is similar to Maffucci's syndrome, without the vascular involvement. Both Maffucci's syndrome and Ollier disease are nonhereditary. The hands are the most common site of involvement for both diseases.

Answer: **True**
Floyd, Troom, p. 127
Hunter, Mackin, Callahan, p. 1433

14. What is the sole source of metacarpophalangeal joint contraction in Dupuytren's disease?

A. Nodule
B. Pretendinous bands
C. Natatory ligament
D. Cords

The most frequently contracted joint in Dupuytren's disease is the metacarpophalangeal joint. With contractures of 30° or more, many patients report a hindrance with daily activities. Metacarpophalangeal joint contracture is caused by the pretendinous bands of the palmar aponeurosis. The cords (spiral/lateral/central) cause proximal interphalangeal joint contractures and the retrovascular cord contributes to contractures at the distal interphalangeal joint. The natatory ligament can cause web-space contractures.

Answer: **B**
Hunter, Mackin, Callahan, p. 983
Refer to Fig. 9-2.

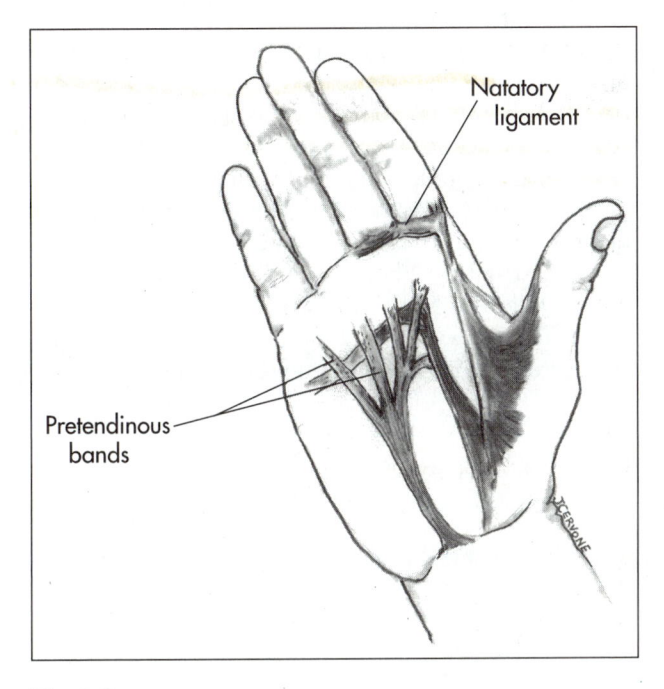

Fig. 9-2

15. A penetrating injury that drives a fragment of epithelium into the subcutaneous tissue can result in a(an):

A. Herpetic whitlow
B. Inclusion cyst
C. Enchondroma
D. Xanthoma

Inclusion cysts are traumatic in origin. These cysts may be present for years and result from a penetrating injury that drives a fragment of epithelium into the subcutaneous tissue. When patients have a decline in function, these cysts are removed. A xanthoma also is known as a giant cell tumor, which is commonly found in the hand. It is a painless, slow-growing tumor that develops in a few months. An enchondroma is the most common primary bone tumor. A herpetic whitlow is a viral infection that frequently is found in dental personnel and usually is treated nonoperatively.

Answer: **B**
Green, pp. 1026, 2225-2227, 2235

16. What is the major advantage of using the McCash open-palm technique for treating Dupuytren's disease?

A. Decreased risk of hematoma
B. Does not require dressing changes
C. Range of motion can be initiated earlier in contrast to primary closure technique
D. Postoperative recovery is accelerated

The open-palm technique for treating Dupuytren's disease is favored by many physicians because of the simplicity and flexibility it allows. The wound closes by secondary intention, it drains well, and skin sloughs are rarely seen; thus, hematomas do not occur. Additional benefits to the patient include decreased pain, decreased edema, and decreased stiffness.

Answer: **A**
Hunter, Mackin, Callahan, p. 996
Green, pp. 563-590
Refer to Fig. 9-3.

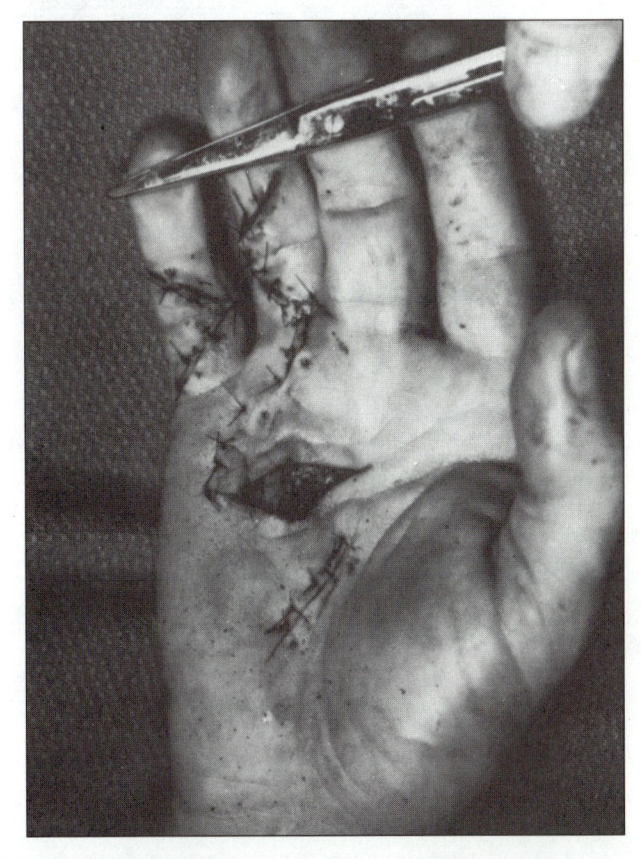

Fig. 9-3 ■ From Hunter JM, Mackin EJ, Callahan AD: *Rehabilitation of the hand: surgery and therapy,* ed 4, St. Louis, 1995, Mosby-Year Book, Inc.

17. What is the most common soft-tissue tumor in children?

A. Ganglion
B. Hemangioma
C. Fibroma
D. Lipoma

Although lipomas and ganglions are common soft-tissue tumors, the hemangioma is more common in children. The lower extremities tend to be more affected than the head, neck, and upper extremities. Hemangiomas are superficial, benign, vascular tumors.

Answer: **B**
Conrad, Enneking, p. 9

18. Reflex sympathetic dystrophy is a serious complication of Dupuytren's disease after surgical release. True or False?

Reflex sympathetic dystrophy is a serious complication of Dupuytren's disease and is best treated if detected early. Cardinal signs of reflex sympathetic dystrophy are severe pain, excessive edema, stiffness, and discoloration. Other signs may include trophic, sudomotor, or vasomotor sympathetic nervous system changes, and fibromatosis. If reflex sympathetic dystrophy is diagnosed, protocol should be modified to focus on resolving the acute reflex sympathetic dystrophy before it becomes chronic; for example, splinting should be modified to reduce tension, or discontinued because aggressive passive range of motion is contraindicated with reflex sympathetic dystrophy. Other complications of Dupuytren's disease following surgical release include wound dehiscence, adhesions, proximal interphalangeal joint flexion contractures, poor flexion, and joint stiffness.

Answer: **True**
Prosser, Conolly, pp. 344-348

Chapter 10
Fractures

Topics to be reviewed in random order are:

- **Anatomy of bones**
- **Primary and secondary healing**
- **Fracture types; complications and therapy**
- **Osteoporosis**
- **Compartment syndrome identification and treatment**
- **Crush injury**
- **Dislocations**
- **Ligamentous injuries**
- **Surgical fixation techniques**

1. **A boxer's fracture is most commonly seen in which digits?**

   A. First and second metacarpals
   B. Second and third metacarpals
   C. Third and fourth metacarpals
   D. Fourth and fifth metacarpals

A metacarpal neck fracture, or boxer's fracture, is most commonly seen in the fourth and fifth metacarpals. This fracture occurs when the clenched fist strikes an object at an oblique angle. The boxer's fracture frequently is treated with a cast or ulnar gutter splint for approximately 3 to 3 1/2 weeks to allow the fracture pain to subside and sufficient healing to occur. Surgical treatment can be performed for cosmetic reasons and to avoid a palmar metacarpal head deformity, which interferes with high-demand grasping activities.

Answer: **D**
Diao, p. 564
Refer to Fig. 10-1.

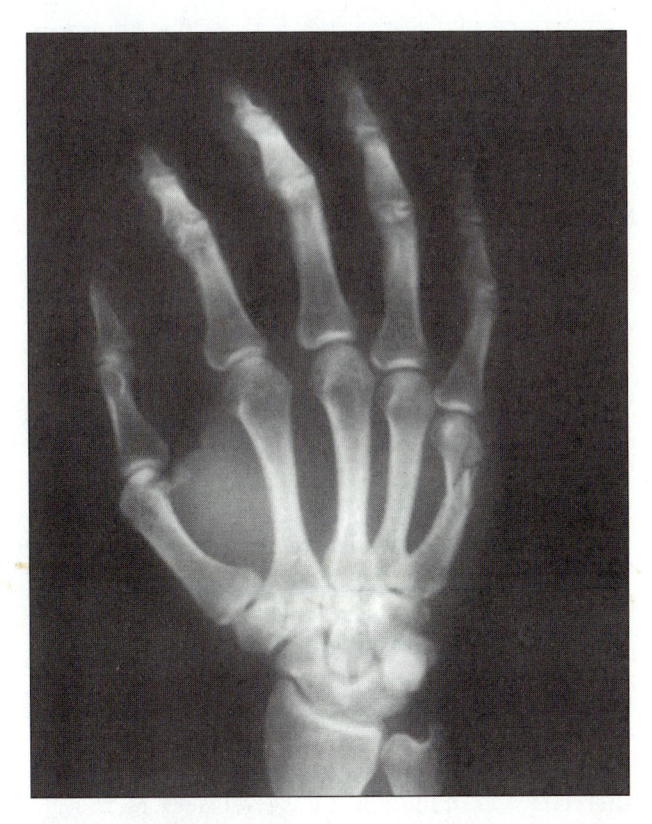

Fig. 10-1 ■ Radiograph of a minimally displaced fracture of the metacarpal neck (boxer's fracture). (From Hunter JM, Mackin EJ, Callahan AD: *Rehabilitation of the hand: surgery and therapy,* ed 4, St. Louis, 1995, Mosby-Year Book.)

2. Stable, internal fixation allows fractures to heal faster. True or False?

Stable, internal fixation allows for a precise restoration of parts, but it does not make fractures heal faster. It does, however, help them heal more precisely; it also allows for primary bone healing. During primary bone healing, direct deposition of bone in the fracture site occurs without the intermediate phase of cartilage formation and without the formation of external callus. The major benefit of stable fixation is that early rehabilitation can be initiated. Stable internal fixation also is a deterrent to the development of a chronically painful, swollen, and stiff hand. Although internal fixation does not necessarily speed fracture healing, it may reduce the time required before the patient can return to productive work or leisure.

Answer: **False**
Freeland, Jabaley, Hughes, p. 28

3. Which joint(s) in the hand, after developing stiffness, causes the most serious functional loss?

A. Distal interphalangeal
B. Proximal interphalangeal
C. Metacarpophalangeal
D. All of the above contribute equally to functional loss

Proximal interphalangeal joint stiffness results in the most serious functional loss. The proximal interphalangeal joint is critical to function and once it is stiffened, its correction is quite difficult. The metacarpophalangeal joint can become stiffened in extension but typically it can be released. The distal interphalangeal joint contributes minimally to the flexion arc; therefore, loss of motion at this level is not as critical.

Answer: **B**
McCollister, p. 1297

4. The stability of a fracture significantly affects the quantity and quality of callus formation. True or False?

The stability of a fracture significantly affects the quantity and quality of callus formation. In general, greater amounts of motion at a fracture site result in a greater amount of callus. It is as if the fracture forms an internal splint. In contrast, very stable fixation with accurate reduction results in very small amounts of callus formation. Immobilization and very stable fixation both have advantages and disadvantages.

Answer: **True**
McCollister, p. 105

5. The cylindrical shaft of a long bone is the:

A. Metaphysis
B. Epiphysis
C. Diaphysis
D. None of the above

The diaphysis is the cylindrical shaft of a bone. The metaphysis is the growing portion of a bone; this is the part between the diaphysis and the epiphysis. The epiphysis is the ossification center at each extreme end of the long bones. When bone growth is complete, the diaphysis is fused with the epiphysis by bony synostosis. Fusion of the epiphysis with the diaphysis occurs approximately 1 to 2 years earlier in females than in males. In general, male bone growth is complete by age 20 and female bone growth is complete by age 18. A radiologist can determine the bone age of a person by studying the ossification center.

Answer: **C**
Taber's
Netter, p. 131
Refer to Fig. 10-2.

hand fractures. The thumb and middle fingers are most commonly involved. Fractures of the distal phalanx often are the result of crushing injuries. Fortunately, fractures of the distal phalanx usually heal without excessive treatment.

Answer: **A**
Hunter, Mackin, Callahan, p. 360

7. **Which of the following is the most serious complication of a proximal phalanx fracture?**

A. Proximal interphalangeal joint extension contracture
B. Metacarpophalangeal joint extension contracture
C. Metacarpophalangeal joint flexion contracture
D. Proximal interphalangeal joint flexion contracture

After a proximal phalanx fracture, development of a fixed proximal interphalangeal joint flexion contracture is the most serious complication because of the associated functional loss. The most effective way to avoid this complication is to splint the proximal interphalangeal joint in full extension to avoid collateral ligament tightness. A dynamic proximal interphalangeal joint extension splint should be initiated at the first sign of flexion deformity. Proximal interphalangeal joint flexion contracture also is a serious complication after middle phalanx fractures.

Answer: **D**
Hunter, Mackin, Callahan, p. 367

8. **Secondary healing occurs in rigidly immobilized fractures. True or False?**

Primary healing occurs in rigidly immobilized fractures and secondary healing occurs when there is motion at the fracture site. When the bone ends are approximated with rigid fixation, primary healing will occur. The callus formed during primary healing is small and therefore mechanically inferior to the callus of a fracture that is allowed to move (not restrained by a fixation device) during healing. When a bone heals secondarily, callus formation is stimulated by motion at the fracture site.

Answer: **False**
Hunter, Mackin, Callahan, pp. 395-396

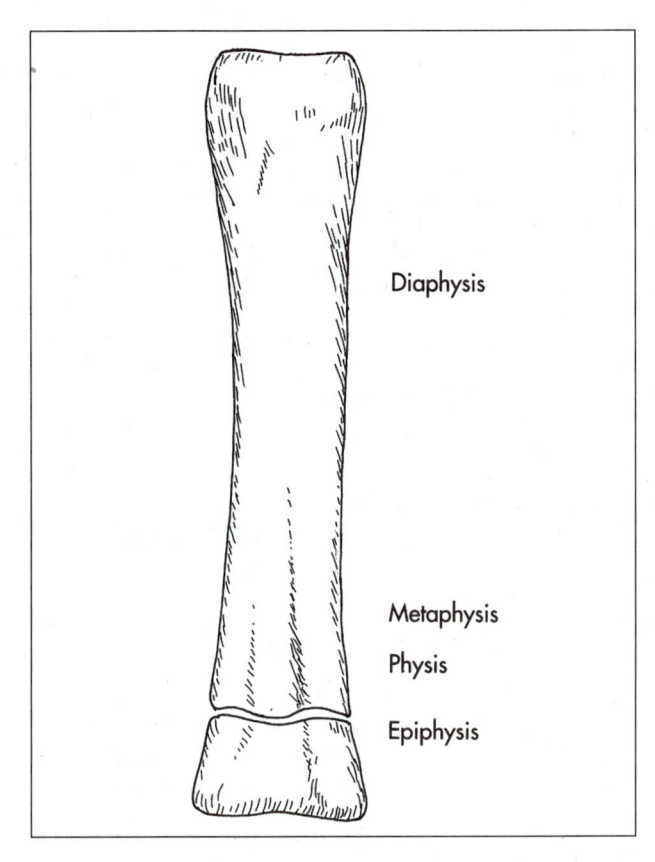

Fig. 10-2 ■ A long bone in a child. (From Hunter JM, Mackin EJ, Callahan AD: *Rehabilitation of the hand: surgery and therapy*, ed 4, St. Louis, 1995, Mosby-Year Book.)

CLINICAL GEM:
The medial epiphysis of the clavicle, which is the last epiphysis of the long bones to appear in the body, develops between the ages of approximately 18 and 20. This epiphysis also is the last to close; closure occurs between the ages of approximately 23 and 25.

6. **Which bone in the hand is most frequently fractured?**

A. Distal phalanx
B. Middle phalanx
C. Proximal phalanx
D. Metacarpal shaft

The most frequently fractured bone in the hand is the distal phalanx, which accounts for 45% to 50% of all

9. What is considered functional flexion for the metacarpophalangeal, proximal interphalangeal, and distal interphalangeal joints, respectively?

   A. 51°, 39°, 32°
   B. 69°, 50°, 21°
   C. 61°, 60°, 39°
   D. 28°, 42°, 30°

Functional flexion averages 61° at the metacarpophalangeal joint level, 60° at the proximal interphalangeal joint level, and 39° at the distal interphalangeal joint level. Functional motion for flexion of the thumb is 21° at the metacarpophalangeal joint level and 18° at the interphalangeal joint level. These measures are based on common activities of daily living. They are not used for addressing individual activities or work skills. They do, however, provide a basic guideline for functional performance of the hand.

Answer: **C**
Hunter, Mackin, Callahan, p. 1185

10. Which of the following distal phalanx fractures is inherently unstable because of the pull of the tendons?

    A. Tuft fracture
    B. Shaft fracture
    C. Base fracture
    D. All the above are inherently unstable

Base fractures usually are unstable because of the pull of the flexor and extensor tendons at the fracture site; they also tend to angulate the fracture with a dorsal apex. Closed fractures usually can be managed with a short Alumafoam splint, which holds the distal phalanx in extension. If the fracture is unstable or open, it is best to treat it with K-wire fixation.

Tuft fractures often are caused by crush injuries and usually are very painful but they are inherently stable. However, if the disruption of the nail and pulp occur with an open fracture, the fracture is likely to be unstable. Shaft fractures usually have minimal displacement and are stable; they also may be either longitudinal or transverse.

Answer: **C**
Hunter, Mackin, Callahan, pp. 361-362
Refer to Fig. 10-3.

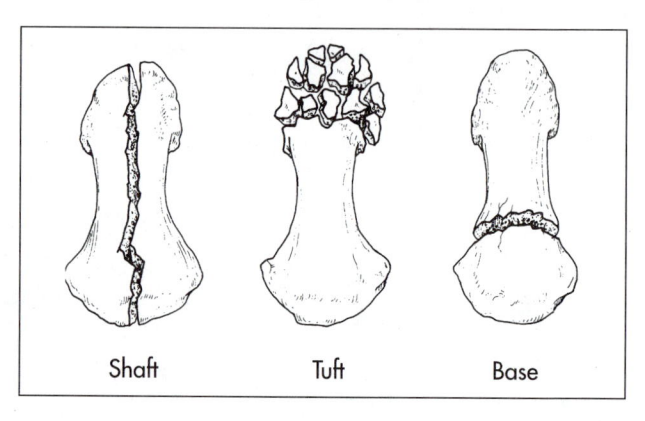

Fig. 10-3 ■ From Hunter JM, Mackin EJ, Callahan AD: *Rehabilitation of the hand: surgery and therapy,* ed 4, St. Louis, 1995, Mosby-Year Book.

11. The term "boxer's fracture" refers to a fracture of the:

    A. Shaft of the proximal phalanx
    B. Shaft of the middle phalanx
    C. Metacarpal neck
    D. Metacarpal base
    E. Distal interphalangeal joint

A boxer's fracture is a fracture involving the metacarpal neck. It usually involves the ring and small fingers and occurs when a clenched metacarpophalangeal joint strikes a solid object. Nonunion almost never occurs but malunion can be a complication. Patients complain of a loss of prominence of the metacarpal head and decreased range of motion and they can palpate the metacarpal head in the palm on occasion. Treatments include closed reduction, closed reduction with percutaneous pin fixation, and/or open reduction (see Fig. 10-1).

Answer: **C**
Green, pp. 698-700

12. A 35-year-old roofer is diagnosed with a boxer's fracture of the fifth metacarpal, with 30° of angulation through the fracture. The patient is anxious to return to work. Which of the following would be the best treatment and splint application?

A. Closed reduction and splint application with the metacarpophalangeal joint flexed at 60° for 3 weeks
B. Closed reduction and splint application with the metacarpophalangeal joint neutral for 3 weeks
C. Application of a static extension splint to the fifth digit with immediate active range of motion
D. Application of a hand-based splint with the metacarpophalangeal joint free for 3 weeks followed by immediate active range of motion

Closed reduction, with either a cast application or use of an ulnar gutter splint positioning the fourth and fifth metacarpophalangeal joints at 60° of flexion, has been a successful treatment of the boxer's fracture of the fifth metacarpal. The splint typically is worn for 3 to 6 weeks. Active range of motion may be initiated as early as 2 weeks. Immediate motion is contraindicated in patients with boxer's fractures because a loss of reduction may occur. However, immediate range of motion may be initiated if the fracture is absolutely stable; as in open reduction internal fixation.

Answer: **A**
Light, Bednar, pp. 303-314
Hunter, Mackin, Callahan, pp. 370-371

13. A patient with osteoporosis has an accelerated loss of bone mass, which leaves the skeleton weakened and more vulnerable to fracture. True or False?

Osteoporosis is insidious in nature. It is a progressive disease that causes an accelerated loss of bone mass, leaving the skeleton weak and vulnerable to fracture. Fractures of the proximal humerus, pelvis, distal radius, and ribs are present in approximately 20 million osteoporotic individuals in the United States. These fractures cause varying degrees of pain, disability, and loss of independence. Impact activities, such as walking, can increase bone mass before age 35 and maintain bone mass after age 35; therefore, it is important to have patients with osteoporosis participate in an exercise program that stresses impact exercise.

Answer: **True**
McCollister, p. 177

14. If the elbow is dislocated in a posterolateral direction, which structure is ruptured in nearly all cases?

A. Distal biceps insertion
B. Triceps tendon
C. Medial collateral ligament
D. Posterior interosseous ligament

A complete disruption of the medial collateral ligament of the elbow is seen in nearly all cases of posterolateral dislocation.

Answer: **C**
Browner et al, p. 1144

15. A Galeazzi fracture is a:

A. Fracture of the distal radial shaft with subluxation/dislocation of the distal radioulnar joint
B. Fracture of the radius and ulna at the same level
C. Fracture of the ulna shaft with disruption of the radiohumeral joint
D. Fracture of the distal ulna with disruption of the distal radioulnar joint

A Galeazzi fracture is a distal radial shaft fracture with subluxation/dislocation of the distal radioulnar joint.

Answer: **A**
Browner et al, p. 1113
Refer to Fig. 10-4.

118   **CHAPTER 10**   Fractures

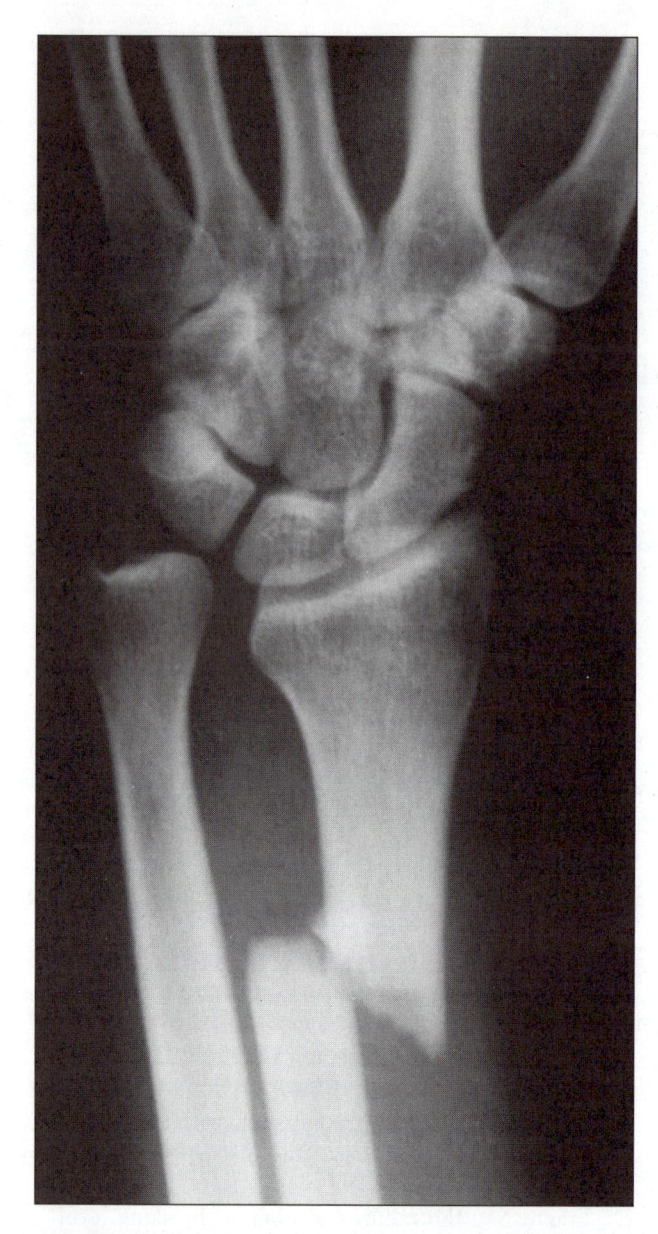

Fig. 10-4 ■ From Cooney WP, Linscheid RL, Dobyns JH: *The wrist: diagnosis and operative treatment*, St. Louis, 1998, Mosby-Year Book.

16. A Monteggia lesion is a:

A. Fracture of the radius and ulna at the same level
B. Fracture of the proximal ulna with dislocation of the radial head
C. Radial head fracture with dislocation
D. Fracture of the distal radius shaft with disruption of the distal radioulnar joint

A Monteggia lesion is a fracture of the proximal ulna with dislocation of the radial head.

Answer: **B**
Browner et al, p. 1117

17. Angulation is more disabling than malrotation with respect to metacarpal shaft fractures. True or False?

Malrotation can be more disabling than angulation because of the tendency for digits to overlap. Some authors have stated that for every degree of malrotation in the metacarpal there are 5° of malrotation at the fingertip.

Answer: **False**
Hunter, Mackin, Callahan, p. 368

> **CLINICAL GEM:**
> When assessing malrotation, examine the patient's nails. If the nail bed is not facing up, malrotation of the digit has occurred.

18. A volar metacarpophalangeal joint capsulectomy is appropriate for all of the following diagnoses, except:

A. Intrinsic muscle contractures
B. Dupuytren's contracture
C. Prolonged immobilization
D. Extension contracture

A capsulectomy is a surgical removal of a capsule; a capsulotomy involves cutting into the capsule. Some authors use these terms interchangeably. **Volar** metacarpophalangeal joint capsulectomies are performed less frequently than dorsal metacarpophalangeal capsulectomies because flexion contractures at the metacarpophalangeal joint level are less common than extensor contractures. Common diagnoses requiring volar capsulectomy include long-standing intrinsic muscle contractures, burns, Volkmann's contracture, Dupuytren's contracture, crush injuries, spasticity, prolonged immobilization, soft-tissue contractures along the volar surface of the metacarpophalangeal joints, and burst injuries to the palm. Postoperative therapy, including edema and pain management, range-of-motion exercises, splinting, and therapeutic modalities, should be initiated within 24 hours after surgery. Splinting of choice is with the metacarpophalangeal joints in full extension for 4 to 6 weeks to maintain gains in surgery. Extension contractures are more common and are treated with **dorsal** metacarpophalangeal joint capsulectomies. Additional common diagnoses requiring dorsal metacarpophalangeal joint capsulectomy are metacarpal fractures, proximal phalanx fractures, crush injuries, nerve palsies, Volkmann's contracture, burns, and Colles' fracture with secondary stiffness (for specific splinting and therapy considerations, see Chapter 15, question 19).

Answer: **D**
Hunter, Mackin, Callahan, pp. 1173, 1174, 1185

19. After a crush injury of the forearm, a patient develops severe forearm pain, exquisite forearm muscle tenderness, and excruciating pain with passive stretching of the fingers and wrist. The most concerning diagnosis is:

A. Compartment syndrome
B. Reflex sympathetic dystrophy (RSD)
C. Tendonitis
D. Fictitious lymphedema

Compartment syndrome after crush injury commonly presents with pain during passive stretch, tenderness over involved muscle, sensory deficits, and weakness. Compartment syndromes can be caused by traumatic insults and crush injuries and can occur after postischemic reperfusion (refill of blood to an area previously lacking blood).

Answer: **A**
Browner et al, pp. 289-298
Hunter, Mackin, Callahan, p. 967

20. The treatment for compartment syndrome is:

A. Pain medication
B. Evaluation of the extremity
C. Sympathetic block
D. Fasciotomy
E. Custom pressure garments

Fasciotomy, on an urgent basis, is indicated for compartment syndrome. Compartment pressure measurement may be beneficial to determine whether release is warranted, but clinical evaluation often provides enough evidence. Normal tissue pressure is between 8 and 10 mmHg. Critical pressures are noted at levels of 30 to 45 mmHg.

Answer: **D**
Browner et al, pp. 285-289, 297-298
Hunter, Mackin, Callahan, p. 967
Refer to Fig. 10-5.

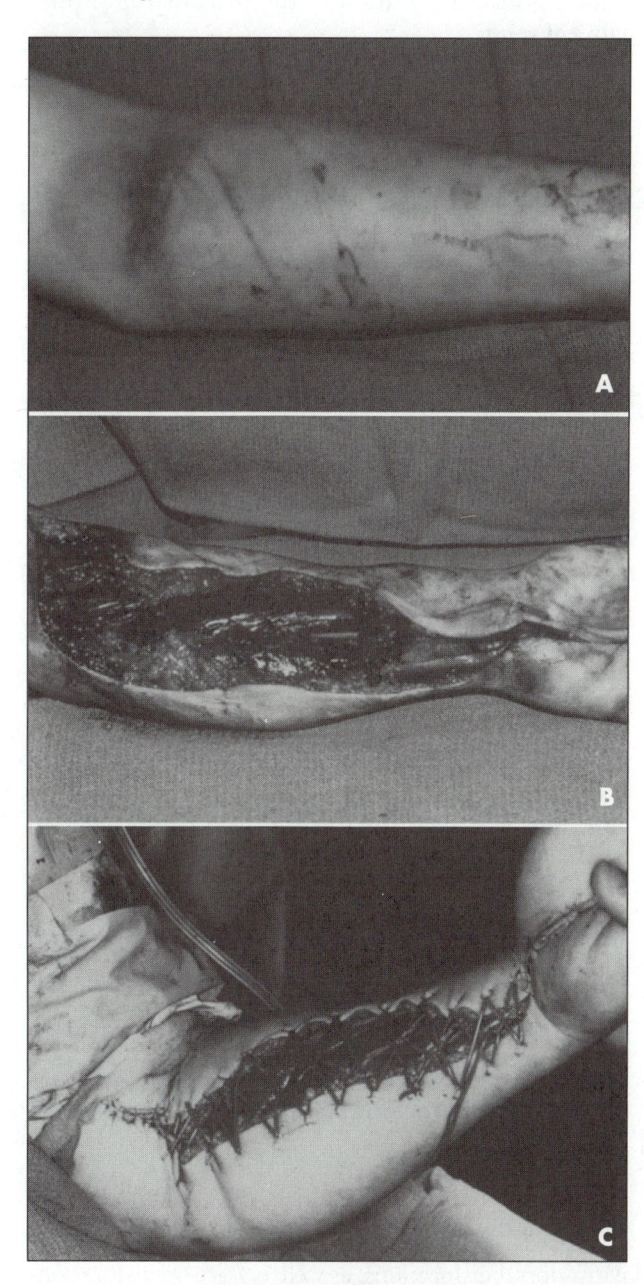

Fig. 10-5 ■ **A,** This young woman developed compartment syndrome after an accident in which her car rolled over and pinned her forearm. **B,** Fasciotomy was performed. **C,** After the swelling receded, the wound was approximated using vessel loops stapled to the skin edges. (From Hunter JM, Mackin EJ, Callahan AD: *Rehabilitation of the hand: surgery and therapy,* ed 4, St. Louis, 1995, Mosby-Year Book.)

120 CHAPTER 10 Fractures

> **CLINICAL GEM:**
> The four "P"s for compartment syndrome include: pain with passive stretch, paresthesias, pallor (pale), and pulselessness.

21. Which structure is most likely to be injured with a dorsal dislocation of the proximal interphalangeal joint?

A. Central slip
B. Volar plate
C. Transverse retinacular ligament
D. Terminal tendon

Dorsal dislocations of the proximal interphalangeal joint usually occur because of hyperextension stress injuries, which result in volar plate damage. These often occur with ball-handling sports. There are three grades of dorsal dislocation injuries (see Chapter 15, question 16 for details).

Answer: **B**
Green, pp. 769-770
Hunter, Mackin, Callahan, p. 383

22. You are treating a patient who is referred to you with a grade two proximal interphalangeal joint dorsal dislocation from a football injury. Orders are to splint, evaluate, and treat. Which splint will you apply to this patient?

A. Dorsal finger splint in 20° to 30° of proximal interphalangeal joint flexion
B. Dorsal finger splint in 50° of proximal interphalangeal joint flexion
C. Dorsal finger splint in 0° of proximal interphalangeal joint flexion
D. No splint. A splint is not indicated for this injury.

Most dorsal dislocations, as well as fracture dislocations of the proximal interphalangeal joint, are treated nonoperatively. For a grade-two injury (Fig. 10-6, *A*), immobilization should be in a dorsal splint (Fig. 10-6, *B*) with 20° to 30° of proximal interphalangeal joint flexion for approximately 7 to 14 days. It is important not to immobilize the proximal interphalangeal joint in too much flexion because this will predispose the joint to the development of a flexion contracture. After immobilization, the finger can be taped to an adjacent finger for additional protection while active exercises are initiated. It is not unusual to have stiffness and swelling for months after this injury.

Grade one can be treated in slight flexion until acute pain subsides. Grade three is treated conservatively as a grade two, unless reduction is not maintained. Surgery is indicated in irreducible dislocations.

Answer: **A**
Green, p. 771
Hunter, Mackin, Callahan, p. 383

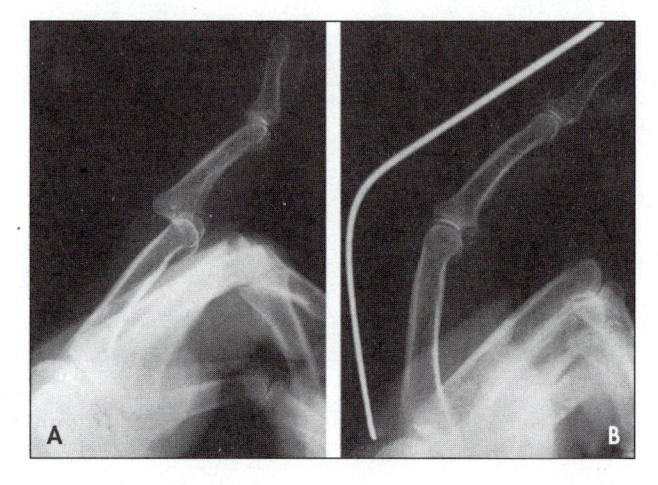

Fig. 10-6, A and B ■ From Hunter JM, Mackin EJ, Callahan AD: *Rehabilitation of the hand: surgery and therapy,* ed 4, St. Louis, 1995, Mosby-Year Book.

23. When a patient sustains a stable midshaft metacarpal fracture, it is important to immobilize the metacarpophalangeal joint and the wrist. True or False?

Not long ago, immobilization of the joint above and below a fracture was required when treating fractures with a closed reduction treatment technique. Currently, we immobilize only the fracture and mobilize the adjacent joints, as well as the musculotendinous units, whenever possible. In this case, mobilization of the metacarpophalangeal joint and the wrist is acceptable while protecting the fracture site. This early motion, in addition to maintaining joint function, helps to prevent adhesions between the fracture callus and adjacent tendons. Early motion is an important aspect of fracture care to prevent fracture disease and obtain optimal results.

Answer: **False**
Freeland, Jabaley, Hughes, p. 12

24. You are treating a patient who is referred to you after a proximal phalanx fracture. The fracture has been fixed internally with mini plates and screws and is considered absolutely stable by the physician. When should range of motion begin?

A. In 24 to 72 hours
B. In 7 to 10 days
C. In 2 weeks
D. In 3 to 4 weeks

For a proximal phalanx fracture that has been internally fixed with **absolute stability**, the patient should be referred to therapy for range of motion within 24 to 72 hours after surgery. Of primary concern for the therapist is managing edema, increasing proximal interphalangeal joint mobility, and avoiding proximal interphalangeal joint flexion contracture. Active and passive range-of-motion exercises are performed regularly. A digital extension splint should be worn in between exercise sessions. If **absolute** fracture stability has not been achieved, active and passive range of motion should not be performed immediately. Absolute fracture stability often is not obtained with open reduction internal fixation. In these cases, range of motion can be initiated as soon as 3 to 7 days if **sufficient** stabilization is obtained; the doctor will give the therapist insight regarding the patient's fracture stability.

Answer: **A**
Hunter, Mackin, Callahan, p. 366

> **CLINICAL GEM:**
> Following is a quick reference chart for range-of-motion initiation after fracture fixation:
>
> | Fracture Fixation | Initiation of Range of Motion |
> |---|---|
> | Absolute stability | 24 to 72 hours |
> | Sufficient stability | 3 to 7 days |
> | Minimal stability | 3 to 6 weeks |

25. Gamekeeper's thumb involves an injury to which structure?

A. Volar plate of the thumb
B. Radial collateral ligament
C. Ulnar collateral ligament
D. None of the above

Injury to the ulnar collateral ligament occurs when the thumb is forced into radial deviation. This injury has been termed "skier's thumb" and "gamekeeper's thumb." If the ulnar collateral ligament is torn completely from the proximal phalanx, it may become situated superficial to the adductor aponeurosis, in which case it would be termed a Stener's lesion. When this occurs, there is no contact between the ligament and its normal insertion and appropriate healing is prevented.

Answer: **C**
Hunter, Mackin, Callahan, pp. 389-390

26. Treatment for a Stener's lesion is:

A. Splinting with the thumb in slight flexion for 2 weeks
B. Continuous immobilization of the thumb for 4 weeks
C. Surgical repair by direct attachment of the ligament
D. All of the above are appropriate treatments

Mild gamekeeper's thumb can be treated with continuous immobilization for 2 weeks. The thumb is placed in slight flexion and care must be taken not to abduct the metacarpophalangeal joint. With moderate gamekeeper's thumb injuries, the patient can be immobilized for 4 weeks in a splint. If a significant fracture is present or if a Stener's lesion is noted, direct ligament repair must be performed. A pin often is placed temporarily across the joint for stabilization until exercises are initiated—approximately 4 to 6 weeks postoperatively.

Answer: **C**
Hunter, Mackin, Callahan, p. 390
Refer to Fig. 10-7.

122 CHAPTER 10 Fractures

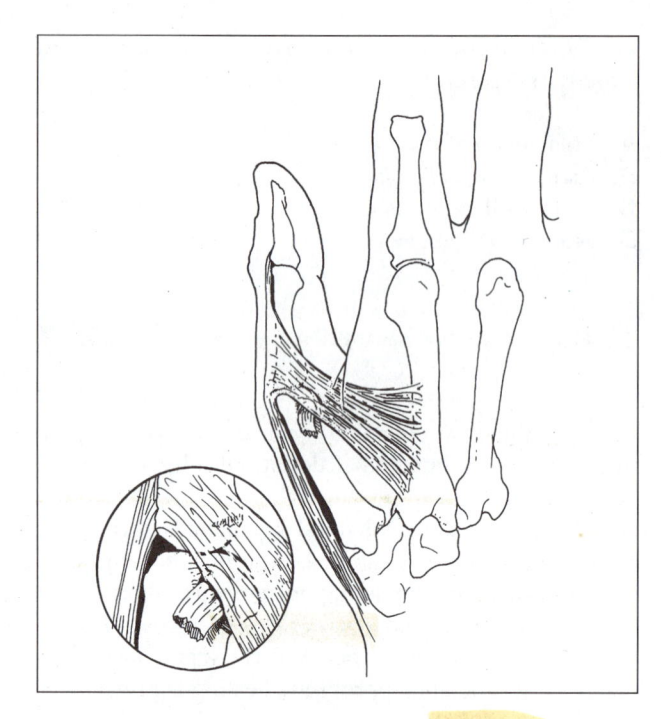

Fig. 10-7 ■ Diagram and enlargement of the Stener's lesion. A hyperabduction force results in complete rupture of the ulnar collateral ligament at its distal insertion, with displacement proximally. The adductor aponeurosis blocks the ligament from returning to its insertion site, thus preventing adequate healing. (From Hunter JM, Mackin EJ, Callahan AD: *Rehabilitation of the hand: surgery and therapy*, ed 4, St. Louis, 1995, Mosby-Year Book.)

CLINICAL GEM:
A tip pinch should be avoided until 8 weeks after gamekeeper's surgery, when progressive resistive exercises are permitted.

27. A _____ thumb fracture occurs through the beak (base) of the metacarpal, with the intact oblique ulnar ligament stabilizing the small fracture fragment. The metacarpal shaft is displaced proximally because of the strong muscle and tendon attached to it.

A. Rolando's
B. Chauffeur's
C. Bennett's
D. None of the above

A Bennett's fracture occurs at the beak (base) of the first metacarpal. The result is a bony failure rather than a ligament disruption. The ulnar oblique ligament remains intact while the metacarpal shaft is displaced by the forces of the abductor pollicis longus, extrinsic thumb extensors, and adductor pollicis. Bennett's fractures can be treated with closed reduction and casting for 4 weeks, closed reduction with percutaneous pinning, or open reduction intenal fixation.

A Rolando's fracture is a comminuted intraarticular fracture at the first metacarpal base. The mechanism of injury is similar to that of a Bennett's fracture. Accurate and anatomic reduction and stable fixation often are not possible because of the many small fragments in this fracture. Treatment options for Rolando's fractures include reduction with cast for 7 to 10 days, followed by early range of motion, skeletal traction, or internal fixation.

Answer: **C**
Hunter, Mackin, Callahan, p. 392
Refer to Fig. 10-8.

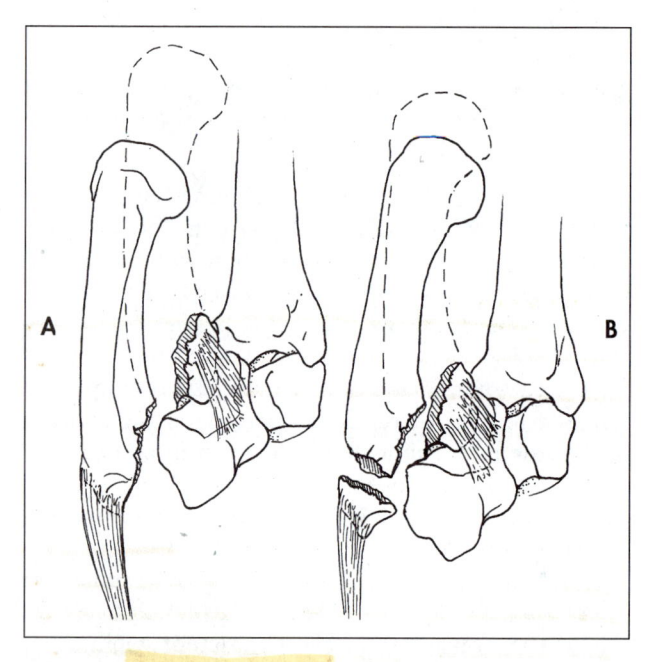

Fig. 10-8 ■ **A,** Bennett's fracture. The fracture occurs through the beak of the metacarpal, with the intact ulnar oblique ligament stabilizing the small fragment. The metacarpal shaft is displaced proximally secondary to the strong muscle and tendon attachments. **B,** Rolando's fracture. This is a T- or Y-shaped intra-articular fracture, frequently with even more comminution than shown here. (From Hunter JM, Mackin EJ, Callahan AD: *Rehabilitation of the hand: surgery and therapy*, ed 4, St. Louis, 1995, Mosby-Year Book.)

28. A reverse Bennett's fracture describes a fracture at the base of the:

A. First metacarpal
B. Second metacarpal
C. Third metacarpal
D. Fourth metacarpal
E. Fifth metacarpal

A fracture dislocation at the base of the fifth metacarpal is analogous to a Bennett's fracture of the thumb and is termed a reversed Bennett's fracture. These fractures tend to be unstable and displace in a manner similar to Bennett's fractures and cause similar functional impairment. The principle dangers of not reducing this fracture dislocation are loss of grip strength and painful arthritis. These fractures often can be managed with closed reduction and percutaneous pinning, but if satisfactory reduction cannot be achieved, open reduction should be performed.

Answer: **E**
Freeland, Jabaley, Hughes, p. 45

29. Which is the least commonly injured carpal bone?

A. Trapezium
B. Pisiform
C. Hamate
D. Trapezoid

The trapezoid (carpal bone) is tightly positioned between the base of the second metacarpal, capitate, scaphoid, and trapezium; therefore, it is the least commonly injured carpal bone; injury of this bone accounts for less than 1% of all carpal injuries. When this bone is injured, it typically is from a high-energy, axially-directed force through the index metacarpal base.

Answer: **D**
Cohen, p. 595
Refer to Fig. 10-9.

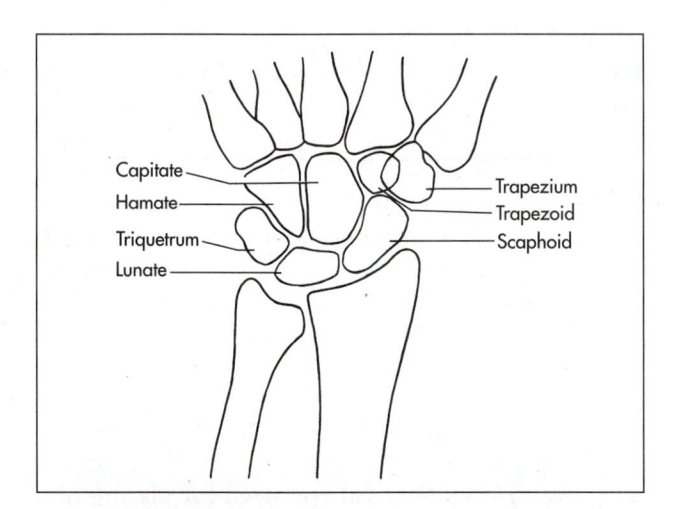

Fig. 10-9 ■ From Hunter JM, Mackin EJ, Callahan AD: *Rehabilitation of the hand: surgery and therapy,* ed 4, St. Louis, 1995, Mosby-Year Book.

30. Which carpal bone fracture is associated with racquet sports?

A. Hamate
B. Capitate
C. Trapezoid
D. Trapezium

The hamate is involved in 2% to 4% of carpal bone fractures. The hook of the hamate protrudes off the hamate into the base of the hypothenar eminence. Hamate hook fractures most commonly occur in people involved in sports using a racquet or clubs (e.g., golf, baseball, racquetball, or tennis). When performing a forceful swing, the base of the club can impinge against the hook of the hamate, causing a fracture. The acute injury often is not recognized and the patient presents late with chronic pain at the base of the hypothenar eminence, weakness of grip, and occasional numbness in the ulnar nerve distribution (see Fig. 10-9).

Answer: **A**
Cohen, p. 591

31. Which of the following is *not* true about Kirschner wires (K-wires)?

A. They are easier to use than mini-fragment plates and screws.
B. They can be placed with minimal soft-tissue dissection.
C. They can be placed percutaneously (through the skin).
D. They provide compression if applied correctly.

Kirschner wires have many advantages when they are used for fracture fixation. They are readily available, easier to use than mini-fragment plates and screws, can be placed with minimal soft-tissue dissection, and can be placed percutaneously. A disadvantage of Kirschner wires is that they do not provide sufficient compression and if applied incorrectly, can actually maintain distraction. They also do not provide rigid internal fixation, which can preclude early motion.

Answer: **D**
Hunter, Mackin, Callahan, p. 357
Refer to Fig. 10-10.

124 CHAPTER 10 Fractures

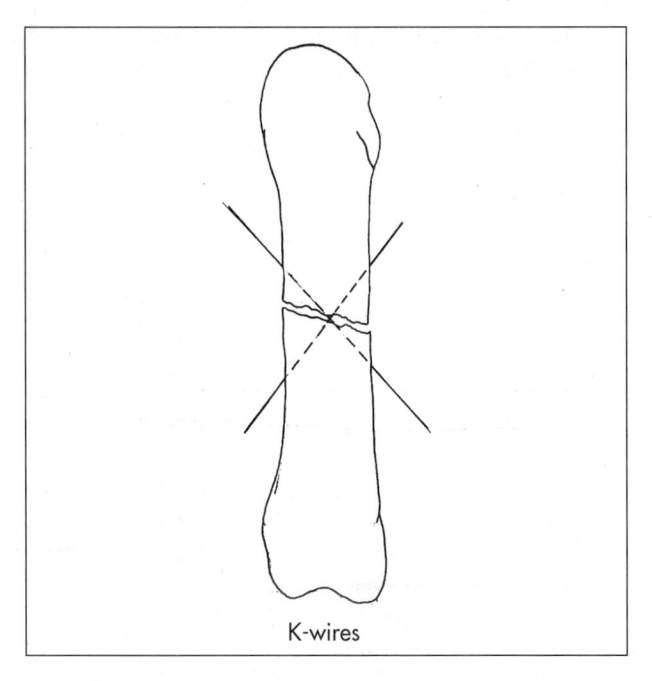

Fig. 10-10 ■ From Hunter JM, Mackin EJ, Callahan AD: *Rehabilitation of the hand: surgery and therapy,* ed 4, St. Louis, 1995, Mosby-Year Book.

32. Match each fracture stabilization technique with its advantages:

Stabilization Technique

1. External fixation
2. Plate and screws
3. Intramedullary device
4. Kirschner pins

Advantages

A. Rigid fixation restores and maintains length
B. Readily available; versatile; easy to insert; requires minimal dissection
C. Preserves length and allows access to bone and soft tissue through percutaneous insertion; direct manipulation of the fracture is avoided
D. No special equipment required; easy to insert; no pins protrude; requires minimal dissection

Answers: **1. C; 2. A; 3. D; 4. B**
Green, p. 705

> **CLINICAL GEM:**
> Disadvantages and therapeutic management of stabilization techniques include:
> • Kirschner pins: lacks rigidity, may loosen, may distract the fracture, causes pin tract infections, and requires external support. Therapist **cannot** begin immediate active range of motion because of lack of absolute stability.
> • Intramedullary device: characterized by rotational instability and rod migration (e.g., rush rod used for humeral fractures). Therapists may begin pendulum exercises within the first week of rush rod fixation.
> • Plate and screws: technically challenging, require special equipment, require extensive exposure, and may require subsequent removal. If absolute stability is obtained, immediate range of motion is initiated; however, if sufficient stability is obtained, active range of motion commences at 3 to 7 days.
> • External fixation: characterized by pin tract infections, osteomyelitis, overdistraction, nonunion, neurovascular injuries, and loosening of the device. Range of motion can be initiated immediately to surrounding joints.

33. After a segmental radius shaft fracture is plated through a volar approach, a patient experiences weakened wrist, finger, and thumb extension. The structure most likely involved is the:

A. Anterior interosseous nerve
B. Radial nerve
C. Posterior interosseous nerve
D. Antebrachial cutaneous nerve

The posterior interosseous nerve, a branch of the radial nerve, enters the forearm through the Arcade of Frohse and the supinator muscle. This nerve is at risk with volar and dorsal surgical approaches to the forearm. Answer B is incorrect because the radial nerve is called the posterior interosseous nerve after it enters the forearm.

Answer: **C**
Hoppenfeld, deBoer, pp. 121, 123, 136

34. After a volar surgical approach for plating of a distal radial shaft fracture, you notice that your patient has no function of the flexor pollicis longus or flexor digitorum profundus to the index and long finger, but sensation is normal. The structure most likely involved is the:

A. Posterior interosseous nerve
B. Median nerve
C. Anterior interosseous nerve
D. Common flexor tendon

The anterior interosseous nerve, a branch of the median nerve, is the motor nerve to the flexor pollicis longus, flexor digitorum profundus of the index and long fingers, and pronator quadratus. This nerve may be damaged during surgical intervention to stabilize distal radius fractures (see Fig. 18-12, question 27).

Answer: **C**
Hoppenfeld, deBoer, p. 124

35. In the adult, displaced both bone forearm shaft fractures are most often treated by:

A. Casting
B. Internal fixation with plates and screws
C. Small intramedullary rods
D. External fixation

Open reduction internal fixation with plates and screws is the standard treatment and gives the best results for displaced fractures of both forearm bones (i.e., radius and ulna fractures).

Answer: **B**
Browner et al, p. 1095

36. Six months after severe both bone forearm shaft fractures are treated with open reduction internal fixation, a patient has total loss of forearm rotation both actively and passively. Bone growth between the two bones is noted on radiograph. This situation is explained by:

A. Plating of the wrong bones
B. Neurological injury to the arm
C. Dislocated distal radioulnar joint
D. Synostosis

Synostosis is a cross union between forearm bones, usually in the middle or proximal forearm. Forearm rotation is absent. Incidence of synostosis is low and its etiology is uncertain, but it may follow severe injury or infection.

Answer: **D**
Browner et al, p. 1121

37. A 35-year-old male carpenter sustains an oblique fracture of the proximal phalanx of his dominant index finger. Methods of fracture fixation commonly employed for this fracture include:

A. Percutaneous transverse pin fixation
B. Cross K-wires
C. Open reduction internal fixation with mini-fragment screws
D. K-wire fixation with supplemental interosseous wiring
E. A, B, and C
F. All of the above

Multiple techniques commonly are employed in the fixation of fractures of phalanges in the hand. All of the above techniques could be used to correct this oblique proximal phalanx fracture. Transverse and short oblique fractures frequently are treated with open reduction internal fixation. The fracture pattern and the surgeon's experience with a given technique may determine the choice of fixation used.

Answer: **F**
McCollister, pp. 350-352

38. A 21-year-old woman sustains a traumatic mallet finger injury with an avulsion fracture involving 10% of the articular surface of the dorsal distal phalanx. Appropriate initial treatment could include:

A. Dorsal extension splinting for 2 months
B. Open reduction internal fixation (ORIF), with a longitudinal K-wire transfixing the joint
C. ORIF, with indirect K-wire fixation of the fragment involving the distal phalanx

D. Dynamic traction splinting combining early active flexion and extension of the distal interphalangeal joint
E. A, B, and C
F. All of the above

Treatment of a mallet finger with a bony fragment often is managed with a standard mallet program, using a dorsal extension splint for 6 to 8 weeks and allowing proximal interphalangeal joint range of motion. If the fragment is large or substantially displaced, internal fixation often is necessary, by either a direct or indirect technique. Postsurgically, the distal interphalangeal joint is immobilized for 6 weeks and active range of motion is initiated when the pin is removed. Night splinting is continued for 2 to 4 weeks or pending reoccurrence of the extensor lag. Answer D, dynamic traction splinting allowing early flexion and extension, would not promote healing of the dorsal fragment to the distal phalanx and therefore would be contraindicated.

Answer: **E**
Schneider, pp. 267-275
Hunter, Mackin, Callahan, pp. 545-548

39. A 32-year-old hospital employee sustains an intraarticular fracture of the proximal interphalangeal joint with dorsal dislocation of the middle phalanx. Appropriate treatment could include:

A. Extension block splinting
B. Percutaneous pin fixation in the form of a dynamic force couple
C. Volar plate arthroplasty
D. Dynamic traction and early motion
E. A, B, and C
F. All of the above

All of the above choices are appropriate treatment techniques for the case presented. Percutaneous pin fixation and application of dynamic traction and/or a dynamic force couple are common techniques for treatment of intraarticular fractures involving the proximal interphalangeal joint. Extension block splinting frequently is employed in fracture dislocations of the proximal interphalangeal joint when the fragment is small and reduction of the joint can be obtained. In late cases or in cases in which extension block splinting alone cannot maintain the reduction, volar plate arthroplasty may be indicated. Active range of motion and splinting programs vary depending on the stability gained in surgery.

Answer: **F**
Schenck, pp. 187-209, 327-337

40. For a severely comminuted fracture involving the entire base of the proximal phalanx, the appropriate treatment would include:

A. Dynamic traction
B. Application of a dynamic external fixator with early active range of motion
C. Application of a force couple splint
D. A and B only
E. None of the above

In severely comminuted fractures of the base of the middle phalanx, early motion and dynamic traction (see Fig. 10-11, *B*) such as described by Robert Schenck can be employed. Application of an external fixator with dynamic traction also has been used successfully. The use of the force couple splint as described by Agee generally is not suitable for such fractures because it does not achieve distraction.

Answer: **D**
Hastings, Ernest, pp. 659-674

41. A 60-year-old jogger falls in a pothole and sustains a fracture dislocation of the proximal interphalangeal joint. He is treated initially with primary arthrodesis because of concomitant arthritis found at the time of surgery. Four months later, the joint is not fused and remains painful, and the finger is pronated 45°. Appropriate treatment would include:

A. A dorsal splint with the finger taped in the reduced position
B. Arthrodesis with a Herbert-Whipple screw
C. Application of an external fixator with bone graft of the proximal interphalangeal joint
D. Tension band wiring with K-wires
E. Interosseous wiring
F. All of the above

For failed internal fixation with a nonunion of the proximal interphalangeal joint, internal fixation with the techniques described in answers B through E has been performed. Some patients may wish to have the finger splinted for a long period of time (answer A) and wait for arthrodesis, despite what appears to be an initial nonunion.

Answer: **F**
Jones, Stern, pp. 267-275

> **CLINICAL GEM:**
> Research has indicated that the use of a bone growth stimulator may assist with fracture healing.

42. Pilon fractures can be treated safely using dynamic traction. True or False?

A pilon fracture is a comminuted intraarticular fracture of the base of the middle phalanx (Fig 10-11, *A*). It can be treated with open reduction internal fixation (ORIF), external fixation, or dynamic traction (Fig. 10-11, *B*). Schenck has popularized the concept of dynamic traction. Using this method, a K-wire is put through the head of the middle phalanx and traction is applied to the phalanx with rubber-band traction attached to a hoop mount on a forearm splint. The patient regularly performs passive range of motion for both flexion and extension in a specified range. Splinting is continued for 6 to 8 weeks. Studies have shown that the skeletal traction technique can be safer and that it produces results equivalent to those of ORIF.

Answer: **True**
Baratz, Divelbiss, pp. 546-557
Hunter, Mackin, Callahan, p. 384

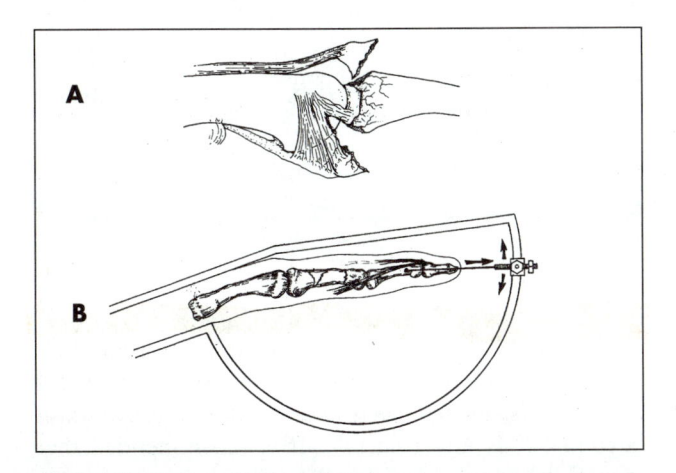

Fig. 10-11 ■ **A**, Pilon fracture. **B**, Dynamic traction. (From Hunter JM, Mackin EJ, Callahan AD: *Rehabilitation of the hand: surgery and therapy,* ed 4, St. Louis, 1995, Mosby-Year Book.)

43. After olecranon osteotomy for repair of a comminuted distal humerus fracture, a patient experiences intermittent paresthesia in her small and ring fingers. The structure likely to be involved is the:

A. Radial nerve in the Arcade of Frohse
B. Ulnar nerve in the cubital tunnel
C. Ulnar nerve in Guyon's canal
D. Ulnar artery

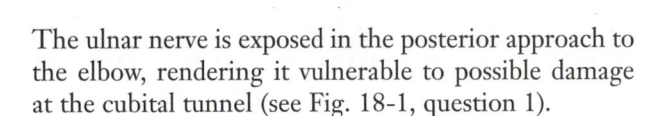

The ulnar nerve is exposed in the posterior approach to the elbow, rendering it vulnerable to possible damage at the cubital tunnel (see Fig. 18-1, question 1).

Answer: **B**
Hoppenfeld, deBoer, p. 80

44. A child is referred to you for therapy after a supracondylar fracture of the humerus. While evaluating the patient you notice that the carrying angle in the injured arm is different from that of the other arm. This child most likely will present with cubitus valgus. True or False?

The carrying angle of the elbow is assessed in the anatomical position. The normal carrying angle measures approximately 5° in males and between 10° to 15° in females. The carrying angle allows the elbow to fit closely to the waist, just superior to the iliac crest. After a medial or lateral supracondylar fracture in a child, in which the distal end of the humerus is subject to either malunion or growth retardation at the epiphyseal plate, the incidence of cubitus varus is more frequent than cubitus valgus. Cubitus valgus is an angle of greater than the normal 5° to 15° described; cubitus varus is a decrease in the carrying angle and is more commonly described as a "gunstock deformity." Cubitus valgus can occur with increased angulation caused by epiphyseal plate damage from a lateral epicondyle fracture.

Answer: **False**
Hoppenfeld, pp. 36, 37
Loth, Wadsworth, p. 145
Refer to Fig. 10-12.

128 CHAPTER 10 Fractures

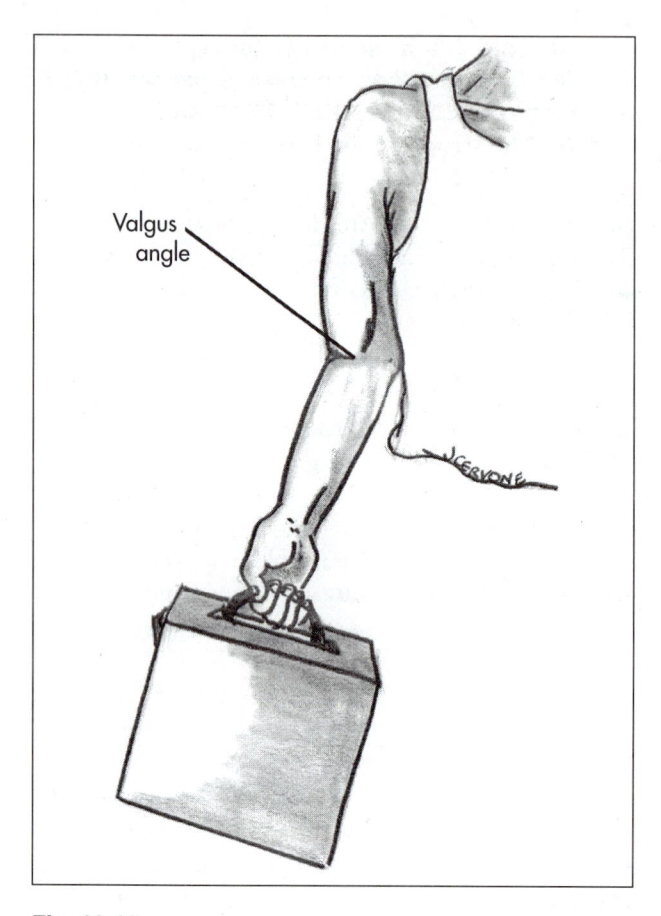

Valgus angle

Fig. 10-12

> **CLINICAL GEM:**
> To remember valgus, recall that the L in valgus correlates with the L in lateral, meaning away from the midline.

45. Which position is selected most often when performing an elbow arthrodesis?

A. 30° of flexion
B. 60° of flexion
C. 90° of flexion
D. 120° of flexion

The position of arthrodesis is selected according to a patient's specific needs. In general, 90° of flexion offers the most functional position. However, if special needs require positioning the hand away from the body, a 30-degree or 60-degree flexion position may be selected.

Answer: **C**
McCollister, pp. 17-34

46. The most significant complication after radial head excision is:

A. Pain at the wrist
B. Regrowth of the radial head
C. Stiffness of elbow flexion
D. Poor cosmetic result

Pain at the wrist caused by ulnar head impaction because of proximal migration of the radius after excision is a significant complication. This migration occurs over time. Weakness of grip, elbow instability, heterotopic bone, and arthritis also are possible complications.

Answer: **A**
Browner et al, p. 1134

47. You are treating a patient after radial head fracture. After extensive therapy, the patient has reached maximum therapeutic improvement, with end range of motion 30° shy of full extension to 130° of flexion. How should this patient be managed?

A. Refer back to doctor for surgical release
B. Continue therapy
C. Recommend massage therapy
D. No treatment is indicated

Functional range of motion of the elbow is 30° to 130° of flexion. A lack of the last 30° of full extension does not tend to be a significant functional deficit. Surgical treatment is not indicated because attaining extension beyond 30° is unpredictable. It is recommended that surgery be avoided for flexion contractures reaching a plateau at less than 45° of extension. At this point, because the patient has plateaued, he or she must adjust to the range-of-motion loss.

Answer: **D**
McCollister, p. 1759
Werner, An, p. 359

> **CLINICAL GEM:**
> Studies have shown that functional forearm rotation is 50° for both pronation and supination.

48. You are treating a patient after a severe elbow fracture and notice progressive loss of motion after initial range-of-motion gains. The patient describes pain and tenderness throughout the elbow region and increased swelling is noted. What do you suspect occurred during the management of this fracture?

A. You were too aggressive in therapy
B. The patient obviously fell and refractured the elbow
C. Heterotopic bone ossification occurred
D. The patient was noncompliant with his home program.

The patient exhibits symptoms of heterotopic bone ossification (HO). The development of HO typically is accompanied by local tissue swelling and hyperemia. Progressive loss of motion can be found after the initial satisfactory achievement of range of motion. The manifestation of these symptoms usually occurs within 1 to 4 months, although symptoms have been noted to develop for up to 1 year after insult. Radiographs can reveal the development of HO within the first 4 to 6 weeks. Direct trauma to the elbow and forearm is the most frequent cause of HO. If surgery for HO is performed, early motion is required. Overaggressive mobilization is contraindicated. Continuous passive motion is advocated to maintain gains made intraoperatively. A dynamic supination-pronation splint often is indicated in the early postoperative stage.

Answer: **C**
Hastings, Graham, pp. 417-421

49. After a minimally displaced shoulder fracture, when can passive range of motion be initiated?

A. In 7 to 10 days
B. In 14 to 21 days
C. In 6 weeks
D. Therapy is not indicated for patients with shoulder fractures.

With a minimally displaced shoulder fracture, sling immobilization is indicated for the first 7 to 10 days. Humeral fracture bracing also is indicated in shaft fractures. Gentle, passive range of motion can be initiated at approximately 7 to 10 days or when the pain has diminished and the patient is less apprehensive. Advancement of the therapy is based on fracture configuration, stability, signs of fracture healing through radiographs, and patient tolerance. Overaggressive rehabilitation can distract a minimally displaced fracture, resulting in a malunion or a nonunion.

Answer: **A**
Basti et al, p. 113

Chapter 11
Arthritis

Topics to be reviewed in random order are:

- Rheumatoid arthritis and osteoarthritis
- Anatomy
- Common deformities
- Joint protection techniques
- Managing arthritis
- Crest syndrome
- Scleroderma
- Arthritis and activities of daily living
- Joint reconstruction and rehabilitation

1. **Rheumatoid arthritis is primarily a disease of the articular cartilage. True or False?**

Rheumatoid arthritis is a generalized disease primarily affecting the synovium. Rheumatoid arthritis affects approximately 3% of the population. Osteoarthritis is a disease that typically affects the articular cartilage. Osteoarthritis is common in adults. Approximately 8% of all adults are estimated to have some degree of osteoarthritis in their hands and feet. Nearly 85% of all people between the ages of 75 and 79 demonstrate evidence of osteoarthritis.

Answer: **False**
Hunter, Mackin, Callahan, p. 1307

2. **The most common collapse deformity in the rheumatoid thumb is the:**

A. Boutonnière deformity
B. Swan-neck deformity
C. Adducted retropositioned thumb
D. All of the above are equally common

The most common collapse deformity of the rheumatoid thumb is a boutonnière deformity. In this deformity, the joint capsule and the extensor apparatus around the metacarpophalangeal joint are stretched by synovitis. The extensor pollicis longus and adductor expansion are displaced ulnarly. The attachment of the extensor pollicis brevis to the proximal phalanx is lengthened and becomes ineffective. The long extensor tendons and extensor insertions of the intrinsics apply their power to the distal joint, producing a hyperextension deformity of this joint. Pinching further accentuates this deformity and a vicious cycle develops; eventually the deformity becomes fixed.

Answer: **A**
Hunter, Mackin, Callahan, pp. 1322-1323
Refer to Fig. 11-1.

132 CHAPTER 11 Arthritis

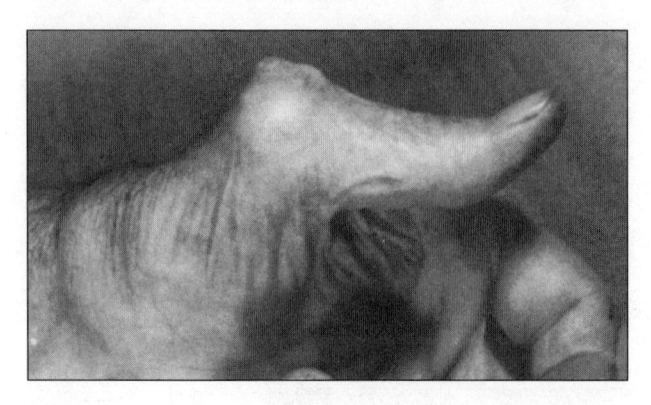

Fig. 11-1 ■ From Hunter JM, Mackin EJ, Callahan AD: *Rehabilitation of the hand: surgery and therapy*, ed 4, St. Louis, 1995, Mosby-Year Book.

3. A patient with rheumatoid arthritis should avoid staying in one position for a prolonged period of time. How often should this patient change positions?

A. Every 10 minutes
B. Every 20 to 30 minutes
C. Hourly
D. Three times a day

Maintaining a static position can put undue stress on underlying structures and lead to joint dysfunction. It is recommended that the patient change his or her position every 20 to 30 minutes. Activities can be alternated to facilitate positional changes; for example, if a patient is reading, a break should be taken after 20 minutes and a stretch should be performed, or the patient should switch to another task, such as folding the laundry.

Answer: **B**
Hunter, Mackin, Callahan, p. 1345

4. Rheumatoid arthritis is a painful disease and a patient with rheumatoid arthritis should expect to have pain for several hours after any activity. True or False?

A patient with rheumatoid arthritis often has a high tolerance for pain. It is important for the patient, however, to monitor his or her activities and to stop when pain or fatigue begins. If discomfort lasts for longer than an hour after an activity, the activity should be modified. In contrast, some patients have a fear of pain, which leads to needless inactivity. A careful balance between rest and use must be employed to allow for maximal function.

Answer: **False**
Hunter, Mackin, Callahan, p. 1348

5. Which of the following is *not* a principle of joint protection?

A. Maintain muscle strength and joint range of motion
B. Avoid positions of deformity
C. Use the weakest joint available for a job
D. Respect pain
E. Avoid prolonged static positions

All the above are principles of joint protection with the exception of using the weakest joint available for a job. It is important to use the strongest joint available to perform a job.

Answer: **C**
Hunter, Mackin, Callahan, pp. 1377-1378

6. During an acute stage of rheumatoid arthritis, how much sleep is recommended in a 24-hour period?

A. 6 to 8 hours
B. 8 to 10 hours
C. 10 to 12 hours
D. 12 to 14 hours

When a patient has a systemic disease, the entire body must be rested—not only the part that hurts. During an acute stage of rheumatoid arthritis, 10 to 12 hours of sleep every 24 hours is recommended. The patient also must be encouraged to balance activity with daytime rest to avoid fatigue. The therapist is responsible for educating the patient to help relieve symptoms in the hand and/or in other parts of the body.

Answer: **C**
Hunter, Mackin, Callahan, p. 1378

7. CREST syndrome is a variant of:

A. Rheumatoid arthritis
B. Osteoarthritis
C. Scleroderma
D. Ollier's disease

Scleroderma is an umbrella term for disorders in which sclerosis of the skin is a predominant feature. Under the general category of scleroderma, there are many classifications. One classification is generalized scleroderma, which includes subcategories of diffuse scleroderma and limited scleroderma. CREST syndrome belongs to the limited scleroderma category. CREST is an acronym that stands for **c**alcinosis, **R**aynaud's phenomenon, **e**sophageal hypomotility, **s**clerodactyly, and **t**elangiectasia.

Answer: **C**
Hunter, Mackin, Callahan, p. 1385

8. When treating a patient with scleroderma, it is important to maintain:

A. Proximal interphalangeal joint flexion
B. Metacarpophalangeal joint flexion
C. Distal interphalangeal joint flexion
D. Carpometacarpal joint flexion

A patient with scleroderma typically presents with the following deformities: metacarpophalangeal joint extension contractures, proximal interphalangeal joint flexion contractures, thumb adduction contractures, and the wrist is contracted in the neutral position. Distal interphalangeal joints often become fixed in mid-range. Therapy must focus on preserving metacarpophalangeal joint flexion and proximal interphalangeal joint extension as primary goals. It also is important to prevent thumb carpometacarpal adduction contractures and, from a functional standpoint, preserving lateral pinch is extremely critical. Lateral pinch is maintained by preserving metacarpophalangeal joint flexion. Loss of lateral pinch represents a tremendous loss of hand function.

Answer: **B**
Hunter, Mackin, Callahan, p. 1387

9. Which of the following is not a risk factor in osteoarthritis?

A. Trauma
B. Obesity
C. Genetic factors
D. All of the above are risk factors in osteoarthritis.

All of the above are risk factors in osteoarthritis. It is important to recognize these risk factors in order to reduce the ones that can be modified. Both trauma and repetitive stress have been implicated as causes of osteoarthritis. Previous vocational or avocational activities also can contribute to symptoms of osteoarthritis. An increased body mass, as in the obese patient, is associated with an increase in the prevalence of osteoarthritis, especially in the knees. Genetic factors have been shown to be noncoincidental in osteoarthritis; these include an autosomal dominant transmission in females and a recessive inheritance in males.

Answer: **D**
Brandt, pp. 25-30

10. In the early stages of osteoarthritis, the cartilage is thicker than normal. True or False?

Most descriptions of the pathology of osteoarthritis focus on the progressive loss of articular cartilage that occurs in the disease. However, in the early stages of osteoarthritis, the cartilage is thicker than normal. This is caused by an increase in water content, which reflects damage to the collagen network of the tissue and results in swelling of the cartilage. Cartilage thickening is associated with an increase in the net rate of synthesis of proteoglycans. With the progression of osteoarthritis, the joint surface thins and the proteoglycan concentration diminishes, leading to a softening of the cartilage. This loss of articular cartilage is the pathologic hallmark of osteoarthritis.

Answer: **True**
Brandt, pp. 35, 36

11. Joint pain from osteoarthritis arises from the articular cartilage. True or False?

The articular cartilage is aneural. Therefore, the joint pain in osteoarthritis must arise from other structures. Joint pain in osteoarthritis can occur from stretching of the nerve endings in the periosteum covering osteophytes, microfractures in subchondral bone, medullary hypertension from the distortion of blood flow by thickened subchondral trabeculae, or synovitis.

Answer: **False**
Brandt, p. 56

12. Bony enlargements of the distal interphalangeal joint are known as:

A. Heberden's nodes
B. Bouchard's nodes
C. Synovial effusions
D. All of the above

Bony enlargements of the distal interphalangeal joints are called Heberden's nodes (Fig. 11-2). Bony enlargements of the proximal interphalangeal joints are called Bouchard's nodes. In some joints, gross deformity is obvious.

Answer: **A**
Brandt, p. 61

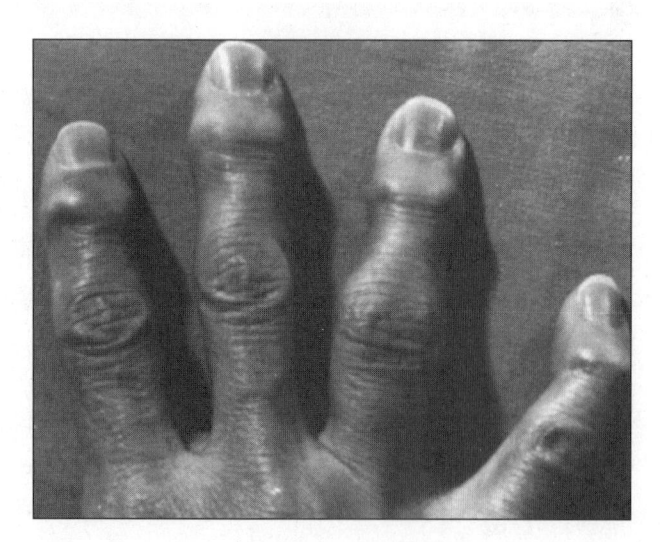

Fig. 11-2 ■ From Hunter JM, Mackin EJ, Callahan AD: *Rehabilitation of the hand: surgery and therapy,* ed 4, St. Louis, 1995, Mosby-Year Book.

13. Which of the following pharmacological management techniques is not indicated in the treatment of osteoarthritis?

A. Acetaminophen
B. Nonsteroidal antiinflammatory drugs
C. Capsaicin
D. Systemic corticosteroid treatments

Systemic corticosteroid treatments are not indicated in the treatment of osteoarthritis. Prolonged systemic use of corticosteroids has significant side effects, which greatly outweigh any possible benefits. However, intraarticular injections of corticosteroids may be beneficial.

The use of nonsteroidal antiinflammatory drugs (NSAIDs) has reduced joint pain and improved mobility for millions of people with osteoarthritis. However, some studies have indicated that a simple analgesic, such as acetaminophen, may be as effective as an NSAID in the treatment of patients with osteoarthritis. Capsaicin is a cream that is applied locally to a painful area. This substance may be useful in symptomatic management of osteoarthritis.

Answer: **D**
Brandt, pp. 135-160

14. Subluxation occurs when joint surfaces are no longer in contact with each other and there is no potential for normal joint motion. True or False?

A subluxation of a joint indicates that the articular surfaces are still in contact but that the joint surfaces are no longer in their normal alignment. A joint that is subluxed often can be manually reduced to its anatomical position but is unable to maintain the position without support. A dislocation occurs when joint surfaces are no longer in contact with each other and there is no potential for normal joint motion. In an arthritic dislocation, the articular surfaces usually are obliterated and the joint cannot be manually reduced. Attempting to splint a dislocation often increases the patient's pain and discomfort. Surgical intervention is indicated for dislocated arthritic joints.

Answer: **False**
Malick, Kasch, p. 118

15. Research tests have shown that _____ pounds of grip and _____ to _____ lbs of pinch are necessary to accomplish most activities of daily living.

A. 10; 1 to 2
B. 15; 8 to 10
C. 20; 5 to 7
D. 5; 1 to 2

Research has shown that a grip strength of 20 lb allows patients to perform most activities of daily living. It also has been shown that a pinch strength of 5 to 7 lb is useful in accomplishing most daily living tasks. However, it must be remembered that patients with rheumatoid arthritis have strength far below these functional levels; it is therefore understandable that they encounter difficulties in accomplishing many daily living tasks.

Answer: **C**
Hunter, Mackin, Callahan, p. 1333

16. A patient is referred to you by his primary care doctor for treatment of his hand pain. During your evaluation you note a scaly, erythematous skin rash. You also note severe nail changes. The patient has flexion deformities of the proximal interphalangeal joints without distal interphalangeal joint hyperextension. He also reports difficulty with grasping activities and intermittent swelling. What might this patient have?

A. Osteoarthritis
B. Boutonnière deformities
C. Psoriatic arthritis
D. None of the above

Psoriatic arthritis, an uncommon form of arthritis, is described in this case. There are similarities between this form of arthritis and rheumatoid or degenerative arthritis. The classic finding in psoriatic arthritis is a scaly, erythematous skin rash. Patients with psoriatic arthritis also have characteristic changes of the nails. These patients tend to present with asymmetric involvement of the hands; asymmetry also can be present unilaterally. The most common deformities seen with this type of arthritis are flexion deformities of the proximal interphalangeal joints, without the corresponding distal interphalangeal joint hyperextension that would be seen in a patient with a boutonnière deformity.

Answer: **C**
Nalebuff, pp. 603-610

17. What is the most commonly ruptured flexor tendon in a patient with rheumatoid arthritis?

A. Flexor pollicis longus
B. Flexor pollicis brevis
C. Flexor digitorum profundus to the index finger
D. Flexor digitorum profundus to the small finger
E. Flexor digitorum superficialis to the ring finger

The most commonly ruptured flexor tendon in patients with rheumatoid arthritis is the flexor pollicis longus. When this flexor tendon ruptures, the patient loses active flexion of the interphalangeal joint of the thumb. Rupture results when the tendon is worn away by a volar osteophyte on the scaphoid that penetrates through the volar wrist capsule. Rupture of the flexor pollicis longus also is known as a "Mannerfelt lesion." Functional loss is variable with this injury.

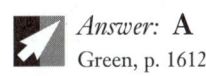

Answer: **A**
Green, p. 1612

18. Which finger is most commonly involved in single extensor tendon ruptures in rheumatoid arthritis?

A. Index finger
B. Middle finger
C. Ring finger
D. Small finger

The small finger is most commonly involved in single extensor tendon ruptures in rheumatoid arthritis (RA). With an isolated rupture of a single tendon, surgical intervention is advised because of the danger that additional ruptures may occur. Surgical treatment of an isolated rupture is relatively easy; surgical repair of multiple tendons is more complicated. Rupture of the extensor pollicis longus also is common in RA.

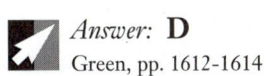

Answer: **D**
Green, pp. 1612-1614

19. The caput ulnae syndrome includes all of the following findings except:

A. Weakness of the wrist and hand
B. Pain with rotation of the distal radioulnar joint
C. Decreased range of motion of the distal radioulnar joint
D. Dorsal prominence of the distal ulna
E. All of the above are findings associated with the caput ulnae syndrome.

The caput ulnae syndrome is described as an end-stage presentation of rheumatoid destruction of the distal radioulnar joint. Findings associated with this syndrome include weakness of the wrist and hand, pain with rotation of the distal radioulnar joint, decreased range of motion of the distal radioulnar joint, dorsal prominence of the distal ulna, bulging of the synovial bursae of the long extensors and extensor carpi ulnaris, and rupture of one or more extensor tendons.

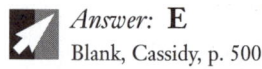

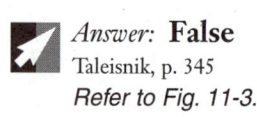

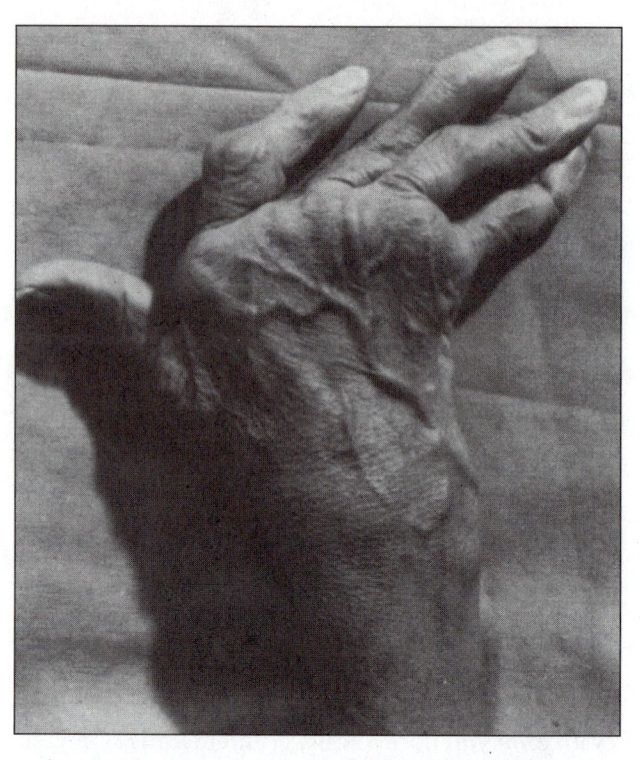

Answer: **E**
Blank, Cassidy, p. 500

Fig. 11-3 ■ From Hunter JM, Mackin EJ, Callahan AD: *Rehabilitation of the hand: surgery and therapy,* ed 4, St. Louis, 1995, Mosby-Year Book.

CLINICAL GEM:
A prominent ulnar head is easily recognized. One way to evaluate caput ulnae syndrome is to manually reduce the ulnar head which resembles the up and down action of a piano key; this finding has been termed the piano-key sign.

CLINICAL GEM:
The typical pattern of deformity in rheumatoid arthritis (RA) is known as a zigzag deformity of the wrist. Carpal supination occurs with a secondary radial shift of the metacarpals followed by an ulnar deviation of the digits. A patient with RA often requires management of the wrist before management of the metacarpophalangeal joints.

20. An ulnar drift of the fingers is commonly seen in rheumatoid arthritis. This disease also causes the metacarpals to shift into ulnar deviation. True or False?

The typical pattern of deformity in rheumatoid arthritis is a palmar subluxation of the radius and the carpus in relation to the ulnar head. The ulnar half of the carpus droops in a palmar direction and the metacarpals shift into radial deviation; this is followed by a shift of the digits into ulnar deviation.

Answer: **False**
Taleisnik, p. 345
Refer to Fig. 11-3.

21. You are evaluating a patient with rheumatoid arthritis. The patient has severe joint deformity and ulnar drift of the fingers and cannot extend his small finger. What might have occurred?

A. Rupture of the extensor tendons to the small finger
B. A radial nerve palsy
C. Subluxation of the extensor tendons to the ulnar aspect of the metacarpophalangeal joint
D. Subluxation of the extensor tendons to the radial aspect of the metacarpophalangeal joint
E. A, B, and C
F. All of the above

The inability to extend the small finger has many possible causes. Radial nerve palsy is an uncommon etiology but it may be the cause if the rheumatoid deformity is around the elbow joint. Rupture of the extensor tendons is not uncommon and occurs at the level of the distal ulna in the condition known as caput ulnae syndrome. Frequently, patients with rheumatoid arthritis have subluxation of the extensor tendons that can preclude extension. Subluxation of the extensor tendons occurs in the ulnar direction at the metacarpophalangeal joint. It is extremely rare for the extensor tendons to sublux to the radial aspect of the metacarpophalangeal joint; therefore, answer D is incorrect.

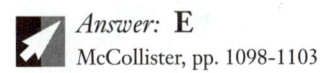

Answer: **E**
McCollister, pp. 1098-1103

22. You are treating a patient who has had metacarpophalangeal joint reconstruction. The following statements are included in the operative note:

The intrinsic tendons are exposed and released. The extensor expansion is opened on the radial side to expose the collateral ligament. The intrinsic tendon is sutured to the radial collateral ligament at its phalangeal attachment, using 4-0 sutures.

What type of surgical repair did this patient undergo?

A. Metacarpophalangeal joint synovectomy
B. Extensor tendon relocation
C. Crossed-intrinsic transfer
D. Metacarpophalangeal joint arthroplasty

Crossed-intrinsic transfers are used as an additional means of restoring finger alignment and preventing recurrent ulnar drift. The intrinsics are released from the ulnar side of the index, long, and ring fingers and transferred to the radial aspect of the adjacent fingers to provide additional radial stability. Some authors have found that this provides effective, long-term correction of ulnar drift in early rheumatoid arthritis. When treating a patient with crossed-intrinsic transfers, it is recommended that the fingers be splinted for 3 weeks before exercises are begun. A dynamic splint may be applied afterward and used for an additional 3 weeks (see Fig. 2-9).

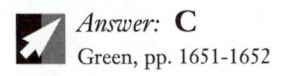

Answer: **C**
Green, pp. 1651-1652

23. The primary treatment of metacarpophalangeal joints during stage one of rheumatoid arthritis is:

A. Metacarpophalangeal joint arthroplasty
B. Wrist fusion followed by metacarpophalangeal joint arthroplasty
C. Splinting
D. Strengthening the intrinsics

Splinting is the main treatment used in stage one of the diseased metacarpophalangeal joint. Patients wear night splints that hold the fingers in relative extension and correct ulnar deviation with finger separators. A resting hand splint also can be used during the day during periods of inflammation. The therapist is responsible for providing the patient with joint protection, adaptive equipment, and general exercise instructions. During stage two of rheumatoid arthritis, decisions regarding hand surgery become more important. In stage two or stage three, synovectomies and soft-tissue reconstructions become options. In stage three and stage four, implant arthroplasty is the procedure of choice.

Answer: **C**
Stirrat, pp. 519-520

24. Indications for Silastic arthroplasty of the metacarpophalangeal joints include:

A. Deformity
B. Pain
C. Desire for cosmetic improvement
D. Joint dislocation
E. All of the above

Pain and severe deformity, which frequently are associated with joint dislocation, are the predominant indications for implant arthroplasties. In addition, patients often are unhappy with the cosmetic appearance of the hand preoperatively and want to improve the appearance of the hand and its function.

Answer: **E**
McCollister, pp. 1118-1126

25. Patients who have swan-neck deformities with end-stage arthritic changes of the metacarpophalangeal joints should have these deformities corrected before metacarpophalangeal arthoplasty. True or False?

The swan-neck deformity must never be surgically corrected before the metacarpophalangeal joint imbalance is corrected. Treatment options vary depending on the stage of the swan-neck deformity.

Answer: **False**
McCollister, pp. 1126-1129

26. A 21-year-old model is injured in a volleyball accident while on vacation in the Caribbean. When she is seen 3 weeks later, the proximal interphalangeal joint of her ring finger shows a fracture with a dorsal dislocation of the proximal phalanx. Which of the following is (are) an appropriate surgical treatment(s)?

A. Open reduction internal fixation
B. Volar plate arthroplasty
C. Proximal interphalangeal joint arthroplasty
D. Arthrodesis of the proximal interphalangeal joint
E. All of the above are appropriate surgical treatments.

All of the above surgical treatments could be employed for this patient. Fractures with substantial comminution or displacement of the joint space frequently require open reduction internal fixation. When the volar plate has been avulsed at its insertion site with comminution, a volar plate arthroplasty may be the only means of restoring stability. In late dislocations of the joint, an arthrodesis or arthroplasty may be necessary to restore a stable, painfree joint and reduce the risk of persistent arthritis.

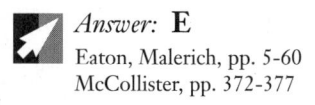

Answer: **E**
Eaton, Malerich, pp. 5-60
McCollister, pp. 372-377

> **CLINICAL GEM:**
> A quick reference for the treatment of proximal interphalangeal joint arthroplasty follows:
> - A digit extension splint is applied at 3 to 5 days postoperatively.
> - Active range-of-motion exercises are initiated 3 to 5 days postoperatively (avoiding lateral forces).
> - Passive range of motion is initiated at 3 weeks.
> - Light strengthening is initiated at 6 weeks.
> - Use of the extension splint is reduced to nighttime only at 6 weeks.

27. A 65-year-old woman is involved in a motor vehicle accident and sustains a severe fracture dislocation of the metacarpophalangeal joint of the index finger, which leads to posttraumatic arthritis. She is treated with metacarpophalangeal arthoplasty of the index metacarpophalangeal joint. Her postoperative therapy program should include:

A. Application of a bulky hand dressing for 3 to 7 days
B. Active metacarpophalangeal joint flexion and extension exercises
C. Splinting, both dynamic and static, of the index finger
D. Splinting of the hand with metacarpophalangeal joints in 90° of flexion for the first 2 weeks
E. A, B, and C
F. All of the above

The postoperative program for Silastic arthroplasty of the metacarpophalangeal joint involves application of a bulky hand dressing or cast for the first 3 to 7 days, followed by a splinting and exercise program. Active and passive metacarpophalangeal joint flexion and extension exercises are performed hourly in the dynamic splint. Both dynamic and static splints are essential for an excellent postoperative result. A static splint is applied at night and a dynamic splint is applied during the day. Initial splinting should be with the fingers in extension, not in flexion, as described in answer D.

Answer: **E**
McCollister, pp. 1120-1126
Hunter, Mackin, Callahan, pp. 1366-1368

> **CLINICAL GEM:**
> After metacarpophalangeal joint arthroplasty, watch digits carefully for pronation or supination deformities and add additional outriggers to the distal phalanx if these develop.

28. It is acceptable for a patient to begin writing 2 weeks after a metacarpophalangeal arthroplasty. True or False?

After a metacarpophalangeal joint arthroplasty, lateral pinch should be avoided because it pushes the fingers in an ulnar direction. In selective cases a working splint can be fabricated in the early postsurgical stage to allow the individual to resume pinch activities earlier than the usual postoperative date of 6 to 8 weeks (Fig. 11-4). A protective writing splint reduces the risk of recurring ulnar drift after reconstruction.

Answer: **False**
Hunter, Mackin, Callahan, pp. 1378-1379

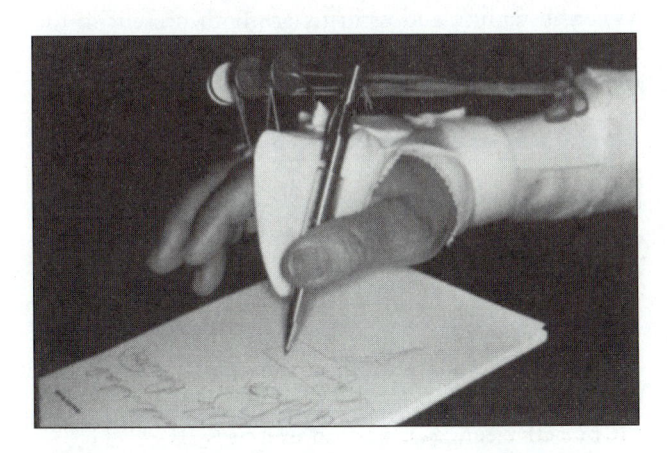

Fig. 11-4 ■ Used with permission from Judy Colditz, OTR/L.

29. You are treating a patient after a metacarpophalangeal joint arthroplasty. What is your range-of-motion goal per metacarpophalangeal joint?

A. Index through small fingers: 90° flexion
B. Index and middle fingers: 45° to 60° flexion; ring and small fingers: 70° flexion
C. Index and middle fingers: 75° to 80° flexion; ring and small fingers: 60° to 70° flexion
D. Index and middle fingers: 30° to 40° flexion; ring and small fingers: 50° to 60° flexion

Range-of-motion goals after metacarpophalangeal joint arthroplasty vary from author to author. In general, a goal of 45° to 60° flexion in the index and middle fingers and 70° flexion for the ring and small fingers are acceptable. Remember, more mobility yields less stability; therefore, it is less important to have extensive motion in the index and middle fingers. More motion should be obtained in the ring and small fingers to allow for grasp; limited motion of the index and middle fingers allows for dexterity and pinch.

Answer: **B**
Hunter, Mackin, Callahan, pp. 1367-1368

30. You are treating a patient with a metacarpophalangeal joint arthroplasty. When can a flexion outrigger be added to the splint postoperatively on this patient?

A. 1 week
B. 3 weeks
C. 6 weeks
D. 10 weeks

A flexion outrigger can be applied 3 weeks after surgery. It is recommended that the flexion outrigger be worn approximately five times a day for 20- to 30-minute intervals to passively stretch the metacarpophalangeal joints. This is done in conjunction with active flexion exercises. Some authors recommend initiating flexion splinting to the metacarpophalangeal joints as early as 2 weeks postoperatively as scar formation will limit motion. The reconstructed joints begin to get tight during the second postoperative week and are very tight by the end of the third week. If range of motion has not been obtained by the end of the third week, it will be difficult to gain further improvement.

Answer: **B**
Hunter, Mackin, Callahan, p. 1368

140 CHAPTER 11 Arthritis

31. In ligament reconstruction tendon interposition arthroplasty of the thumb, the tendon most commonly used to reconstruct the palmar oblique ligament is:

A. Abductor pollicis longus
B. Extensor pollicis brevis
C. Extensor pollicis longus
D. Flexor carpi radialis
E. Flexor carpi ulnaris

During reconstruction of the thumb basal joint (first carpometacarpal joint), the flexor carpi radialis is the preferred tendon for reconstructing the palmar oblique ligament when instability exists. This technique is known as ligament reconstruction tendon interposition arthroplasty of the basal joint of the thumb.

Answer: **D**
Burton, Pellegrini, p. 11

32. Which of the following procedures is frequently used for treating a patient with pantrapezial arthritis at the base of the thumb?

A. Excision of the trapezium and ligament reconstruction tendon interposition arthroplasty
B. Hemiresection of the trapezium and use of a metacarpal resurfacing Silicone implant
C. Arthrodesis of the trapezial first metacarpal joint
D. All of the above

Pantrapezial arthritis refers to all joints surrounding the trapezium. All of the above techniques are used to reconstruct the basal joint when arthritis involves the first metacarpal joint and trapezium. However, when arthritis also exists between the scaphoid and trapezium, and between the trapezium and trapezoid, hemiresection of the trapezium or arthrodesis of the trapezial first metacarpal joint alone may not adequately relieve the patient's pain.

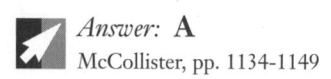

Answer: **A**
McCollister, pp. 1134-1149

> **CLINICAL GEM:**
> Some surgeons use Silicone implant arthroplasty to reconstruct the basal joint. The Silicone implant arthroplasty technique is not used as frequently as other reconstructive procedures.

33. The most common procedure associated with ligament reconstruction tendon interposition arthroplasty of the thumb for basal joint arthritis is:

A. Arthrodesis of the first metacarpophalangeal joint
B. Arthrodesis of the interphalangeal joint of the thumb
C. de Quervain release
D. Trigger finger release
E. None of the above

de Quervain tenosynovitis commonly occurs in patients who have basal joint arthritis. However, instability of the first metacarpophalangeal joint is the most common associated condition and it requires either stabilization or arthrodesis, depending on the degree of instability. When instability and arthritis are both present in the metacarpophalangeal joint, arthrodesis is the treatment of choice.

Answer: **A**
Burton, Pellegrini, p. 11

34. Appropriate rehabilitation of the thumb after carpometacarpal joint implant arthroplasty includes:

A. Immediate mobilization of the joint
B. Immobilization of the thumb for 1 week followed by active range-of-motion exercises
C. Cast immobilization of the thumb for 4 weeks followed by use of a protective splint for 2 weeks
D. Cast immobilization of the thumb and index finger for 6 weeks
E. None of the above

After most implant arthroplasties of the thumb, cast immobilization is recommended for 3 to 4 weeks, followed by the use of thumb spica splinting for an additional

2 weeks. Active range-of-motion exercises are initiated 3 to 4 weeks postoperatively when the cast is removed.

Answer: **C**
McCollister, pp. 1134-1145

> **CLINICAL GEM:**
> A quick reference for rehabilitation after ligament reconstruction tendon interposition arthroplasty follows:
> • A cast is applied for the initial 3 to 4 weeks
> • A thumb spica splint is applied after cast removal
> • Active range of motion of the thumb and wrist is initiated at 3 to 4 weeks
> • Gentle passive range of motion of the carpometacarpal joint is initiated at 6 weeks
> • The splint is discontinued at 6 weeks (and used as needed)
> • Light resistance is initiated at 8 weeks

> **CLINICAL GEM:**
> Ensure your patients that it is not uncommon to experience discomfort for 6 to 12 months after ligament reconstruction tendon interposition surgery.

35. Ligaments in the rheumatoid wrist typically loosen on the ulnar aspect of the radiocarpal joint, allowing a radial displacement of the proximal carpal row. When this occurs, the result is ulnar deviation of the hand on the forearm. True or False?

When ligaments loosen on the radial aspect of the radiocarpal joint, ulnar displacement of the proximal carpal row will occur. **Radial deviation** of the hand occurs secondarily on the forearm. An associated subluxation of the distal radioulnar joint often occurs, causing a loss of stability on the ulnar aspect of the wrist. A palmar subluxation of the proximal row on the radius also is commonly seen.

Answer: **False**
Hunter, Mackin, Callahan, pp. 1325-1326
Refer to Fig. 11-5.

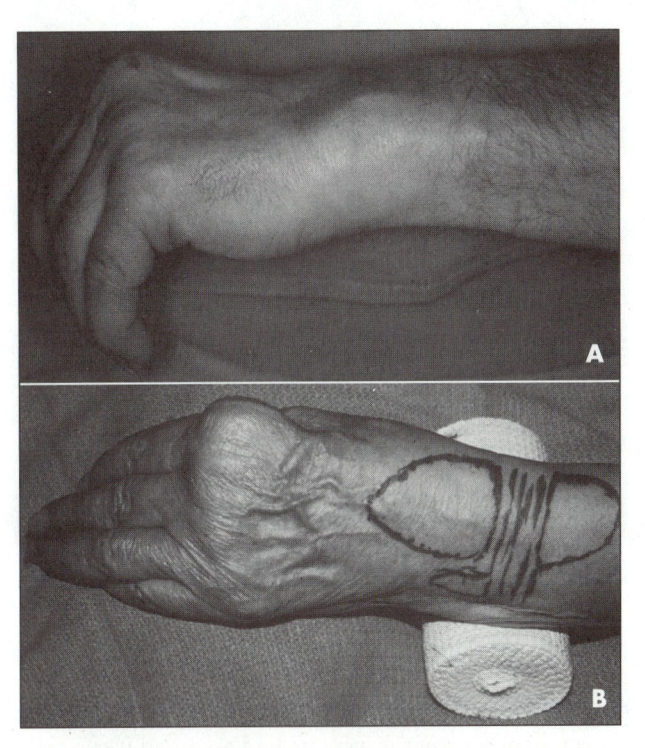

Fig. 11-5 ■ **A**, Ulnar aspect of hand and carpus, palmarly subluxed and supinated relative to the forearm bones. **B**, Apparent radial deviation of the wrist as a result of ulnar translation of the carpus relative to the radius. The *outlined area* illustrates soft-tissue swelling, which is characteristic of extensor tenosynovitis. (From Cooney WP, Linscheid RL, Dobyns JH: *The wrist: diagnosis and operative treatment,* St. Louis, 1998, Mosby-Year Book.)

36. A total wrist arthrodesis is an excellent procedure for a patient with rheumatoid arthritis and is used frequently. True or False?

A total wrist arthrodesis is not frequently performed on a patient with rheumatoid arthritis (RA) for several reasons. First, patients with RA maintain relatively good function in a relatively painfree range after synovectomy and stabilization. Second, maintenance of wrist motion allows for tendon excursion in patients who require tendon transfers or repairs. Third, the involvement of other joints, including the elbow, shoulder, and contralateral hand and wrist, hampers function of these patients significantly with a fusion of one wrist. Total wrist arthrodesis is reserved for the completely destroyed, painful wrist in young, vigorous patients—particularly in one who has less involvement of other joints.

Answer: **False**
Taleisnik, p. 387

37. Postoperative treatment of a 61-year-old woman who has undergone Silastic implant arthroplasty of the wrist should include:

A. Cast immobilization for 3 to 4 weeks
B. Cast immobilization for 7 to 10 days
C. Nighttime splinting for 3 years to prevent a recurrence of deformity
D. Bulky dressing with immediate active range-of-motion exercises

After a wrist implant arthroplasty, immobilization in a bulky hand dressing or plaster shell cast for 3 to 4 weeks postoperatively, to ensure that the ligaments and the capsule have time to heal, commonly is employed. After a period of cast immobilization, a custom splint frequently is used intermittently for an additional 3 to 4 weeks. Long-term nighttime splinting frequently is performed for metacarpophalangeal joint arthroplasty but is rarely necessary for wrist arthoplasty–and it certainly is not indicated for a 3-year period.

Answer: **A**
McCollister, pp. 1106-1112

> **CLINICAL GEM:**
> A quick reference for rehabilitation of wrist arthroplasties follows:
> - Cast immobilization for 3 to 4 weeks
> - Wrist support splint applied after cast removal
> - Active range of motion to the wrist at 3 to 4 weeks
> - Gentle passive range of motion to the wrist at 6 weeks
> - Light strengthening at 8 weeks
> - Splint used as needed at 6 to 8 weeks

38. Which type of joint replacement has shown the highest complication rate?

A. Basal joint
B. Metacarpophalangeal joint
C. Elbow joint
D. Knee joint

Of all major total joint arthroplasties, elbow arthroplasty has the highest complication rate. Complications include infection, dislocation, loosening of components, malalignment, nonunion, delayed union, and instability. In the future, elbow arthroplasty designs may include smaller components that save bone stock, provide alternatives to cement fixation, or allow for a biological implant such as an allograft.

Answer: **C**
Green, p. 1706

Chapter 12
Reflex Sympathetic Dystrophy

Topics to be reviewed in random order are:

- Evaluation of reflex sympathetic dystrophy
- Stages of reflex sympathetic dystrophy
- Classifications of reflex sympathetic dystrophy
- Reflex sympathetic dystrophy in children
- Stellate ganglion blocks
- Modalities and treatment for reflex sympathetic dystrophy

1. Match the reflex sympathetic dystrophy stage with the appropriate characteristics:

Stage

1. Stage I
2. Stage II
3. Stage III

Characteristics

A. Trophic skin changes and widespread osteoporosis; brawny edema; increased stiffness
B. Skin atrophy; severe joint stiffness; muscle wasting
C. Pain; pitting edema; joint stiffness; accelerated growth of hair and nails

Answer: **1. C; 2. A; 3. B**
Hunter, Mackin, Callahan, pp. 782-784
Wong, Wilson, pp. 319-341
Refer to Fig. 12-1.

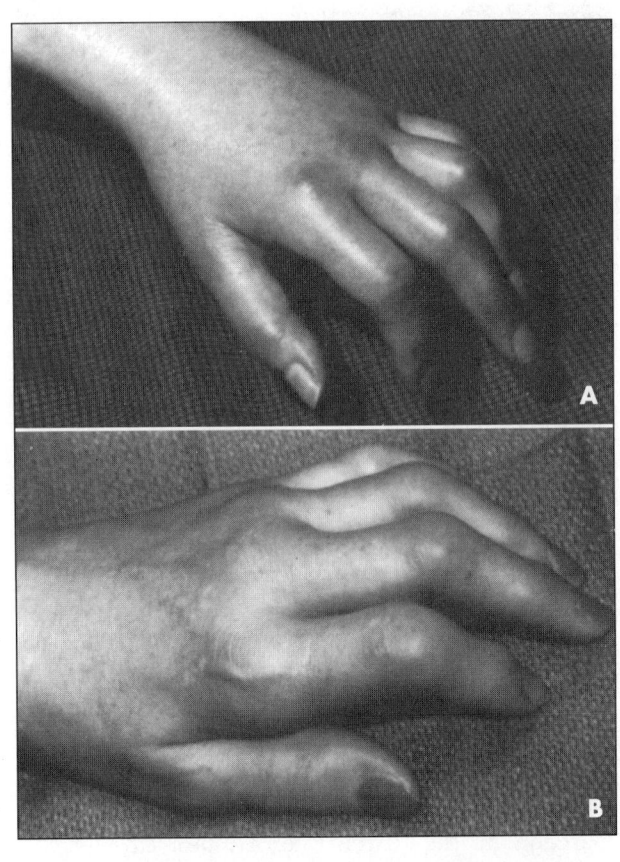

Fig. 12-1 ■ **A,** In stage I of reflex sympathetic dystrophy, swelling usually is soft and puffy, with redness over joints. **B,** Stage II is characterized by brawny edema with stiffness, as evidenced by a flattening of extensor and flexor wrinkles. (From Lankford LL, Thompson JE: *Reflex sympathetic dystrophy, upper and lower extremity: diagnosis and management.* In American Academy of Orthopaedic Surgeons: instructional course lectures, vol 26, St. Louis, 1977, C.V. Mosby.)

Continued

144 CHAPTER 12 Reflex Sympathetic Dystrophy

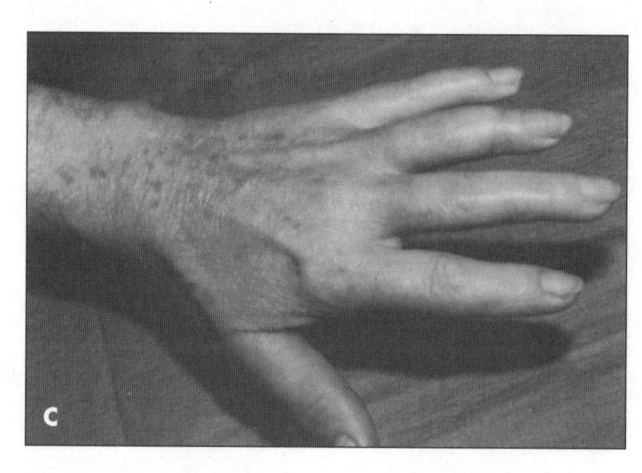

Fig. 12-1, cont'd ■ **C,** Stage III is characterized by atrophy of skin and subcutaneous tissue, which produces a glossy appearance of the skin. (From Lankford LL, Thompson JE: *Reflex sympathetic dystrophy, upper and lower extremity: diagnosis and management.* In *American Academy of Orthopaedic Surgeons: instructional course lectures,* vol 26, St. Louis, 1977, C.V. Mosby.)

> **CLINICAL GEM:**
> The length of each reflex sympathetic dystrophy stage varies from author to author. However, the following is generally accepted when staging reflex sympathetic dystrophy:
> Stage I: 0 to 3 months; Stage II: 3 to 9 months; Stage III: 9 months or longer.

2. Which of the following conditions is/are associated with reflex sympathetic dystrophy?

A. Fracture
B. Cerebrovascular accident
C. Soft-tissue injury
D. Immobilization
E. All of the above

Conditions associated with reflex sympathetic dystrophy can be grouped into three categories: (1) peripheral; (2) central; and (3) other. In the peripheral category, abnormalities include fracture, malignancy, immobilization, infection, dislocation, or myocardial infarction. In the central category, problems include cerebrovascular accident, cerebral tumor, head injury, or spinal cord injury. In the other category, associations include diabetes, genetic and idiopathic conditions, and/or medication.

Answer: **E**
Dumitru, p. 91

3. The diagnosis of reflex sympathetic dystrophy depends primarily on:

A. Triple-phase bone scan
B. Sweat test
C. Thermography
D. History and physical exam

In the evaluation of patients with reflex sympathetic dystrophy, the patient's history and the physical exam usually provide the diagnosis; the laboratory data often are normal. A few nonspecific diagnostic tests may aid in the diagnosis and also serve to rule out other disease states. A triple-phase bone scan may be helpful. Typically, the third phase of the triple-phase bone scan helps with the diagnosis of reflex sympathetic dystrophy. The sweat test is not diagnostic and may vary from patient to patient. Thermography can indicate various temperatures but is nonspecific and of questionable prognostic significance. Many conditions can show skin temperature changes; therefore, thermography is not considered a reliable test.

Answer: **D**
Dumitru, pp. 95-96
Hunter, Mackin, Callahan, p. 789

4. "Classic" findings of upper-extremity reflex sympathetic dystrophy on electrodiagnostic studies are:

A. Prolonged nerve conduction velocities of the upper extremity
B. Generalized decreased SNAP amplitudes
C. Fibrillation potentials and positive sharp waves on the electromyogram of the hand muscles
D. Prolonged median and ulnar F waves
E. The tests typically are normal, unless there is a concomitant nerve injury.

Electrodiagnostics essentially are normal in reflex sympathetic dystrophy, except when there is damage to the peripheral nervous system during the initial injury.

Answer: **E**
Dumitru, p. 96

5. You are treating a patient with a sprained finger. She has excessive pain, swelling, discoloration, and temperature changes in the involved digit. Which

classification of reflex sympathetic dystrophy would best describe her symptoms?

A. Minor causalgia
B. Minor traumatic dystrophy
C. Shoulder-hand syndrome
D. Major traumatic dystrophy
E. Major causalgia

This patient would be classified in the minor traumatic dystrophy category because her injury did not specifically involve damage to a nerve and was from a minor initial trauma. A minor causalgia involves a purely sensory nerve in the distal extremity, such as the palmar cutaneous branch of the median nerve. Shoulder-hand syndrome involves the whole extremity and is caused by a proximal trauma, a painful visceral lesion, or a cerebrovascular accident. Major traumatic dystrophy occurs after a major hand trauma without specific nerve injury. Major causalgia involves an injury to a major mixed nerve proximal to the extremity and is the most severe form of reflex sympathetic dystrophy.

Answer: **B**
Green, pp. 630-632
Hunter, Mackin, Callahan, pp. 784-786

6. Which of the following is not one of the four cardinal signs of reflex sympathetic dystrophy?

A. Pain
B. Swelling
C. Discoloration
D. Temperature changes
E. All of the above are cardinal signs.

The four cardinal signs and symptoms of reflex sympathetic dystrophy are pain, swelling, stiffness, and discoloration. Secondary signs include osseous demineralization, sudomotor changes, temperature changes, vasomotor instability, palmar fibromatosis, and pilomotor activity.

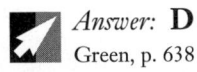

Answer: **D**
Green, p. 638

7. When is the earliest time that osteoporosis might be noted in a patient with reflex sympathetic dystrophy?

A. 3 weeks
B. 12 weeks
C. 6 months
D. Osteoporosis is not noted in patients with reflex sympathetic dystrophy.

Osteoporosis is not present before 3 weeks in patients with reflex sympathetic dystrophy and often is not seen until the fifth week (stage I). During stage II, demineralization increases and spotty demineralization in the carpal bones changes to a more widespread homogenous appearance. In stage III, osteoporosis is profound.

Answer: **A**
Hunter, Mackin, Callahan, pp. 782-783
Refer to Fig. 12-2.

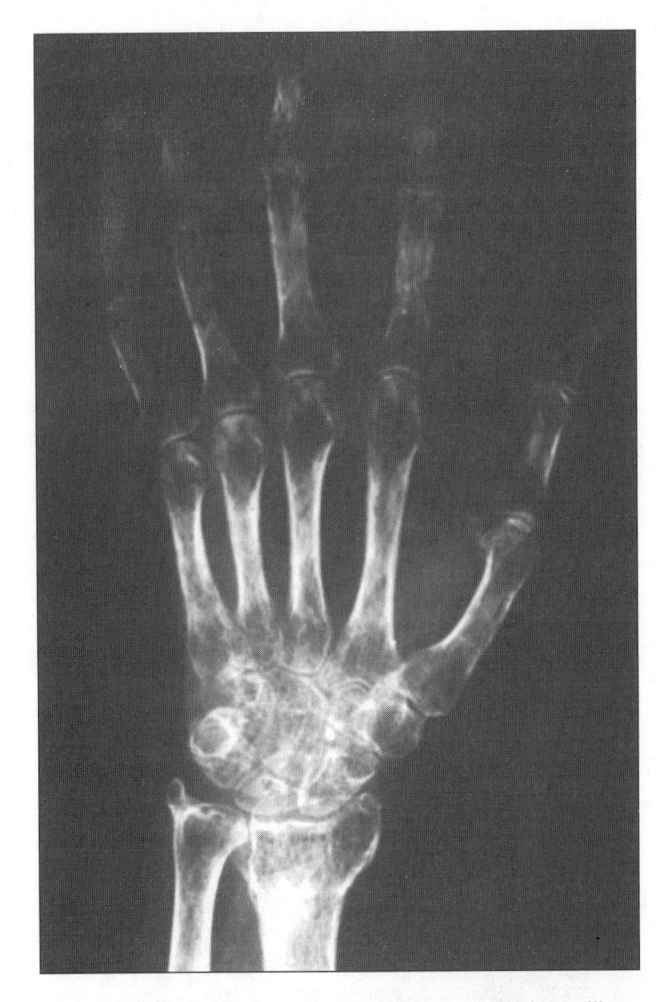

Fig. 12-2 ■ Near the end of stage II and in the early part of stage III, osteoporosis has become uniform and very intense throughout all bones of the hand and wrist. (From Lankford LL, Thompson JE: *Reflex sympathetic dystrophy, upper and lower extremity: diagnosis and management.* In American Academy of Orthopaedic Surgeons: instructional course lectures, vol 26, St. Louis, 1977, C.V. Mosby.)

8. Neuromuscular electrical stimulation may be used to help gain range of motion in patients with reflex sympathetic dystrophy. True or False?

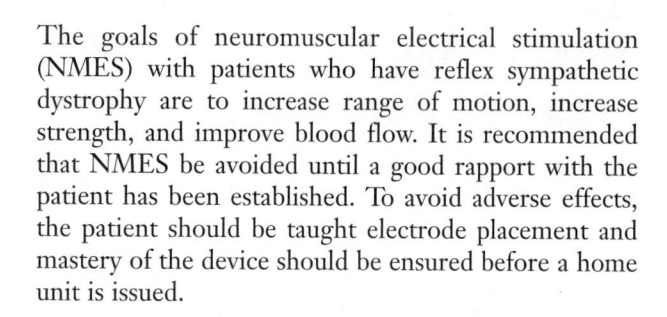

The goals of neuromuscular electrical stimulation (NMES) with patients who have reflex sympathetic dystrophy are to increase range of motion, increase strength, and improve blood flow. It is recommended that NMES be avoided until a good rapport with the patient has been established. To avoid adverse effects, the patient should be taught electrode placement and mastery of the device should be ensured before a home unit is issued.

Answer: **True**
Hareau, p. 368

9. When using transcutaneous electrical nerve stimulation for patients with reflex sympathetic dystrophy, the burst mode is recommended to avoid accommodation. True or False?

The burst mode avoids accommodation of fibers, allowing prolonged use of the machine. Transcutaneous electrical nerve stimulation (TENS) can be a beneficial adjunct to therapy; however, if the patient becomes dependent on the device, its use should be gradually discontinued. There is controversy in the literature regarding the effects of TENS on sympathetic activity. Other TENS settings that have been used successfully in the treatment of reflex sympathetic dystrophy include conventional and brief intense settings. Additional research is needed in this area.

Answer: **True**
Hareau, p. 378
Hunter, Mackin, Callahan, p. 821

> **CLINICAL GEM:**
> High-voltage galvanic stimulation is helpful in managing edema in patients with reflex sympathetic dystrophy. It also provides a residual transcutaneous electrical nerve stimulation effect.

> **CLINICAL GEM:**
> Vasodilation occurs with the use of burst transcutaneous electrical nerve stimulation (TENS), whereas vasoconstriction occurs with the use of brief intense TENS. Therefore, a patient's vascular status should be assessed in order to pick the most appropriate TENS.

10. Which modality is most helpful in treating a patient with reflex sympathetic dystrophy who presents with a vasodilated hand?

A. Thermal biofeedback
B. Fluidotherapy
C. Burst transcutaneous electrical nerve stimulation
D. Hot pack
E. All of the above

When a patient is vasodilated, he or she presents with a red, swollen, and warm hand. The treatment goal for this patient is to create vasoconstriction. Thermal biofeedback is advocated to treat the vasodilated or vasoconstricted condition. Other vasoconstrictors include ice and brief intense TENS. All other answers above are used to promote vasodilation in a patient presenting with vasoconstriction.

Answer: **A**
Hunter, Mackin, Callahan, pp. 805, 823

11. Splinting of patients with reflex sympathetic dystrophy should:

A. Not be performed
B. Be of low force to avoid exacerbation of pain
C. Be of moderate force to overcome contractures
D. Be of high force in short intervals

Splinting is a helpful adjunct in the treatment of reflex sympathetic dystrophy as long as it is used with a low force to avoid pain exacerbation. Low-load dynamic or static progressive splinting is proposed to alleviate discomfort through stimulation of large-diameter fibers if used at the appropriate force levels.

Answer: **B**
Hunter, Mackin, Callahan, p. 827

12. A therapist may cause pain through gentle touch in patients with reflex sympathetic dystrophy. True or False?

Traditionally, therapists are "high touch" clinicians who use their hands to facilitate healing. However, the hands-off approach is best when treating patients with reflex sympathetic dystrophy. If contact is used, continuous, firm "touch" is recommended because light touch or gentle stimuli can increase temporal summation of pain.

Temporal summation can occur with three-second interval tactile stimulation or with monofilament testing performed at three-second intervals. To avoid causing this phenomena, do not repetitively remove hands from the surface of the skin during massage or tactile stimulation. When treating reflex sympathetic dystrophy, the patient should remain in control of all movements to help reduce anxiety and pain. Minimal manipulation of the symptomatic extremity is important. To avoid touching the patient's painful extremity during passive range-of-motion exercises, a self-inflatable splint (long arm air cast) allows continuous pressure over the extremity and avoids direct hand contact.

Answer: **True**
Hardy, pp. 143-145
Hareau, p. 379
Hunter, Mackin, Callahan, p. 825
Refer to Fig. 12-3.

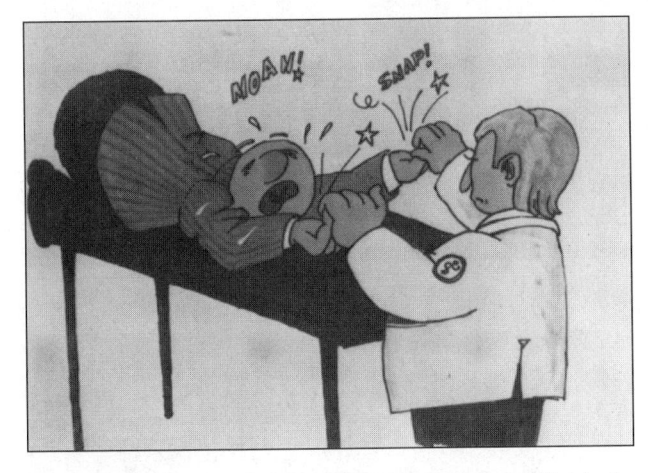

Fig. 12-3 ■ Painful manipulations should be strictly avoided in the treatment of reflex sympathetic dystrophy because these patients are hypersensitive to pain and any painful manipulation creates a "vicious pain cycle." (From Hunter JM, Mackin EJ, Callahan AD: *Rehabilitation of the hand: surgery and therapy,* ed 4, St. Louis, 1995, Mosby-Year Book.)

13. You have a patient who has difficulty grooming and washing her face because of reflex sympathetic dystrophy. All of the following should be included in your initial plan of care, except:

A. Instructing the patient to walk daily
B. Range-of-motion exercises with proximal joints, progressing distally
C. Informing the patient that intense pain is expected during range-of-motion exercises
D. Stress-loading program

The therapist should never elicit pain while achieving gains in range-of-motion exercises; therefore, answer C is incorrect. Initial goals are to teach relaxation techniques and gain the patient's trust. Next, gentle range-of-motion exercises, proximal to distal, are begun. A walking protocol should be incorporated to help increase range of motion and circulatory flow because this is necessary for muscle performance. Muscles deprived of oxygen fatigue easily and eventually do not contract. A stress-loading program is appropriate when treating patients with reflex sympathetic dystrophy.

Answer: **C**
Hareau, p. 368
Hardy, Hardy, p. 145

14. In patients with reflex sympathetic dystrophy, it is helpful to treat edema preventatively because interstitial fluid volume can increase 30% to 50% above normal before it is visibly noted. True or False?

It is helpful to begin edema control in a preventative fashion because interstitial fluid volume can increase 30% to 50% before visual detection. Edema should be controlled early and management should be continuous, with the use of various pressure techniques. Edema management techniques include elevation, active exercise, retrograde massage (in patients with reflex sympathetic dystrophy, it is important to maintain continuous contact to avoid temporal summation of pain), intermittent compression, and edema control garments.

Answer: **True**
Hunter, Mackin, Callahan, p. 824

CHAPTER 12 Reflex Sympathetic Dystrophy

15. Continuous passive motion is contraindicated in patients with reflex sympathetic dystrophy. True or False?

Continuous passive motion can be used safely in patients with reflex sympathetic dystrophy as long as it is used in a painfree range. It is helpful in reducing pain through stimulation of large, diameter fibers.

Answer: **False**
Hunter, Mackin, Callahan, p. 828

16. Which is the least common form of reflex sympathetic dystrophy?

A. Minor causalgia
B. Minor traumatic dystrophy
C. Shoulder-hand dystrophy
D. Major traumatic dystrophy
E. Major causalgia

Shoulder-hand dystrophy is the least common form of reflex sympathetic dystrophy. This dystrophy typically starts with pain and stiffness in the shoulder, which spreads to the entire extremity. Causes of shoulder-hand dystrophy include: proximal trauma to the shoulder, neck, or rib cage; visceral organ pathology; strokes; stomach ulcers; and Pancoast tumors in the lung. Patients present with fusiform (tapering at both ends) swelling in the fingers, with the digits stiffened in extension. Therapists must be careful not to confuse this diagnosis with "frozen shoulder syndrome." In a shoulder-hand dystrophy, the degree of pain, swelling, stiffness, dysfunction, and osteoporosis is much greater than in frozen shoulder syndrome.

Interestingly, minor traumatic dystrophy is the most common clinical form of reflex sympathetic dystrophy. This form is most common because it does not involve a specific nerve and also because minor traumas are more common than major traumas.

Answer: **C**
Hunter, Mackin, Callahan, pp. 784-786, 797

17. The stress-loading program for patients with reflex sympathetic dystrophy:

A. Should be avoided during the early stages because it can increase the patient's pain.
B. Is a passive program directed and administered by the therapist.
C. Consists of active exercises that require stressful use of the entire upper extremity with minimal joint motion.
D. Uses exercises such as scrubbing, carrying, and passive stretching.

Stress-loading is a program that consists of active exercises that require stressful use of the entire upper extremity with minimal joint motion. It uses scrubbing (Fig. 12-4, *A*) and carrying (Fig. 12-4, *B*) activities. It is not a passive program and is best used early in the rehabilitation of patients with reflex sympathetic dystrophy. According to Watson and Carlson, this is the treatment of choice; however, pain and swelling may increase before effectiveness is noted.

Answer: **C**
Carlson, Watson, pp. 149-153

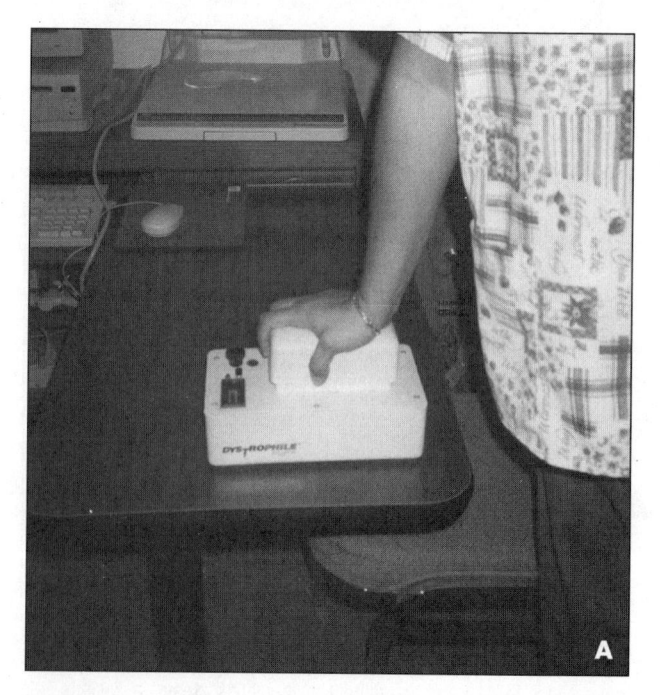

Fig. 12-4
Continued

CHAPTER 12 Reflex Sympathetic Dystrophy 149

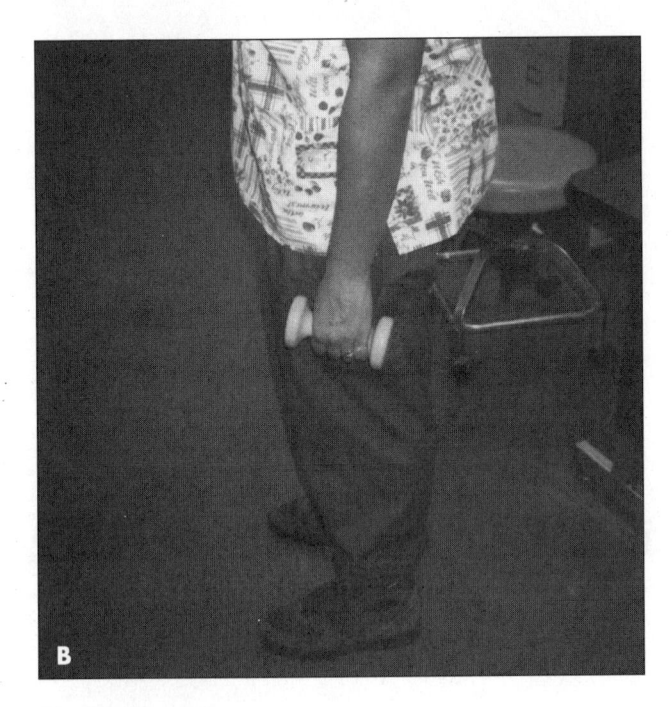

Fig. 12-4, cont'd

18. All patients with reflex sympathetic dystrophy have severe pain. True or False?

Some patients with reflex sympathetic dystrophy may not have any pain. When pain does occur, it has two basic components, which are sensory-discriminative and affective-motivational. Evaluation of pain is important because it provides a baseline by which to measure progress. A body diagram should be included for the patient to complete.

Answer: **False**
Hunter, Mackin, Callahan, p. 818

19. Which of the following statement(s) is/are true about sympathetic blockade in the cervical/thoracic region?

A. It is also called a stellate ganglion block.
B. Patients notice an immediate change in the condition of their hands or extremities.
C. The development of a Horner's syndrome is a sign of a successful block.
D. All of the above are true.

After sympathetic blockade (stellate ganglion block), patients notice immediate changes in the condition of their hands or extremities. A patient should be observed for 1 hour after injection to monitor vital signs for complications and to assess the block outcome. Successful sympathetic blockade is indicated by the development of an ipsilateral Horner's syndrome (Fig. 12-5) with conjunctival redness, a temperature increase of the ipsilateral upper extremity of 2°, and enophthalmos (see Chapter 4, question 22 for definitions).

Answer: **D**
Lennard, pp. 254-259
Hunter, Mackin, Callahan, p. 797

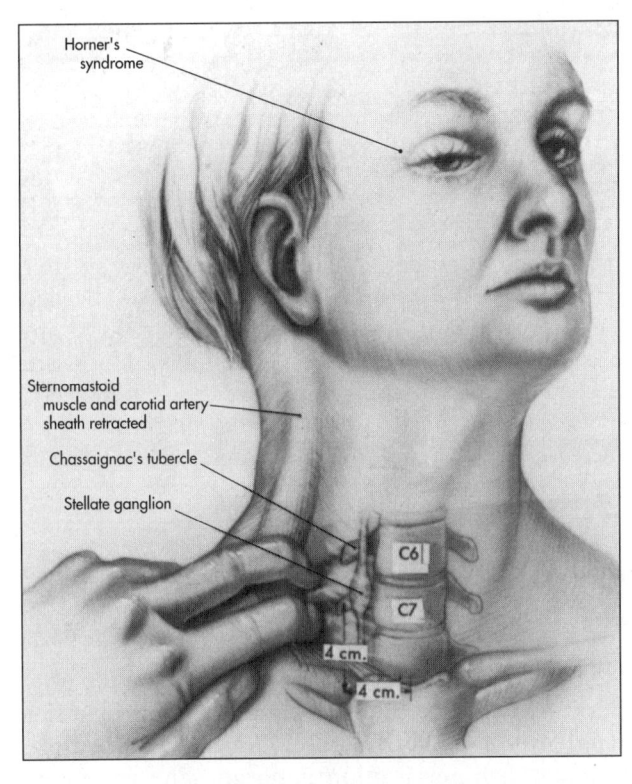

Fig. 12-5 ■ Modified from Lankford LL, Thompson JE: *Reflex sympathetic dystrophy, upper and lower extremity: diagnosis and management.* In American Academy of Orthopaedic Surgeons: instructional course lectures, vol 26, St. Louis, 1977, C.V. Mosby.

20. After a stellate ganglion nerve block, when should therapy be initiated?

A. Immediately
B. 24 hours later
C. 3 to 5 days later
D. Therapy is not indicated; the block will resolve the symptoms.

Therapy should begin immediately after the block is administered. During this painfree state, gentle passive exercises can be performed as long as they do not exacerbate symptoms. Active functional use of the hand is emphasized during this time.

Answer: **A**
Hunter, Mackin, Callahan, p. 831

21. What is the average number of blocks needed to assist in the reversal of an abnormal sympathetic reflex?

A. One to two
B. Four to five
C. 10 to 15
D. More than 20

It is rare for a patient to have a complete reversal after only one block. The average number of blocks needed for a reversal of an abnormal sympathetic reflex is approximately four or five. Occasionally more blocks are needed to reverse the disease process. Sympathetic blockade is most effective when the diagnosis is detected early, such as within the first 3 to 4 months of onset.

Answer: **B**
Hunter, Mackin, Callahan, p. 797

22. A patient presents in your clinic with pain, tenderness, swelling, stiffness, and discoloration in the hand after a Colles' fracture. During a radiograph, osseous demineralization is noted. The patient is sent for a sympathetic blockade and afterward has a significant reduction in pain. What is the diagnosis for this patient?

A. Carpal tunnel syndrome
B. Fictitious lymphedema
C. Madelung's disease
D. Reflex sympathetic dystrophy

If a patient has a significant resolution of signs and symptoms after a sympathetic blockade, the diagnosis of reflex sympathetic dystrophy is confirmed. Symptom resolution may not be long-lasting; more than one block often is needed. A stellate ganglion block is a reliable, specific test for reflex sympathetic dystrophy. Other testing modalities are nonspecific tests for reflex sympathetic dystrophy.

Answer: **D**
Hunter, Mackin, Callahan, pp. 788-790

23. Reflex sympathetic dystrophy in children:

A. Involves females more than males
B. Can be treated with conservative treatment, including cognitive and behavioral treatments, transcutaneous electrical nerve stimulation, tricyclic antidepressants, and/or neural blockade
C. Is best treated with corticosteroids
D. B and C
E. A and B

The mean age of children who have reflex sympathetic dystrophy was found to be 12.5 years and 84% were females. Children's responses to treatment for reflex sympathetic dystrophy are highly variable and difficult to predict. Therapy has been reported by many to be the mainstay of treatment. Transcutaneous electrical nerve stimulation has been described as a highly effective treatment. Sympathetic blocks are appropriate when the patient has a clear clinical diagnosis of reflex sympathetic dystrophy. Some patients respond to a multidisciplinary program that includes therapy and behavioral management. Most children with reflex sympathetic dystrophy do not benefit from the use of corticosteroids.

Answer: **E**
Wilder et al, pp. 910-919

24. Select the terms that are synonymous with reflex sympathetic dystrophy.

A. Causalgia
B. Algodystrophy
C. Posttraumatic dystrophy
D. Sudeck's atrophy
E. Pourfour del petit syndrome
F. Shoulder-hand syndrome
G. Postinfarctional sclerodactyly
H. Complex regional pain syndrome

All the above, A through H, are synonymous with the term reflex sympathetic dystrophy.

Answer: **A through H**
Lyckle van der Laan, Goris, p. 379

25. Which term was implemented in 1993 to replace the term reflex sympathetic dystrophy?

- **A.** Causalgia
- **B.** Sympathetic maintained pain
- **C.** Complex regional pain syndrome
- **D.** Sympathetically independent pain

In Orlando in 1993, the American Pain Society determined the need for a revision of the taxonomic system. The new nomenclature, complex regional pain syndrome (CRPS), was developed to replace the terms reflex sympathetic dystrophy (RSD) and causalgia.

Two types of CRPS have been recognized: type one corresponds to RSD and type two corresponds to causalgia. The terms sympathetic maintained pain (SMP) and sympathetically independent pain (SIP) were not considered separate disorders but descriptors of types of pain. SMP and SIP can be found in a variety of pain disorders, including CRPS types one and two.

Answer: **C**
Wong, Wilson, pp. 319-325

Chapter 13

Tendons

Topics to be reviewed in random order are:

- **Tendon anatomy**
- **Flexor and extensor tendon zones**
- **Tendon healing**
- **Nutritional pathways**
- **Surgical and suture techniques**
- **Rehabilitation of tendon injuries**
- **Widely accepted protocol techniques**
- **Tenolysis**

1. Match each extensor zone with its correct definition:

Zone

1. Zone I
2. Zone II
3. Zone III
4. Zone IV
5. Zone V
6. Zone VI
7. Zone VII
8. Zone VIII

Definition

A. Extensor retinaculum
B. Central slip
C. Distal to extensor retinaculum to just proximal to the metacarpophalangeal joint
D. Terminal tendon
E. Proximal to extensor retinaculum
F. Triangular tendon (middle phalanx)
G. Sagittal bands
H. Distal to sagittal bands and proximal to central slip

Answers: **1. D; 2. F; 3. B; 4. H; 5. G; 6. C; 7. A; 8. E**

Thomas, Moutet, Guinard, p. 309
Hunter, Schneider, Mackin, p. 547
Refer to Fig. 13-1.

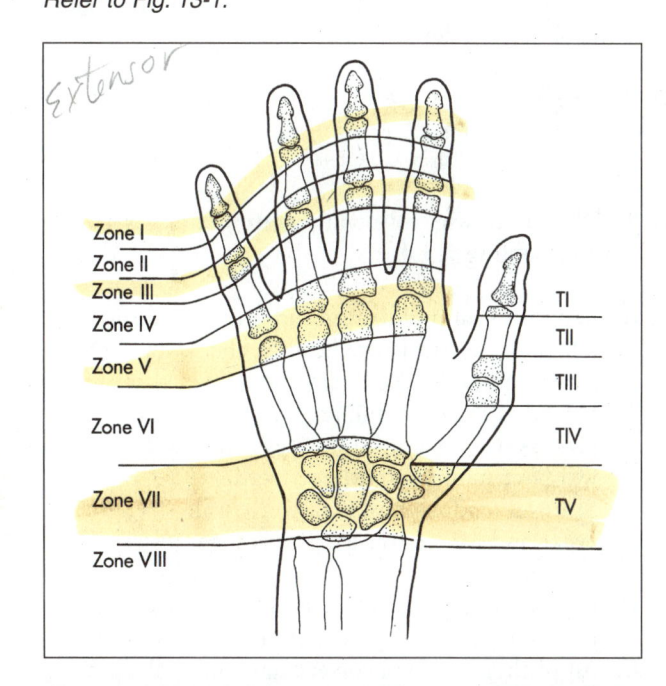

Fig. 13-1 ■ From Wilson RL: *Management of acute extensor tendon injuries.* In Hunter JM, Schneider LH, Mackin EJ, editors: *Tendon surgery in the hand,* St. Louis, 1987, Mosby.

CLINICAL GEM:
Zones I, III, V, and VII (excluding the thumb) all correspond with joints:
- Zone I - distal interphalangeal joint
- Zone III - proximal interphalangeal joint
- Zone V - metacarpophalangeal joint
- Zone VII - wrist joint

CLINICAL GEM:
The thumb generally is classified into five extensor zones (TI; TII; TIII; TIV; and TV; see Fig. 13-1).

2. How many pulleys are in the thumb?

A. two
B. three
C. four
D. five

The thumb has one oblique pulley overlying the proximal phalanx and two annular pulleys. The A1 pulley is just proximal to the metacarpophalangeal joint and the A2 pulley is at the volar plate of the distal interphalangeal joint. The most important pulley in the thumb is the oblique pulley.

Answer: **B**
Hunter, Schneider, Mackin, p. 269
Hunter, Mackin, Callahan, pp. 418-419

3. Which of the following statements regarding tendon healing is false?

A. Tendons heal by intrinsic and extrinsic means. The more intrinsic the healing, the fewer the adhesions.
B. If tendon repair is not stressed, the healing process may take up to 8 weeks and the tendons will have minimal tensile strength.
C. Stressed tendons heal and gain tensile strength faster and have fewer adhesions than unstressed tendons.
D. Repair strength usually decreases by 30% to 50% between 1 and 2 days after repair (unstressed).
E. All of the above are correct statements about tendons.

Statement D is incorrect. One or two days after repair, the tendon is at its strongest. Repair strength in the unstressed tendon usually decreases by 10% to 50% between 5 and 21 days after repair.

Answer: **D**
Hunter, Schneider, Mackin, p. 354

4. Match each flexor zone with its correct description:

Zone
1. Zone I
2. Zone II
3. Zone III
4. Zone IV
5. Zone V

Description
A. The A1 pulley to the insertion of the flexor digitorum superficialis
B. Proximal to the carpal tunnel
C. From the insertion of the flexor digitorum superficialis at the middle phalanx to the flexor digitorum profundus at the distal phalanx
D. From the distal end of the carpal tunnel to the first annular ligament
E. The carpal tunnel

Answers: **1. C; 2. A; 3. D; 4. E; 5. B**
Hunter, Mackin, Callahan, p. 420
Refer to Fig. 13-2.

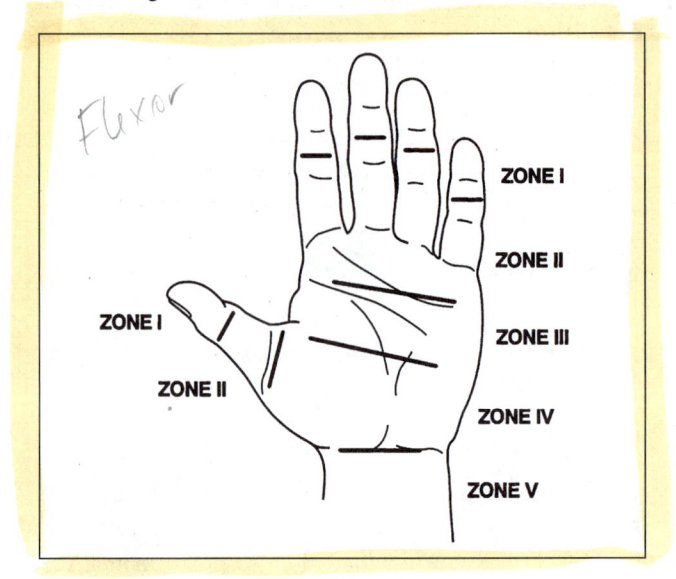

Fig. 13-2 ■ From Hunter JM, Mackin EJ, Callahan AD: *Rehabilitation of the hand: surgery and therapy,* ed 4, St. Louis, 1995, Mosby-Year Book.

5. Intrinsic tendon healing suggests that surrounding peritendinous adhesions allow healing of the tendon. True or False?

The **extrinsic** healing theory suggests that peritendinous adhesions allow healing of the tendon. The sequence of healing by extrinsic means is through the ingrowth of capillaries and fibroblasts during the first 4 days after the injury, followed by the formation of collagen at 4 to 21 days and scar remodeling after 21 days. The theory of **intrinsic** healing suggests that healing occurs in the absence of cells and tissue extrinsic to the tendon. Intrinsic healing occurs between the tendon ends. Tendon healing probably is a combination of extrinsic and intrinsic cellular activity. Theoretically, if more intrinsic healing occurs, fewer adhesions are formed.

Answer: **False**
Hunter, Mackin, Callahan, p. 419

6. What is the major nutritional pathway for extensor tendons underneath the extensor retinaculum?

A. Vascular perfusion
B. Synovial diffusion
C. Vincula
D. All of the above are equally involved in extensor tendon nutrition.

Synovial diffusion is the major nutritional pathway for the extensor tendons beneath the extensor retinaculum. Extensor tendons also receive their blood supply through vascular mesenteries or mesotendons. Vascular perfusion through the mesotendons provides 30% of nutrition, and synovial diffusion, the major nutritional pathway, provides 70%.

Answer: **B**
Hunter, Mackin, Callahan, pp. 520-521

7. Which flexor zone was referred to by Bunnell as "no man's land"?

A. Zone I
B. Zone II
C. Zone III
D. Zone IV
E. Zone V

Bunnell coined the term "no man's land" for the zone II portion of the flexor system because of the extreme difficulty in obtaining a good result with primary repair of tendons lacerated in this area. More recently, the classically termed "no man's land" is now termed "some man's land" (see Fig. 13-2).

Answer: **B**
Green, p. 1836

8. The vincula are folds of mesotendon carrying blood supply to the flexor tendons. True or False?

One way flexor tendons receive their blood supply is from the vincula, which are folds of the mesotendon. The vincular system exits on the dorsal surface of the tendons and is supplied by transverse communicating branches of the common digital artery. If the vincula are uninjured after tendon damage, clinical results are better than in cases in which the vincula are injured.

Answer: **True**
Green, p. 1826
Hunter, Schneider, Mackin, pp. 278-285
Hunter, Mackin, Callahan, p. 413
Refer to Fig. 13-3.

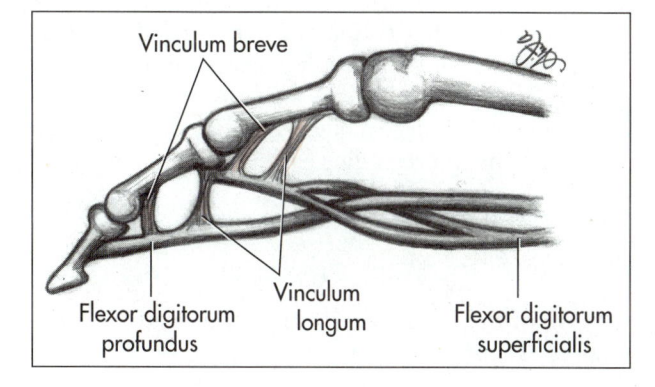

Fig. 13-3

9. Early motion programs of controlled stress for flexor tendon repairs are used to decrease tendon adhesions. According to Duran, how much tendon glide is needed to prevent adhesions from forming?

A. 2 to 3 mm
B. 3 to 5 mm
C. 4 to 5 mm
D. 5 to 6 mm

Duran recommends 3 to 5 mm of tendon glide to minimize tendon adhesion, and Gelberman indicates that 3 to 4 mm of tendon glide decreases gap formation in flexor tendon repairs.

Answer: **B**
Green, p. 1830
Hunter, Schneider, Mackin, p. 335

10. A core suture alone can withstand early active motion without gap formation or rupture. True or False?

Active motion puts forces on the repair site that are greater than a core suture can withstand alone. With the addition of a running epitenon suture, tensile strength of the repair is increased and early active motion can be performed more safely. It is important to note that this data is generated from cadaver tendons and does not account for the decreased pullout strength of the tendon ends (which occurs 4 to 10 days after surgery), the effect of cyclic stress, gap formation, or the effect of tendon sheath dissection. Some authors indicate that a core suture with epitendinous repair is not able to tolerate full fisting and recommend modified fisting instead. More research is needed in this area in order to provide our patients with safe early active motion programs. Refer to question 28 in chapter 13 for more information regarding early active motion.

Answer: **False**
Hunter, Schneider, Mackin, p. 322

11. All of the following are true about suture techniques except:

A. The strength of a tendon repair is roughly proportionate to the number of suture strands crossing the repair.
B. A six-strand repair is technically difficult for the physician.
C. A peripheral epitendinous suture reduces tendency toward gap formation.
D. All of the above are true about suture techniques.

All of the above comments are applicable to suture techniques. The number of strands crossing the repair site is roughly proportional to the strength of the tendon repair; thus a two-strand repair is weaker than a four- or six-strand repair. Four- and six-strand repairs increase strength, but add technical difficulty for the surgeon and increase the volume of suture material in the repair site. With horizontal mattress, or running locked peripheral epitendinous sutures with four- and six-strand repairs, therapists enjoy the relative safety of both passive and light active digital motion during the entire healing process in an unswollen digit. A peripheral epitendinous suture repair assists in increasing repair strength and reduces the tendency toward gap formation at the repair site. The therapist must consult the surgeon regarding the type of repair used on the patient.

Answer: **D**
Hunter, Schneider, Mackin, p. 354

12. Camper's chiasm is where the:

A. Central slip inserts
B. Two flexor digitorum superficialis slips reunite
C. Flexor digitorum profundus splits
D. Terminal tendon inserts

Camper's chiasm is where the two flexor digitorum superficialis slips reunite. This intersection of fibers is similar to the intersection of the neurofibers of the chiasm opticum of the second cranial nerve. The chiasma of Camper (also called the chiasma tendinum of Camper or Camper's chiasm) forms a plate underneath the flexor profundus and can be lifted off the periosteum and the capsule of the proximal interphalangeal joint.

Answer: **B**
Hunter, Mackin, Callahan, p. 417
Hunter, Schneider, Mackin, pp. 245, 250
Spinner, p. 63
Refer to Fig. 13-4.

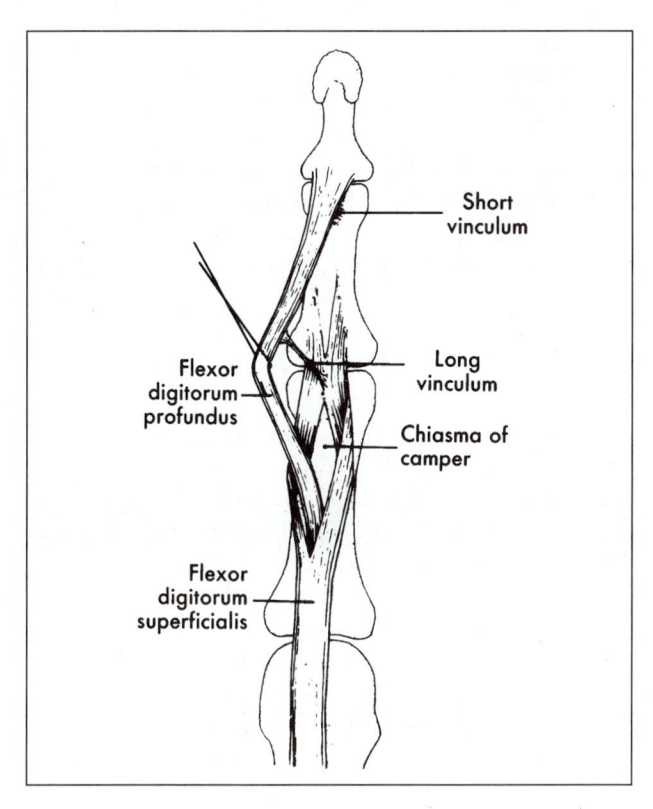

Fig. 13-4 ■ From Schneider LH: *Flexor tendon injuries,* Boston, 1985, Little Brown. Reproduced by permission.

13. When does a tendon have the least tensile strength after it is surgically repaired?

A. 4 to 5 days
B. The first day
C. 10 to 14 days
D. 16 to 21 days

A tendon has the least tensile strength 4 to 5 days after surgical repair secondary to softening of the tendon ends. Its tensile strength is greater on the first day after repair. From days 5 to 21, tensile strength increases as the collagen matures and cross-linking continues. Recent studies indicate that a decrease in tensile strength may not occur with early *active* motion programs such as those used at the Indiana Hand Center.

Answer: **A**
Strickland, pp. 30-41
Hunter, Mackin, Callahan, p. 438

14. The flexor digitorum superficialis in the small finger is absent in which percentage of the population?

A. 5%
B. 21%
C. 42%
D. 60%

The flexor digitorum superficialis of the small finger is variable and is absent in 21% of the population. It is important to note, however, that when the flexor digitorum superficialis and flexor digitorum profundus are lacerated, it is necessary to repair both tendons. Advantages of repairing and maintaining both tendons include maintenance of the vincular blood supply, retention of a smooth gliding surface for the flexor digitorum profundus, and the reduced possibility of hyperextension deformities at the proximal interphalangeal joint.

CLINICAL GEM:
Some authors report that the flexor digitorum superficialis has a slip to the flexor digitorum profundus; not allowing for independent flexor digitorum superficialis glide; mimicking the absence of the flexor digitorum superficialis tendon.

Answer: **B**
Hunter, Mackin, Callahan, pp. 420-421

15. Which muscle is able to extend the interphalangeal joint of the thumb despite a rupture of the extensor pollicis longus?

A. The extensor pollicis brevis
B. The abductor pollicis longus
C. The abductor pollicis brevis
D. All of the above

Despite an extensor pollicis longus rupture, the interphalangeal joint can be extended by the intrinsic muscles through their contribution to the dorsal apparatus. The abductor pollicis brevis contributes to interphalangeal joint extension. The most disabling impairment after a rupture of the extensor pollicis longus is extension loss at the metacarpophalangeal joint. Retroposition, which is the ability to lift the thumb off the table into the extended position, also is lost.

Answer: **C**
Hunter, Mackin, Callahan, p. 551

16. A pullout suture using a button is a helpful procedure in which scenario?

A. When the distal flexor digitorum profundus stump is extremely short after laceration
B. When both tendons are cut in zone II
C. When both slips of the flexor digitorum superficialis are cut and epitendinous repair is not appropriate
D. None of the above

When a patient sustains a laceration of the flexor digitorum profundus and the distal stump is short or nonexistent, the tendon must be repaired to the distal phalanx. The suture is pulled through both the radial and ulnar aspects of the bone, exiting through the nail plate, and tied over the nail with a button (Fig. 13-5). The pullout suture and button are removed 4 to 6 weeks after repair. Rehabilitation with the button is the same as rehabilitation without the button for zone-I tendon repairs.

Answer: **A**
Hunter, Mackin, Callahan, pp. 423-424

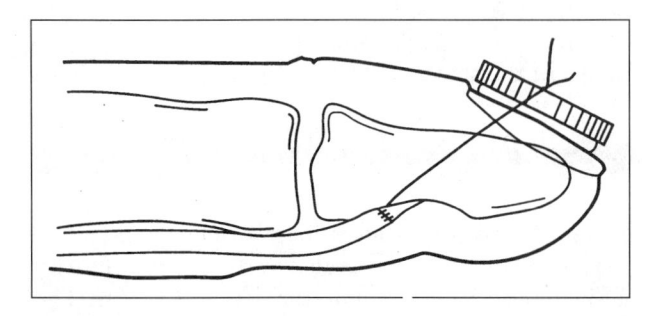

Fig. 13-5 ■ From Hunter JM, Mackin EJ, Callahan AD: *Rehabilitation of the hand: surgery and therapy,* ed 4, St. Louis, 1995, Mosby-Year Book.

> **CLINICAL GEM:**
> Although a Kleinert program can be used with the application of the hook onto the button, it often is easier to use a Duran protocol for this repair. Evans has developed a specific protocol for zone-I repairs. For details on this protocol, consult Hunter, Mackin, Callahan, pages 454 and 455.

17. A 21-year-old lawn worker complains of an inability to flex his ring finger after his pull-start lawn mower backfired. Radiographs confirm an intraarticular fracture of the distal phalanx with rupture of the profundus insertion. The fragment involves less than 10% of the articular surface of the distal phalanx. Appropriate treatment would include:

A. Cast immobilization of the hand in a functional position
B. Dynamic flexion-assist splinting for 3 weeks to see whether the tendon heals in the appropriate position
C. Repair of the flexor tendon after excision of the fragment and Bunnell pullout-wire technique
D. All of the above

Repair of the flexor tendon using a Bunnell pullout-wire is the appropriate technique in this case. Often a fragment involving less than 10% of the articular surface can be excised and the tendon can be repaired directly into the defect. Splint immobilization and/or casting are not indicated until after the flexor tendon has been repaired.

Answer: **C**
Schneider, pp. 277-285

18. Which protocol emphasizes controlled passive motion to treat flexor tendon injuries?

A. Kleinert
B. Duran
C. The Washington regime
D. McLean

Duran and Houser described a controlled passive motion program for flexor tendons in 1975 and 1978. In this program, they permitted proximal interphalangeal and distal interphalangeal joints to be passively exercised to impart tendon glide of the repaired tendons. In contrast, Hernandez, Emery, and Kleinert developed a technique in the late 1950s that has been widely adopted with many variations. With this technique, elastic bands are attached to the patient's fingers and the patient is permitted to actively extend the fingers within the confines of the splint as the elastic band passively returns the fingers to the palm.

Answer: **B**
Strickland, p. 71

19. Patients who "cheat" on their passive mobilization programs usually rupture their tendons. True or False?

Hand therapists often observe their patients "cheating" on their passive mobilization programs by actively flexing either during the passive exercises or inadvertently flexing between their exercise sessions. Contrary to our fears, many of these patients do exceptionally well. This raises the question of whether light active flexor muscle contraction is beneficial.

Answer: **False**
Hunter, Schneider, Mackin, p. 336

20. Your patient is a 30-year-old woman status post flexor digitorum profundus repair in zone I of the middle finger. You note decreased tendon glide 7 weeks after surgery. You decide to teach home exercises to increase tendon glide. Which exercise provides the maximum profundus tendon excursion?

A. Straight fist
B. Full fist
C. Hook fist
D. All of the above provide equal profundus excursion

The full-fist position provides maximum profundus tendon excursion. The straight-fist position provides maximum superficialis tendon excursion. The hook-fist position provides maximum differential gliding between the flexor digitorum profundus and flexor digitorum superficialis tendons. Maximum tendon and joint motion can be obtained with tendon gliding exercises.

Answer: **B**
Wehbe, p. 164
Hunter, Mackin, Callahan, p. 443
Refer to Fig. 13-6.

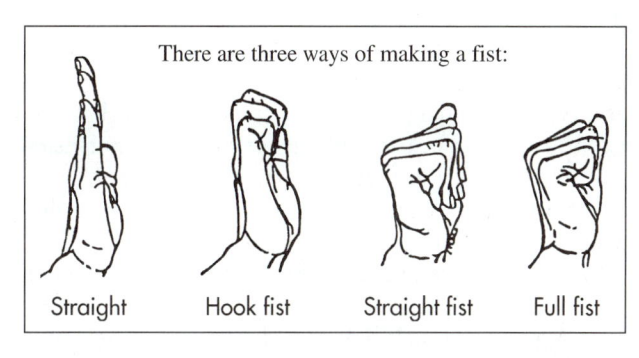

Fig. 13-6 ■ From Hunter JM, Mackin EJ, Callahan AD: *Rehabilitation of the hand: surgery and therapy,* ed 4, St. Louis, 1995, Mosby-Year Book.

21. In traditional management of an extensor tendon zone-III acute closed injury (no surgery performed), the patient is treated with which protocol?

A. Immobilization of the proximal interphalangeal joint at 0° for 3 weeks
B. Immobilization of the proximal interphalangeal joint at 0° for 6 weeks
C. Immobilization of the proximal interphalangeal joint slightly flexed to 10° for 3 weeks
D. Immobilization of the proximal interphalangeal joint slightly flexed to 10° for 6 weeks

Most authors recommend that traditional management of a zone III acute closed injury be managed with uninterrupted immobilization of the proximal interphalangeal joint at 0° for 6 weeks. Injuries requiring surgical repair are mobilized earlier—sometimes as early as 3 to 4 weeks—with protective splinting between exercise sessions. It is critical for the splint to be positioned with the proximal interphalangeal joint at absolute 0 to avoid gapping of the tendon in an elongated position.

Answer: **B**
Hunter, Mackin, Callahan, pp. 576-579

160 CHAPTER 13 Tendons

22. One method of treating a central slip extensor tendon surgical repair (zone III) is to begin early proximal interphalangeal joint motion within 1 week. True or False?

Thomes and Thomes advocate an early motion protocol using a hand-based dynamic extension splint with a lumbrical stop for central slip tendon repairs. The splint positions the metacarpophalangeal joint at 20° of flexion with the proximal interphalangeal joint at neutral to slight hyperextension. Evans advocates short arc motion using template splints for proximal and distal interphalangeal joint exercise sessions and resting the proximal interphalangeal joint and distal interphalangeal joint at absolute 0° between exercising.

In general, both protocols allow for 30° of proximal interphalangeal joint flexion during the first 2 weeks, with a progression of 10° for each following week, providing that no extensor lag develops. Some authors advocate no range-of-motion restrictions at the proximal interphalangeal joint as early as week 4; others advocate some degree of caution until week 6.

Answer: **True**
Thomes, Thomes, p. 195
Hunter, Mackin, Callahan, p. 383

23. Distal interphalangeal joint flexion exercises can be advocated within the first week after a central slip extensor tendon surgical repair. True or False?

Distal interphalangeal joint flexion exercises, with the proximal interphalangeal joint at absolute zero, are advocated within the first week unless the lateral bands are involved. If the lateral bands are involved, distal interphalangeal joint flexion is delayed until approximately the fourth week after surgery.

Answer: **True**
Maddy, Meyerdierks, p. 207
Hunter, Mackin, Callahan, p. 578

24. You are treating a patient with an extensor tendon repair to the ring finger in zone VI, just distal to the extensor retinaculum. Which of the following would be an appropriate splint?

A. Forearm-based splint, with wrist in extension, including the ring finger only
B. Hand-based splint extending the ring finger only
C. Forearm-based splint, with wrist in extension, including the middle, ring, and little fingers
D. Forearm-based splint, with wrist in slight flexion, including the middle, ring, and little fingers

---

A zone VI repair just distal to the extensor retinaculum requires a forearm-based splint with the wrist in 30 to 40 of extension and with the middle, ring, and little fingers extended. Many static and dynamic splinting protocols with varying degrees of wrist and digit extension are used. It is important to consider the juncturae tendinum, which are interconnections between the extensor communis on the dorsum of the hand. If the repair is proximal to the juncturae tendinum (Fig. 13-7), as in this situation, it is necessary to splint the affected and adjacent digits in extension to eliminate stress on the repair site. If the repair is distal to the juncturae tendinum, only the affected digit must be splinted, and the adjacent fingers can be splinted with the metacarpophalangeal joints at 30° of flexion and interphalangeal joints free. This position reduces stress at the repair site as it permits advancement of the proximal end of the severed tendon.

Answer: **C**
Thomas, Moutet, Guinard, p. 310
Hunter, Mackin, Callahan, p. 588

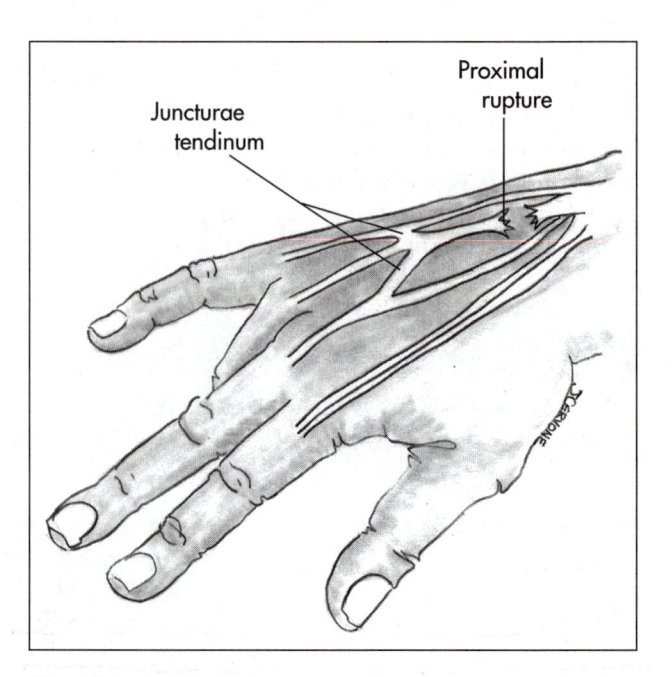

Fig. 13-7

25. A patient you have been treating status post flexor tendon repair is preparing for another surgery. This patient has joint contractures that have not responded to therapy, an extensive amount of scar tissue, and an obvious loss of the pulley system as indicated by bowstringing. Which surgical procedure is most likely indicated for this patient?

A. Tenolysis
B. Reconstruction of the pulleys
C. Placement of a silicone tendon implant with reconstruction of the pulleys
D. Surgery is not a good option for this patient.

Placement of a Silicone tendon implant would be a preparatory stage to allow for the formation of a favorable bed for tendon grafting. This procedure, which is a two stage reconstruction, is indicated when the patient's original trauma was from a crushing injury and is characterized by an underlying fracture or overlying skin damage; when a patient displays excessive scarring of the tendon bed; when prior surgery has failed; when complications from a healed infection occur; when there is significant loss of the pulley system; or when joint restrictions with contractures are not responsive to therapy.

In 1965, Hunter first published his personal experience with the tendon implant. In stage one, the Silicone implant is placed in the hand and the pulley system is reconstructed. The implant is left in place for 3 months to allow a new bed to form. In stage two, the implant is removed and a long tendon graft is placed in the newly-formed sheath. This procedure is demanding and requires the postoperative care of a skilled hand therapist.

Answer: **C**
Hunter, Schneider, Mackin, pp. 518-521

26. The use of immediate active motion is a new technique that is widely accepted in clinical practice. True or False?

The use of immediate active motion is not a new or widely accepted technique. It is, however, a subject of renewed interest. Stronger suture techniques that are designed for active motion have now been developed. Early active motion with current popular suture techniques has not been recommended because most clinicians believe that these repairs do not provide enough tensile strength (with adequate safety margins) to tolerate the forces of full active motion.

Answer: **False**
Evans, Thompson, p. 266

27. A 6-year-old patient is referred to you for splinting 3 days after surgery for flexor tendon repair. Which of the following protocols would be most appropriate in this situation?

A. Immobilization splinting for 3 to 4 weeks
B. Kleinert protocol with traction to the fingers
C. Duran protocol with protected dorsal blocking splint
D. Early active motion protocol

Immobilization protocols are the treatment of choice for patients younger than 10 years of age, patients with cognitive deficits, or patients who for any other reason are clearly unable or unwilling to participate in a rehabilitation program. Frequently the patient is casted for 3 to 4 weeks postoperatively. He or she may, however, be referred for an early dorsal blocking-type splint with complete immobilization. When the splint is applied, it should be a dorsal forearm-based splint with the wrist in 10° to 30° of flexion, metacarpophalangeal joints at 40° to 60°, and interphalangeal joints in full extension. At 3 to 4 weeks, the splint is modified to bring the wrist to a neutral position and the patient exercises in the splint hourly. At 4 to 6 weeks, the dorsal blocking splint is discontinued and gentle blocking exercises and isolated gliding exercises are initiated.

Answer: **A**
Hunter, Mackin, Callahan, pp. 442-443

28. The finger and wrist positions recommended by Evans while performing the early active motion "place and hold" component for repaired flexor tendons in zone I or II are:

A. Wrist in slight flexion, metacarpophalangeal joints at 70° flexion, proximal interphalangeal joints at 60° flexion, and distal interphalangeal joints at 30° flexion
B. Wrist at 20° extension, with metacarpophalangeal joints at 83° flexion, proximal interphalangeal joints at 75° flexion, and distal interphalangeal joints at 40° flexion
C. Wrist flexed 20° with metacarpophalangeal joints at 80° flexion, proximal interphalangeal joints at 75° flexion, and distal interphalangeal joints at 40° flexion

D. Wrist at 10° extension, with metacarpophalangeal joints at 43° flexion, proximal interphalangeal joints at 40° flexion, and distal interphalangeal joints at 80° flexion

The position Evans recommends for the early active place and hold technique for zone I and II flexor tendon repairs using the minimal active muscle tendon tension or short arc motion (SAM) is: wrist at 20° extension, metacarpophalangeal joints at 83° flexion, proximal interphalangeal joints at 75° flexion, and distal interphalangeal joints at 40° of flexion (Fig. 13-8, *A*). The therapist places the fingers and the wrist in the SAM position and the patient is asked to gently maintain the placed position with minimal tension. The therapist can measure the tension with a force gauge (Fig. 13-8, *B*). A force of 15 to 20 g allows the force application tension to be reliable and repeatable, minimizing the risk of rupture using a standard two-strand with epitendinal suture (modified Kessler) technique. This protocol must be initiated within 24 to 48 hours postoperatively because presumably it is safer to move a tendon at this time than at day 5 or 10, when adhesions have formed.

Answer: **B**
Evans, Thompson, pp. 275-277
Hunter, Schneider, Mackin, pp. 337, 362-391

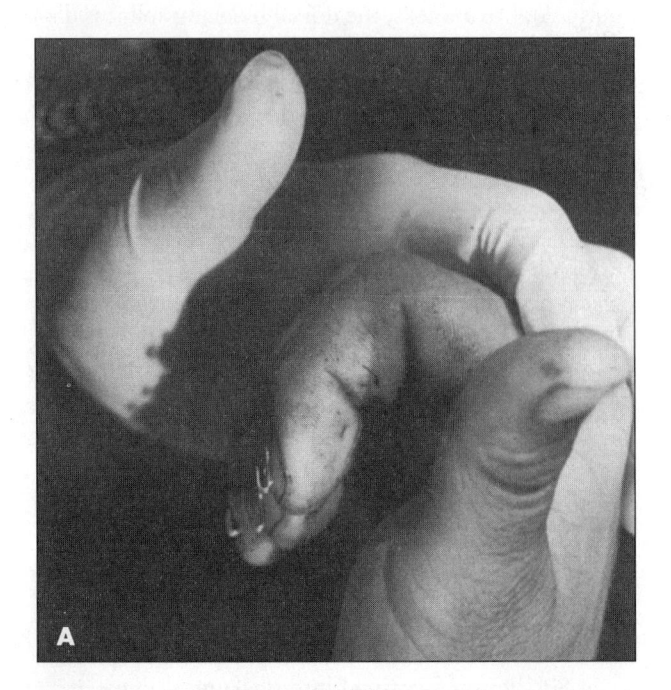

Fig. 13-8 ■ **A,** According to the MAMTT protocol, the active hold positions the digits in moderate flexion (MPJ 83°, PIPJ 75°, DIPJ 40°). (From Evans RB, Thompson DE: The application of force to the healing tendon, *J Hand Ther* 6:276, 1993.) *Continued*

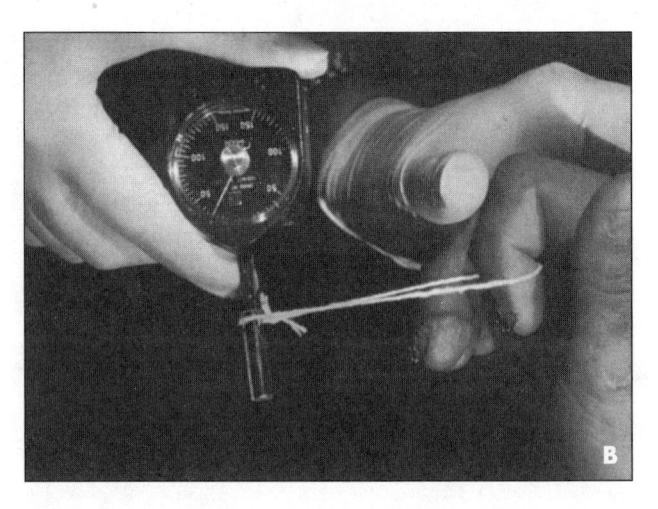

Fig. 13-8 ■ **B,** Tension is limited to 50g of force, which is measured with the Haldex gauge. (From Evans RB, Thompson DE: The application of force to the healing tendon, *J Hand Ther* 6:276, 1993.)

> **CLINICAL GEM:**
> The therapist must take a patient's edema into consideration. Edema can increase the force at the repair site with active motion. Therefore, the therapist should carefully evaluate a patient's edema before initiating the short arc motion program. If edema is present, a modified position requiring less flexion at the MPJ, PIPJ, and DIPJ is indicated.

> **CLINICAL GEM:**
> Remember to always communicate with the hand surgeon about tendon repair. It is essential to know how many strands cross the repair site as well as whether an epitenon suture was used.

29. A patient is referred to you for treatment of extensor tendon subluxation of the ring finger. During the evaluation, you notice that the patient is able to hold the involved finger in the fully extended position only when it is placed there. When starting from the fisted position, the patient is unable to achieve full extension of the involved digit. The extensor lag with active extension is approximately 35°. Which structure might be involved?

A. Extensor digitorum communis
B. Transverse retinacular ligament
C. Sagittal band
D. Central tendon

This patient is unable to extend the metacarpophalangeal joint actively; however, the patient is able to sustain active metacarpophalangeal extension, which indicates that the extensor tendon is intact. The structure that is damaged in this case is most likely the sagittal band because the patient is able to hold the digit in the fully extended position once the tendon is relocated over the metacarpophalangeal joint. Rupture is, most often, of the radial sagittal band and is common in the long finger where the extrinsic extensor tendon may dislodge from its weak attachment to the underlying sagittal fibers. The result is an ulnar displacement of the extensor tendon. Conservative, nonoperative treatment includes splinting of the wrist with the metacarpophalangeal joints in neutral for 4 weeks; frequently this is successful for an acute injury. However, surgery is indicated with complete rupture of the sagittal band and for chronic, recurrent cases (see Fig. 2-8 and question 12 in chapter 2).

Answer: **C**
Hunter, Mackin, Callahan, p. 531

30. You are treating a patient referred for evaluation and treatment after a football injury that resulted from grabbing his opponent's shirt. While evaluating the patient, you notice he is unable to bend the distal interphalangeal joint of his ring finger. The appropriate treatment plan for this patient is:

A. Electrical stimulation to facilitate tendon glide of the scarred flexor digitorum profundus tendon
B. Ultrasound of the tendon to improve flexor glide
C. A strengthening regime
D. Referral to a hand surgeon for Jersey finger repair
E. None of the above

A Jersey finger occurs in high-velocity injuries such as those that involve grabbing an opponent's shirt in rugby or football. The distal phalanx of the finger is passively hyperextended while the other fingers remain flexed. Therapy treatment for this patient would not be indicated because the flexor tendon is not intact. Surgical intervention should be considered.

Answer: **D**
Tubiana, Thomine, Mackin, p. 217

31. A 35-year-old office worker sustained a laceration over the palmar aspect of her ring finger at the middle phalanx. She initially was treated with sutures in the emergency room and was told that there was no underlying structural damage to the hand and that she should follow-up with her primary care doctor for suture removal. After 4 weeks post repair, the patient was referred to hand therapy because of decreased strength. She complained to the hand therapist that her grip is weak and that it was hard for her to fully extend her metacarpophalangeal joint. The therapist noted that the patient was unable to flex her distal interphalangeal joint. The patient was then referred to a hand surgeon. Which procedure would the hand surgeon most likely plan?

A. Long finger flexor digitorum superficialis transfer to ring finger flexor digitorum profundus with lumbrical release
B. Flexor digitorum profundus tendon repair using modified Kessler technique
C. Distal interphalangeal fusion
D. Flexor digitorum profundus tendon repair using modified Kessler technique with lumbrical release
E. Flexor digitorum profundus tendon repair with distal interphalangeal joint fusion

Flexor digitorum profundus tendons lacerated proximal to the insertion of or through the long vincula can retract all the way into the wrist. In this case, the patient likely experienced weakness and difficulty with metacarpophalangeal joint extension because of lumbrical tightness secondary to proximal flexor digitorum profundus migration. Two and one-half weeks after such an injury, the muscle is fibrosed and attempts to repair the severed tendon ends would likely result in quadrigia. In this situation, the lumbrical-plus deformity can be corrected with a lumbrical release and the flexor digitorum profundus can be easily reconstructed with a transfer of the flexor digitorum superficialis from an adjacent finger. Distal interphalangeal fusion can be considered in cases of missed flexor digitorum profundus laceration when prolonged rehabilitation should be avoided (e.g., for manual laborers or elderly patients).

Answer: **A**
Green, pp. 1853-1868

32. You are treating a patient with an extensor pollicis longus tendon repair in zone V. How much flexion is desired at the interphalangeal joint to

produce a 5-mm passive glide of the extensor pollicis longus?

A. 20°
B. 40°
C. 60°
D. 80°

When treating an extensor pollicis longus repair in zone IV or V with a dynamic splinting protocol, the wrist is splinted in extension with the carpometacarpal joint in neutral, the metacarpophalangeal joint at 0, and the interphalangeal joint at 0 with dynamic extension (Fig. 13-9, *A*). The distal joint is actively flexed to 60° to produce a 5-mm passive glide at the extensor pollicis longus tendon (Fig. 13-9, *B*). The traction then returns the distal phalanx to the resting position at 0.

Answer: **C**
Hunter, Schneider, Mackin, p. 388

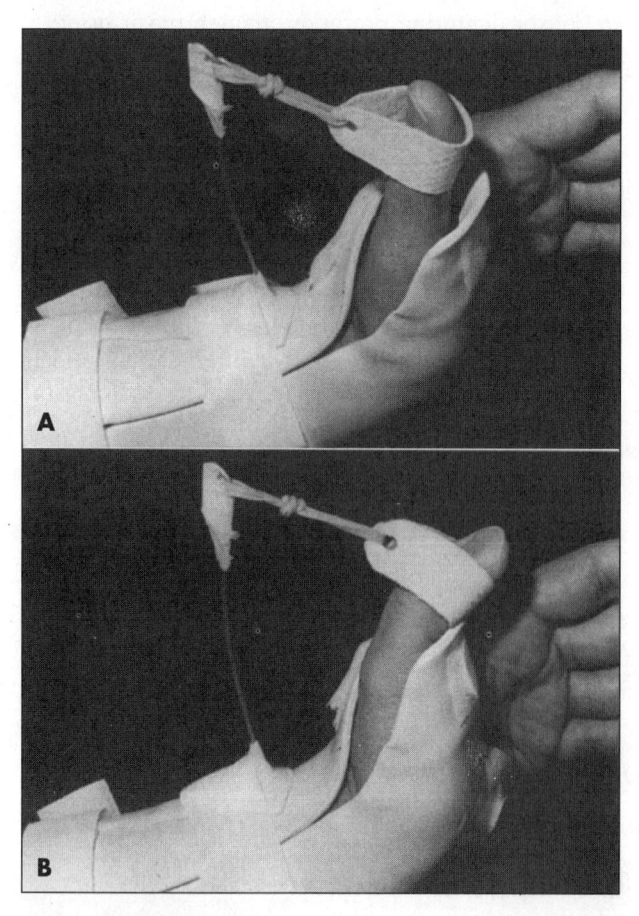

Fig. 13-9, A and B ■ From Evans RB, Burkhalter WE: A study of the dynamic anatomy of extensor tendons and implications for treatment, *J Hand Surg* 11A:777, 1986.

33. In which flexor zone should the wrist be splinted in neutral?

A. Zone I
B. Zone II
C. Zone III
D. Zone IV
E. Zone V

After surgical repair of a flexor tendon in zone IV, the wrist should be splinted at a near neutral position with the metacarpophalangeal joints at 70° of flexion. If the wrist is splinted in flexion, bowstringing can occur. If the wrist is splinted in extension, rupture may occur (see Fig. 13-2).

Answer: **D**
Hunter, Mackin, Callahan, p. 424

34. It is important to include all fingers in dynamic traction when treating flexor tendon injuries with a Kleinert-type protocol. True or False?

There are several theories about including or not including all the fingers in dynamic traction. Some therapists propose keeping all of the fingers in traction with flexor digitorum superficialis repairs because passive flexion is easier to obtain and inadvertent flexion of adjacent fingers is avoided. Other therapists hope that by leaving the adjacent, uninvolved fingers free the patient is more likely to have uninvolved finger flexion, allowing him or her to "cheat" in a helpful fashion. A choice of one protocol over another depends on the surgeon's preference as well as the therapist's comfort level with treating the diagnosis.

Answer: **False**
Hunter, Mackin, Callahan, p. 455

35. A patient is referred to you 3 days after extensor tendon repair in zone VI. Orders are to evaluate, treat, and splint. Which of the following protocols is best suited for this patient?

A. Treatment by immobilization with the wrist at 40° to 45° extension, with 0° to 20° metacarpophalangeal joint flexion and 0° interphalangeal joint flexion

B. Dynamic splint with wrist at approximately 40° to 45° extension, with the metacarpophalangeal and interphalangeal joints resting at 0 in the slings
C. Same splint as in answer B with the application of immediate, minimal active muscle tendon tension as described by Evans
D. All of the above

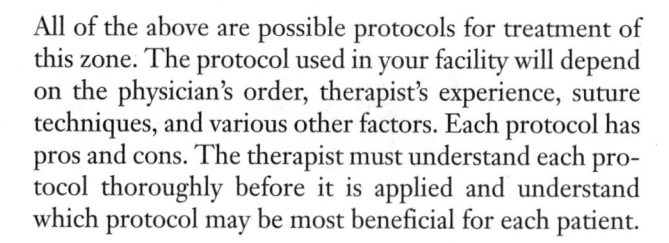

All of the above are possible protocols for treatment of this zone. The protocol used in your facility will depend on the physician's order, therapist's experience, suture techniques, and various other factors. Each protocol has pros and cons. The therapist must understand each protocol thoroughly before it is applied and understand which protocol may be most beneficial for each patient.

Answer: **D**
Hunter, Mackin, Callahan, pp. 590-596

36. When is the earliest that a tenolysis should be considered after flexor tendon repair?

A. 6 weeks
B. 12 weeks
C. 24 weeks
D. 36 weeks

The proper timing for tenolysis after tendon repair is controversial. Studies on chicken tendons conclude that waiting a minimum of 12 weeks is optimum for the procedure. Other authors recommend waiting as long as 6 to 9 months after tendon repair. Most important to consider are the prerequisites for tenolysis. All fractures should be healed, wounds should have reached tissue equilibrium with soft and pliable skin, joint contractures must be overcome, near normal passive range of motion must be achieved, and satisfactory sensation must be present. Another important factor is that a tenolysis must be performed on an extremely compliant patient who understands what is involved in the surgery and what is expected of him or her in rehabilitation.

Answer: **B**
Hunter, Schneider, Mackin, pp. 443-444

> **CLINICAL GEM:**
> It is important to consult with the surgeon regarding tendon integrity after tenolysis before initiating therapy. If the tendon is frayed, a frayed tendon protocol must be initiated. Consult Hunter, Mackin, and Callahan, pages 463 through 473, for tenolysis protocols.

37. The extensor indicis proprius and extensor digiti minimi tendons usually run on the ulnar side of the extensor digitorum communis tendon. True or False?

The extensor digitorum communis and the two independent extensor tendons pass underneath the extensor retinaculum on the back of the wrist. Both the extensor indicis and the extensor digiti minimi have independent muscles that allow independent function of the second and fifth digits, respectively. Both tendons run on the ulnar side of the extensor digitorum communis tendon.

Answer: **True**
Hunter, Schneider, Mackin, p. 547

38. You are treating a patient after flexor tendon repair in zone II. At 3 weeks, active range of motion is assessed. The patient is able to actively complete a fist. How should the program progress?

A. Continue splinting
B. Discontinue splinting and begin active range-of-motion program
C. Begin blocking exercises to further increase tendon glide
D. Initiate strengthening program because the patient has full range of motion

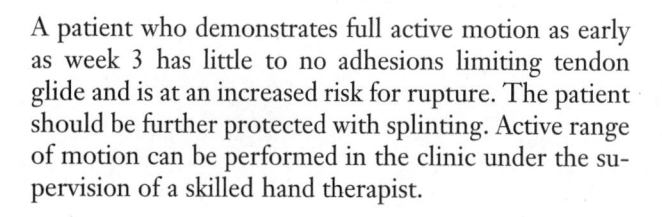

A patient who demonstrates full active motion as early as week 3 has little to no adhesions limiting tendon glide and is at an increased risk for rupture. The patient should be further protected with splinting. Active range of motion can be performed in the clinic under the supervision of a skilled hand therapist.

In contrast, if the patient exhibits little to no tendon glide at 3 weeks after surgery, a more aggressive program should be initiated. The heavily scarred patient may be able to start active or resistive exercises earlier under the close supervision of a skilled hand therapist. Protocols are helpful for an inexperienced therapist but with time a therapist must make such judgments without relying on protocols to optimize treatment.

Answer: **A**
Hunter, Mackin, Callahan, p. 455

Chapter 14

Biomechanics and Tendon Transfers

Topics to be reviewed in random order are:

- Common levers
- Biomechanical terms
- Muscle biomechanics
- Blix curve
- Tendon transfers, pathology, and treatment
- Splinting
- Terminology
- Resting length
- Radian
- Tendon excursions
- Rehabilitation after tendon transfer

1. Match the biomechanical term to its correct description:

Biomechanical Term

1. Stress
2. Shear stress
3. Mechanical advantage
4. Axis

Description

A. Occurs when one force acting on a lever has doubled the moment arm of the opposing force
B. Force per unit area
C. Occurs in tissue that is subjected to two opposing forces that are not exactly in line
D. Two bones moving around each other at a joint and one line that does not move in relation to either bone

Answers: 1. B; 2. C; 3. A; 4. D
Brand, Hollister, pp. 3-6

2. In relation to a muscle contraction, the resting length is the:

A. Distance between the maximal stretch and the maximal contracture of a fiber.
B. Maximal stretch of a muscle fiber.
C. Optimal position for a muscle to generate a strong contraction.
D. A and B are correct.
E. A and C are correct.

The resting length is the length that a sarcomere, or a muscle fiber, assumes when a limb is in its resting and balanced condition. Resting length is approximately equal to the distance between the maximal stretch and the maximal contracture of a fiber. The optimal strength of active contraction is obtained when the muscle is in the middle of its normal excursion (neutral). At the two extremes of maximal stretch and maximal contraction, the ability of a muscle to form an active contraction is close to 0. In contrast, when a muscle

167

is at resting length, it has the maximal power to perform a strong contraction of a fiber.

> *Answer:* **E**
> Brand, Hollister, p. 14
> Tubiana, Thomine, Mackin, pp. 44-46

3. Match each term to the correct description:

Term

1. Force
2. Friction
3. Static friction
4. Coulomb friction
5. Radian

Description

A. Frictional force resulting between two surfaces that move relative to one another
B. Defined as that which will cause acceleration.
C. A unit of angular measurement
D. A friction force produced when two surfaces do not move relative to one another
E. Resisting force parallel to and resulting from direct contact between two surfaces

> *Answer:* 1. B; 2. E; 3. D; 4. A; 5. C
> Brand, Hollister, pp. 5,6
> Giurintano, p. 84

4. Which of the following statement(s) is (are) true of a sarcomere?

A. It is the basic contractile unit.
B. It shortens during contraction.
C. It is composed of interacting myosin and actin.
D. All of the above

A sarcomere is the basic contractile unit of muscle tissue in muscle fiber. It is composed of two overlapping filaments: the thick myosin filament and the thin actin filament. There is an overlap and interdigitation of actin and myosin molecules with a subsequent shortening of the sarcomere during active contraction.

> *Answer:* **D**
> Brand, Hollister, pp. 14-16
> Tubiana, Thomine, Mackin, pp. 42-45
> *Refer to Fig. 14-1.*

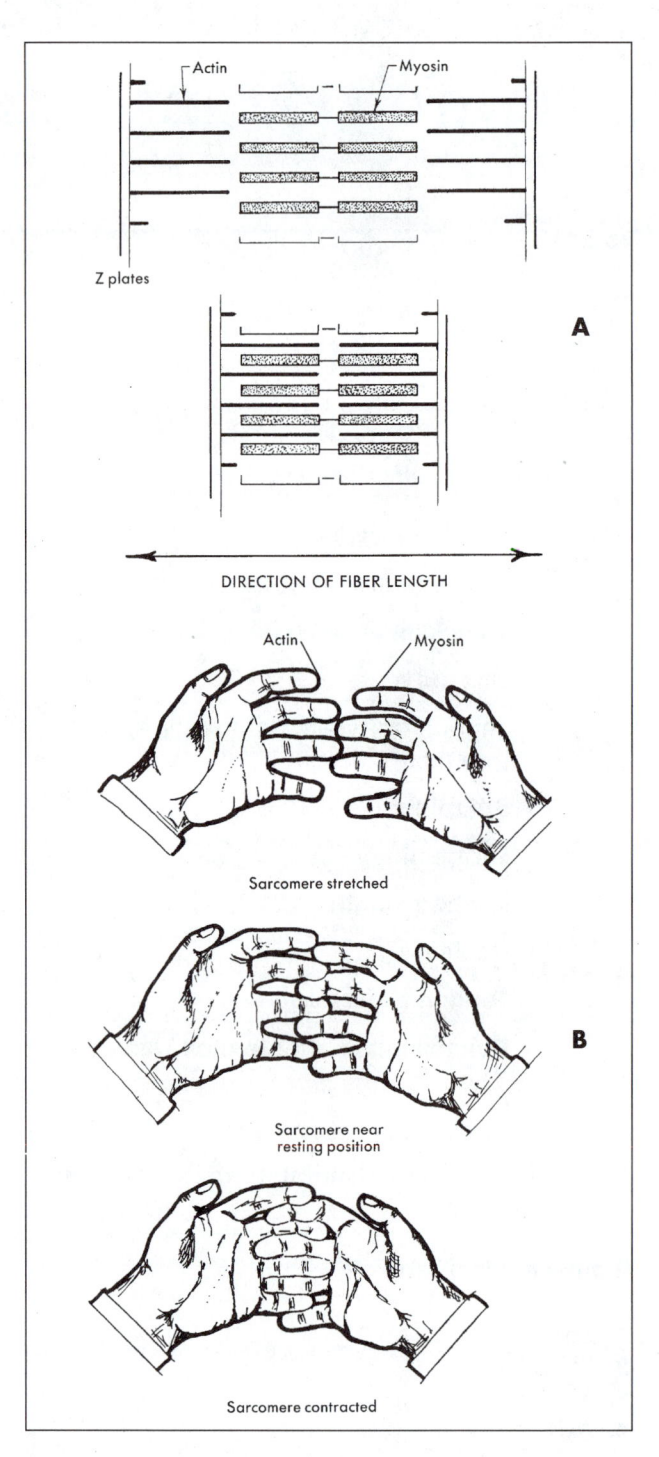

Fig. 14-1 ■ **A,** Sarcomeres when muscle fiber is stretched (*top*) and when it is contracted (*bottom*). **B,** Contraction of a sarcomere is similar to a pair of hands with interdigitating fingers (the fingers of one hand are actin and those of the other are myosin). (From Brand PW, Hollister A: *Clinical mechanics of the hand,* ed 2, St. Louis, 1993, Mosby-Year Book.)

5. Match each term to its definition:

Term

1. Creep
2. Work
3. Drag
4. Hysteresis
5. Stress relaxation

Definition

A. Shear stresses resulting from the action of a fluid on a surface
B. Energy required to move a force through a distance
C. A decrease in stress after a material is initially strained and then held at a constant for a long time
D. A stretched, elastic material springing back to its original shape when stress is removed
E. Tissue permanently remaining in a lengthened state after being stretched and held under moderate tension for a long time

Answers: 1. E; 2. B; 3. A; 4. D; 5. C
Brand, Hollister, pp. 6-9

6. The most common lever found in the human body is the:

A. First-class lever
B. Second-class lever
C. Third-class lever
D. Force arm

A lever is defined as a rigid bar revolving around a fixed point or fulcrum. The force arm is the distance between the fulcrum and the applied force and the resistance arm is the distance between the fulcrum and the resistance. A first-class lever is characterized by a fulcrum between the force and the resistance, as in a teeter-totter, scissors, or anatomically, the triceps. A second-class lever is the resistance between the fulcrum and the force, as in a wheelbarrow or a nutcracker. In a third-class lever, the force is applied between the fulcrum and the resistance (e.g., the biceps). **The third-class lever is the most common lever found in the human body.**

Answer: **C**
Brand, Hollister, pp. 62-66
Holderman

7. Which of the following types of stress typically occurs in a tendon or ligament?

A. Shear stress
B. Compression stress
C. Tension stress
D. Strain

Tension stress occurs when applied forces are colinear and act in opposite directions. Tendons use tension stress to produce joint movement and ligaments use tension stress to provide joint stability.

Sprains, strains, ruptures, and avulsions may occur if opposing forces exceed the ability of the materials to resist them. A strain is the deformation of an object or tissue. Compression stress is present when a force presses perpendicular to a surface or when forces act toward each other. Compression and pressure are defined as force per unit area (i.e., pounds per square inch or psi). Shear stress is caused by forces that are parallel to a surface but are not exactly in line or colinear. Shear can occur within tissues beneath the skin or between skin and external forces (e.g., splints).

Answer: **C**
Brand, Hollister, pp. 1,3

8. The clinical significance of applying heat to tissues before stretching exercises is related to the biomechanical principle of:

A. Viscosity
B. Elasticity
C. Plastic change
D. Creep

All of the above can affect the outcome of stretching or lengthening exercises. Creep occurs when a tissue gradually changes its structure and remains in a lengthened state after being stretched and held under tension for a long time. Rising temperature may increase the amount of creep. Maximizing creep is the goal of stretching tissues.

Viscosity is the property of a material that causes it

to resist movement. Viscosity does not prevent motion, it retards it; for example, a thick fluid offers greater resistance than a thin fluid and is thus more viscous.

Elasticity is the property that enables a material or tissue to return to its exact original shape after the removal of all stress; it allows a tissue to be deformed and then return to its resting state. Elastic tissues hinder the motion of a joint or tendon by maintaining the tissues' initial state. Collagen is elastic and can resist stretch.

Plastic change occurs when a tissue is stretched beyond its elastic limit and may be permanently deformed. Tendon attenuations, ruptures, avulsions, and stress fractures are examples of plastic change; these tissues never return to their original shape.

Answer: **D**
Brand, Hollister, pp. 5-7, 94-105

9. Which of the following variables is not measurably related to muscle tension capability?:

A. Physiological cross sectional area
B. Actin/myosin fibril ratio
C. Muscle fiber length
D. Mass

There are three measurable variables for each muscle: (1) mass, which is directly proportional to volume; (2) muscle fiber length, which is proportional to the potential for excursion; and (3) the physiological cross sectional area, which is muscle volume divided by its mean fiber length and is proportional to total maximum tension.

The actin/myosin fibrils entwine within muscle sarcomeres as the fingers of one hand might interdigitate and overlap with the fingers of the other hand. When the sarcomere unit is activated by a motor nerve impulse, the actin and myosin exercise a strong attraction to one another, pulling together into deeper interdigitations. These fibrils are the basis of all muscle contractions but are not measurable with regard to strength of contraction.

Answer: **B**
Brand, Hollister, pp. 13-16, 26-28

10. Muscle tissues are best described by the term elasticity rather than viscoelasticity. True or False?

Elasticity allows soft tissues to be deformed and then immediately return to their resting shape. Viscoelasticity is a combination of both viscous and elastic properties and is characterized by hysteresis, which allows a material to spring back to its original shape more slowly when tension is removed. All muscles have a certain tone, even in the absence of apparent nerve stimulation. This tone is a combination of the elasticity of a muscle and the connective tissue that surrounds it. The term viscoelasticity is better suited to describe muscle tissue than elasticity because muscle behaves differently when it is subjected to fast movement than when it is subjected to slow movement.

Answer: **False**
Brand, Hollister, pp. 6,7,21,94-98,115

11. A radian is approximately how many degrees?

A. 30°
B. 57°
C. 73°
D. 91°

Tendon excursion can be calculated geometrically through radians. A radian is an angle that is created when the radius lies along the circumference of the circle and is joined by a line at each end in the center of the circle. This angle is always equal to 57.29°, or 1 radian.

It is important to understand the concept of radians when calculating extensor tendon excursions. For example, when the metacarpophalangeal joint is moved 1 radian (57.29°), the metacarpophalangeal joint motion of 57.29° will yield a 10-mm extensor tendon excursion. Therefore, as suggested by Duran and Gelberman, to obtain the 5 mm of excursion to minimize extrinsic adhesions, a joint must be moved through .05 radian, or 28.64° of rotation (flexion). It is important to know that joints have various tendon excursions, depending on their size. A small joint with a smaller moment arm produces less tendon excursion.

Answer: **B**
Hunter, Mackin, Callahan, p. 569
Brand, Hollister, pp. 67-68
Refer to Fig. 14-2.

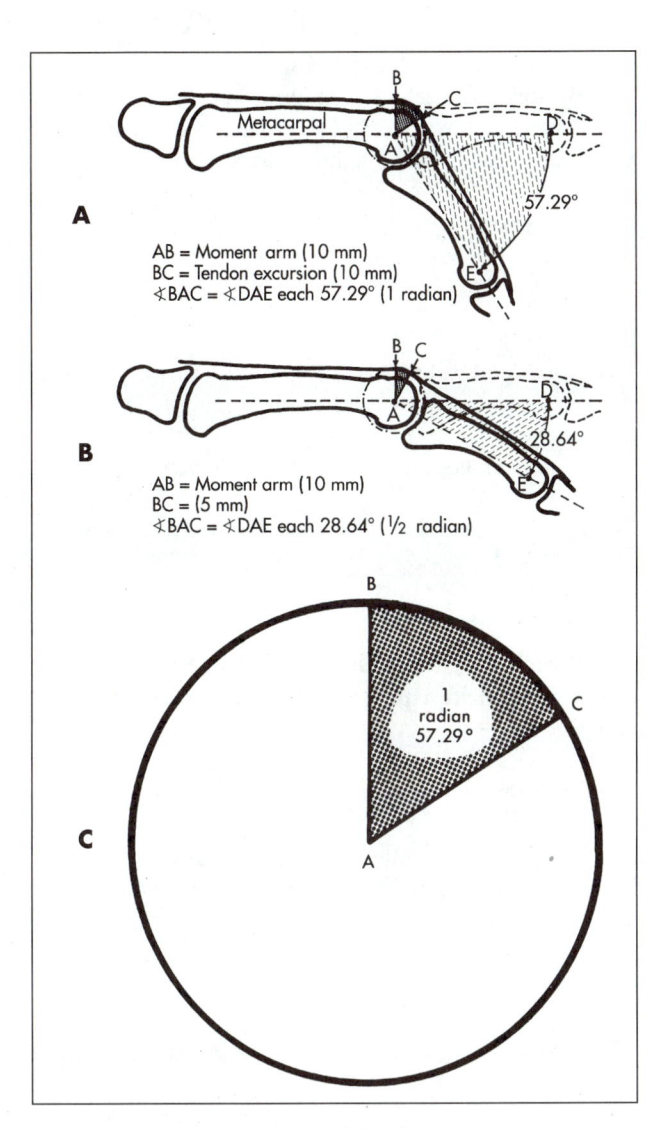

Fig. 14-2 ■ **A,** If the head of the metacarpal is considered in terms of a circle, the moment arm of the extensor tendon is equal to the radius of that circle. If metacarpophalangeal joint motion equals 57.29°, or 1 radian, tendon excursion is equal to the moment arm, or AB=BC. If the moment arm equals 10 mm, angular change of 57.29° affects 10 mm of extensor tendon excursion. **B,** Angular change of 0.5 radian or 28.3° affects the 5 mm of extensor tendon excursion recommended for the early passive motion program. **C,** A radian is the angle that is created when the radius that lies along the circumference of a circle is joined by a line at each end in the center or axis of the circle. Angle BAC equals 1 radian, or 57.29°. (*A* From Evans RB, Burkhalter WE: A study of the dynamic anatomy of extensor tendons and implications for treatment, *J Hand Surg* 11A:776, 1986. *B* and *C,* From Hunter JM, Mackin EJ, Callahan AD: *Rehabilitation of the hand: surgery and therapy,* ed 4, St. Louis, 1995, Mosby-Year Book.)

12. A muscle will always drop a grade (on a manual muscle test scale of zero to five) on a manual muscle test after tendon transfer. True or False?

A widely quoted rule in the past was that when a muscle-tendon unit was transferred, its strength would drop one level; however, this generalization is not accepted today. Diminished effectiveness of muscles after transfer is more likely to be a function of scar adhesion, drag (force resulting from action of a fluid on a surface), and/or imperfect re-education than of actual loss of muscle tension capability. However, if a muscle has been weakened by disease or paralysis it is unwise to expect a better performance after transfer.

Answer: **False**
Brand, Hollister, p. 30

13. The strongest muscle that crosses the wrist is the:

A. Extensor carpi radialis brevis
B. Flexor carpi ulnaris
C. Extensor carpi radialis longus
D. Flexor digitorum profundus

The flexor carpi ulnaris is the strongest muscle that crosses the wrist. The loss of the flexor carpi ulnaris results in more than a 50% weakening of the wrist, which is functionally detrimental to the patient.

The extensor carpi radialis brevis is the strongest and **most** efficient wrist extensor; the extensor carpi radialis longus has the greatest capacity for sustained work. The flexor digitorum profundus flexes the distal interphalangeal joint and may assist as a weak wrist flexor.

Answer: **B**
Brand, Hollister, pp. 189, 267, 276, 311-315
Hunter, Mackin, Callahan, p. 523

14. You have a patient who underwent a proximal row carpectomy in which the scaphoid, lunate, triquetrum, and tip of the radial styloid were excised. After surgery and rehabilitation, this patient is expected to achieve normal strength. True or False?

Grip strength deficits will be marked because of the length-tension alterations of muscles that cross the wrist. Strength will average between 50% and 80% of the opposite hand.

Answer: **False**
Wright, Michlovitz, pp. 149-151

172 CHAPTER 14 Biomechanics and Tendon Transfers

15. The Blix curve depicts two curves of muscle tension, one by active contraction and the other by passive recoil. True or False?

When a muscle is stretched, it stores potential energy, in a similar way as an elastic band. When it is released, the muscle contracts. Passive recoil is an elastic passive contracture that is not controlled by the nervous system but is an important component of total muscle tension. The Blix curve (Fig. 14-3) depicts two different tension curves—one of active contracture (contractile tension) and the other of elastic (passive) stretch and passive recoil in the same fiber.

Answer: **True**
Brand, Hollister, pp. 17,18
Tubiana, Thomine, Mackin, pp. 42-44

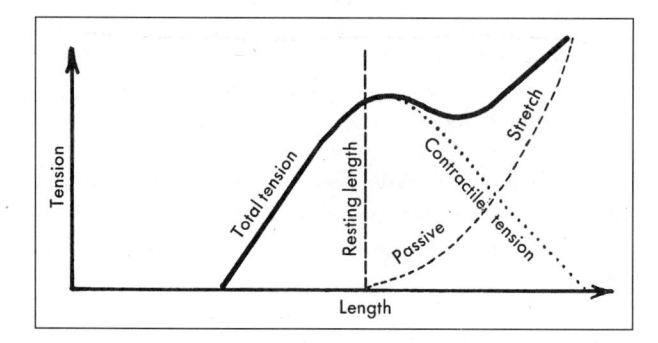

Fig. 14-3 ■ From Brand PW, Hollister A: *Clinical mechanics of the hand,* ed 2, St. Louis, 1993, Mosby-Year Book.

16. The motor muscles of the wrist have a tendinous excursion of approximately 3.5 cm. True or False?

Tendon excursion depends on muscular contractions. Other factors that influence tendon excursion are adherence of muscles to the aponeurosis, the freedom of a tendon gliding with its paratenon, the changes in direction around a pulley, and the crossing of one or more articulations. Tendon excursion for the wrist is approximately 3.5 cm. The common extensors of the fingers along with the long flexor of the thumb have an excursion of approximately 4 to 5 cm. The tendons of the long flexors of the fingers have the greatest excursion of all of the muscles in the hand—approximately 7 cm.

Answer: **True**
Tubiana, Thomine, Mackin, p. 53

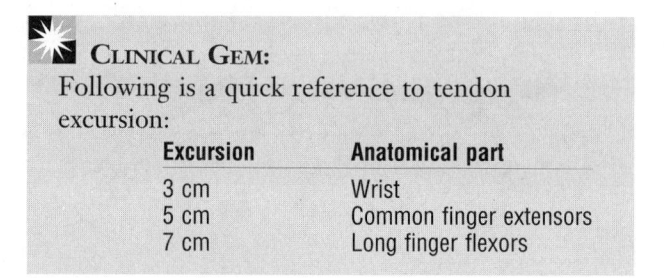

> **CLINICAL GEM:**
> Following is a quick reference to tendon excursion:
>
> | Excursion | Anatomical part |
> |-----------|-----------------|
> | 3 cm | Wrist |
> | 5 cm | Common finger extensors |
> | 7 cm | Long finger flexors |

17. Which of the following transfers augments finger flexion in a person with high median nerve palsy?

A. Extensor carpi radialis longus to flexor digitorum profundus
B. Pronator teres to flexor digitorum profundus
C. Brachioradialis to flexor digitorum profundus
D. Extensor indicis proprius to flexor digitorum profundus

The extensor carpi radialis longus and extensor carpi ulnaris are most often used to power the flexor digitorum profundus and flexor pollicis longus, respectively, after high median nerve palsy. A fairly balanced hand may be obtained after transfer. The pronator teres is median-nerve innervated and, therefore, unsuitable for this transfer. The brachioradialis is difficult to re-educate and usually is not transferred in median nerve palsy. The extensor indicis proprius tendon is commonly used for transfer but is not strong enough to provide real power for finger flexion, thumb adduction, or replacement of the first dorsal interosseus muscle.

Answer: **A**
Brand, Hollister, pp. 214-215, 322-323

18. Match each opposition transfer with the surgeon(s) for which it is named.

Surgeon

1. Royle-Thompson
2. Huber
3. Bunnell
4. Phalen/Miller
5. Camitz

Opposition Transfer

A. Extensor carpi ulnaris to thumb through the pisiform/flexor carpi ulnaris pulley
B. Ring finger flexor digitorum superficialis to thumb through the pisiform/flexor carpi ulnaris pulley
C. Palmaris longus to thumb
D. Ring finger flexor digitorum superficialis to thumb metacarpophalangeal joint
E. Abductor digiti minimi to thumb metacarpophalangeal joint

Answers: **1. D; 2. E; 3. B; 4. A; 5. C**
Green, pp. 1419-1440

19. Which tendon transfer would best replace the flexor pollicis longus after a high median nerve injury?

A. Extensor carpi radialis longus
B. Extensor carpi radialis brevis
C. Flexor carpi radialis
D. Brachioradialis

A hand with a high median nerve palsy lacks the flexor pollicis longus, flexor digitorum superficialis, flexor digitorum profundus to the index and middle fingers, palmaris longus, flexor carpi radialis, and the pronators. Major functional losses include opposition, flexion of the interphalangeal joint of the thumb, and distal interphalangeal joints of the index and middle fingers. An excellent transfer to regain thumb interphalangeal joint flexion is the brachioradialis to the flexor pollicis longus. The extensor carpi radialis longus to the flexor digitorum profundus of the index and middle fingers also is a useful transfer with this nerve palsy. Opposition transfers are presented in the previous question.

Answer: **D**
Hunter, Schneider, Mackin, p. 215

20. A patient presents to your clinic with classic "wrist drop." Which nerve is injured?

A. Median nerve
B. Ulnar nerve
C. Musculocutaneous nerve
D. Radial nerve

In a patient with a radial nerve paralysis, the forearm is pronated in the classic "wrist drop" position. The patient's grip strength is substantially reduced because the inactive wrist extensors create an unstable wrist and minimize the finger flexor's power. The patient also displays an inability to extend the fingers of the metacarpophalangeal joints, which prevents the grasp and release of large objects.

Answer: **D**
Hunter, Mackin, Callahan, p. 753

21. In a high radial nerve palsy, wrist extension always should be restored by transferring the pronator teres tendon into both the extensor carpi radialis longus and extensor carpi radialis brevis tendon insertions. True or False?

The extensor carpi radialis longus has a smaller moment arm for wrist extension than the extensor carpi radialis brevis, unless radial deviation also occurs. It is better to put the pronator teres into only the extensor carpi radialis brevis, or the patient will be forced into radial deviation every time he or she tries to extend the wrist. If one muscle has multiple insertions, all of the muscles will always move together. In high median and ulnar palsy, for example, the extensor carpi radialis longus may be used to power all of the finger flexors. If one finger flexes, all will flex. If one is prevented from flexion by stiffness, none of the fingers will be able to flex.

Answer: **False**
Brand, Hollister, pp. 75, 183

22. You are treating a patient with a radial nerve palsy and you note that he is able to supinate. You recall your anatomy and remember that the supinator is innervated by the radial nerve. Why is this patient still able to supinate?

A. Pronator teres can act as a supinator
B. Flexor carpi radialis can act as a supinator
C. Biceps brachii can act as a supinator
D. Palmaris longus can act as a supinator

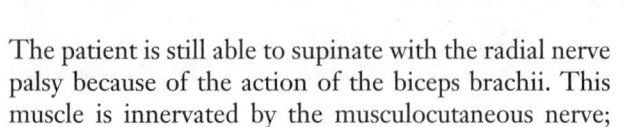

The patient is still able to supinate with the radial nerve palsy because of the action of the biceps brachii. This muscle is innervated by the musculocutaneous nerve; therefore, supination is not lost even with the loss of the supinator muscle. To eliminate the biceps and assess the supinator, the therapist should extend the elbow completely before evaluating the supinator's function.

Answer: **C**
Hunter, Mackin, Callahan, p.754

23. What muscle is most commonly used to restore extension of the wrist after radial nerve palsy?

A. Flexor carpi radialis
B. Flexor carpi ulnaris
C. Pronator teres
D. Palmaris longus

One "standard" set of tendon transfers for radial nerve palsy is the pronator teres (PT) to the extensor carpi radialis brevis (ECRB), the flexor carpi ulnaris to the extensor digitorum communis (EDC) two through five, and the palmaris longus (PL) to the extensor pollicis longus (EPL) (see part A of the following Clinical Gem). However, the best combination of transfers has not been agreed upon.

Some authors feel that the sublimis tendon is a more ideal tendon for finger extensors, and the use of the third FDS tendon to the EDC, the fourth FDS to power the EPL and extensor indicis proprius (EIP), and the flexor carpi radialis to power the extensor pollicis brevis (EPB) and abductor pollicis longus (APL) is an alternative method of transfer. The PT is used to power the extensor carpi radialis longus and the ECRB (Clinical Gem part B).

Another set of authors uses the following combinations: the pronator teres (PT) to the ECRB; the flexor carpi radialis (FCR) to the EDC; and the PL to the EPL (Clinical Gem part C). These three sets of tendon transfers currently are considered the most feasible alternatives.

Answer: **C**
Green, pp. 1406, 1408

> **CLINICAL GEM:**
> A quick reference to radial nerve tendon transfers:
>
> (A)
> PT → ECRB
> FCU → EDC
> PL → EPL
>
> (B)
> PT → ECRB, ECRL
> Middle FDS → EDC
> Ring FDS → EPL and EIP
> FCR → EPB and APL
>
> (C)
> PT → ECRB
> FCR → EDC
> PL → EPL

24. After a radial nerve tendon transfer, in which position should the arm be immobilized?

A. Elbow flexed to 90°; forearm pronated; wrist extended 30° to 45°; metacarpophalangeal joints neutral; and interphalangeal joints free
B. Elbow flexed to 30°; forearm supinated; wrist extended 30° to 45°; metacarpophalangeal joints at neutral; and interphalangeal joints free
C. Elbow flexed to 70°; forearm supinated; wrist extended 50° to 60°; metacarpophalangeal joints at neutral; and interphalangeal joints free
D. Elbow flexed to 90°; forearm pronated; wrist at neutral; metacarpophalangeal joints at neutral; and interphalangeal joints free

After tendon transfers of the wrist and digital extensors, the extensors of the arm should be immobilized in a cast for 4 weeks. The position of immobilization is with the elbow flexed to 90°, the forearm pronated naturally, the wrist extended 30° to 45°, the metacarpophalangeal joints extended to neutral, and the interphalangeal joints free. If transfers were completed for the thumb, the thumb also is immobilized, with the interphalangeal joint and metacarpophalangeal joint completely extended, and the thumb abducted and extended at the carpometacarpal joint.

The purpose of a long-arm cast is to prevent supination of the forearm and protect the pronator teres transfer. This position takes tension off of the tendon transfers, allowing healing to occur without overstretching or rupturing transfers. Four weeks after surgery, re-education exercises are initiated. A custom-made, removable splint is fabricated at this time to protect transfers between exercise sessions. The splint is used for an additional 3 to 4 weeks.

Four weeks after surgery, the focus should be on metacarpophalangeal joint flexion to avoid debilitating extension contractures. In the second week of rehabilitation (five weeks postoperatively), the focus should be on the tendon transfers themselves. Re-education is challenged most when finger flexors are transferred to finger extensors. Exceptional patient concentration and cooperation are needed to achieve extension of the digits when sublimis transfers are used. Seven weeks after surgery, dynamic splinting can be initiated if there is a need to increase flexion of the metacarpophalangeal joint. At eight weeks after surgery, protective splinting is discontinued and resistive exercises are initiated.

Answer: **A**
Hunter, Mackin, Callahan, p. 758

25. You are evaluating a patient with a nerve palsy. During your evaluation, the patient reveals a positive Froment's sign. Which nerve is injured?

A. Median
B. Radial
C. Ulnar
D. Musculocutaneous

A positive Froment's sign occurs in a patient with an ulnar nerve palsy. A Froment's test is performed by putting a piece of paper between the thumb and the radial side of the index finger, using the lateral pinch. When grasping the paper, the thumb interphalangeal joint hyperflexes to hold or stabilize the paper because of the imbalance from lost intrinsic muscles. Usually lost are: half of the flexor pollicis brevis, the first dorsal interosseous, and the adductor pollicis muscles.

Answer: **C**
Hunter, Mackin, Callahan, p. 733
Refer to Fig. 14-4.

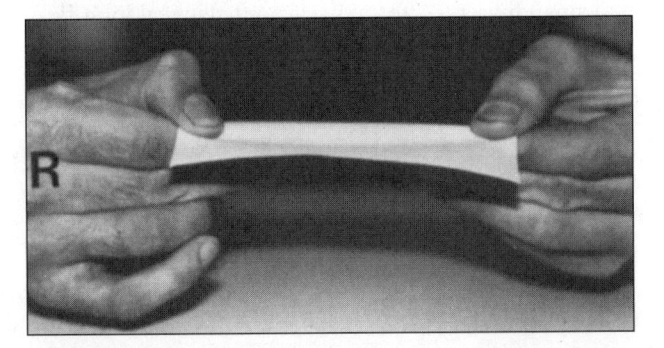

Fig. 14-4 ■ Right hand demonstrates a positive Froment's sign. (From Hunter JM, Mackin EJ, Callahan AD: *Rehabilitation of the hand: surgery and therapy,* ed 4, St. Louis, 1995, Mosby-Year Book.)

26. You are treating a patient 6 months after a complete ulnar nerve laceration 3 inches proximal to the wrist. The patient does not exhibit clawing. Why doesn't the patient exhibit clawing?

A. Patient stretches regularly
B. Patient has a Riche Cannieu anastomosis
C. Patient has made an internal splint using stronger tendons to overcome the clawing
D. None of the above

A Riche Cannieu anastomosis is a connection between the motor branch of the ulnar nerve and the recurrent branch of the median nerve in the hand. This anomalous neural pattern permits a hand to present without deformity, even with a complete ulnar nerve palsy. There is no clawing in the digits if the median nerve innervates all of the lumbricals and interossei through the Riche Cannieu anastomosis.

Answer: **B**
Green, p. 1450

27. Successful treatments for the intrinsic minus hand include:

A. Dorsal metacarpophalangeal joint blocking splints
B. Flexor digitorum superficialis to A1 pulley attachment
C. Flexor digitorum superficialis to lateral bands attachment
D. All of the above

The intrinsic minus hand deformity is called claw hand because the extensor tendons overact in an attempt to extend the fingers. The ulnar paralyzed intrinsic muscles are unable to stabilize the metacarpophalangeal joints on the flexor side. Anything that limits extension of the metacarpophalangeal joints, including splinting, capsulodesis, or even a scar on the palm, can assist the long extensors in extending the proximal interphalangeal joints. Unless they are controlled, almost all cases of low ulnar palsy develop into a progressive deformity because the unopposed extensor pull stretches the volar plate, skin, and other soft tissues over time. There often is a delay in correcting the clawing because the deformity is not apparent at first. If the flexor digitorum superficialis is attached to the A1 pulley, it serves as a tenodesis to hold the metacarpophalangeal joints just short of full extension. Likewise, the flexor digitorum superficialis may be attached to the lateral bands so that it becomes a proximal interphalangeal joint extensor and metacarpophalangeal joint flexor.

Answer: **D**
Brand, Hollister, pp. 189, 203-204

28. Which of the following procedures uses a "lasso" technique to correct clawing in ulnar nerve palsy?

A. Huber
B. Camitz
C. Royle-Thompson
D. Zancolli

The Zancolli technique uses the flexor digitorum superficialis in a "lasso" procedure through a transverse incision at the level of the distal palmar crease. The proximal pulley (A1) of the flexor sheaths are exposed and the flexor digitorum superficialis tendons are used in sections and divided into two slips for each finger. Each tendon slip is volarly retained to the deep transverse metacarpal ligament and looped through the A1 pulley and sutured to itself. The metacarpophalangeal joint is pulled down into approximately 45° of flexion. This transfer should be carried out to all four fingers because weakness is not limited to the clawing fingers.

All of the other transfers listed above are used for median nerve palsy to restore opposition.

Answer: **D**
Green, p. 1455

29. Which function(s) is/are lost after low ulnar nerve palsy?

A. Lateral or key pinch
B. Proficient grip
C. Tip pinch
D. All of the above functions are lost after low ulnar nerve palsy.

With a low ulnar nerve palsy, a patient displays a loss of flexion of the proximal phalanges from paralysis of the interossei and other intrinsic muscles. Clawing results from the extrinsic muscles hyperextending the proximal phalanges and from the pull of the proximally innervated flexor digitorum profundus, which contributes to poor grasp. A flat metacarpal arch, which also contributes to poor grasp, may be noted with ulnar nerve palsy because of the paralysis of the opponens digiti quinti and the decreased range of the little finger metacarpophalangeal joint. Loss of lateral or key pinch of the thumb is caused by paralysis of the adductor pollicis muscle. The patient also loses distal stability and rotation for tip pinch between the thumb and index finger. This loss is caused by paralysis of the first dorsal and second palmar interossei as well as the adductor pollicis muscle.

Answer: **D**
Green, p. 1449-1450

30. When treating a patient with an ulnar nerve peripheral neuropathy, which splint should be applied?

A. Passive metacarpophalangeal joint flexion splint to the ring and small fingers
B. Passive metacarpophalangeal joint flexion splint to the index and middle fingers
C. Passive metacarpophalangeal joint extension splint to the index and small fingers
D. Passive metacarpophalangeal joint extension to the ring and small fingers

After ulnar nerve injury, the splint should focus on restoring the longitudinal arch by providing a means of passive metacarpophalangeal joint flexion to the ring and small fingers. After metacarpophalangeal joint flexion is established, the intact extrinsic finger extensors are actively able to extend the interphalangeal joints of the fourth and fifth fingers, reducing the risk of interphalangeal joint flexion contractures. If the patient already has interphalangeal joint contractures, serial casting is an effective means of improving passive range of motion. Prevention is the best means of intervention when treating a patient with ulnar nerve paralysis or any nerve palsy (see Fig. 15-15 [1]).

Answer: **A**
Hunter, Schneider, Mackin, p. 97

Chapter 15
Splinting

Topics to be reviewed in random order are:

- **Purpose of static and dynamic splints**
- **Assorted static and dynamic splints**
- **Arches of the hand**
- **Creases of the hand**
- **Splint precautions**
- **Serial splinting and casting**
- **Low- versus high-profile splinting**
- **Galveston brace**
- **Fracture bracing**
- **Splinting for specific diagnoses**

1. Match each arch of the hand with the correct definition.

Arch

1. Longitudinal arch
2. Distal transverse arch
3. Proximal transverse arch

Definition

A. Consists of the distal row of carpal bones. It is rigid and acts as a stable pivot point for the wrist and long finger flexor muscles.
B. Deepens with flexion of the fingers, is mobile, and passes through the metacarpal heads.
C. Allows distal interphalangeal joints, proximal interphalangeal joints, and metacarpophalangeal joints to flex.

Answers: **1. C; 2. B; 3. A**
Coppard, Lohman, pp. 22, 23
Refer to Fig. 15-1.

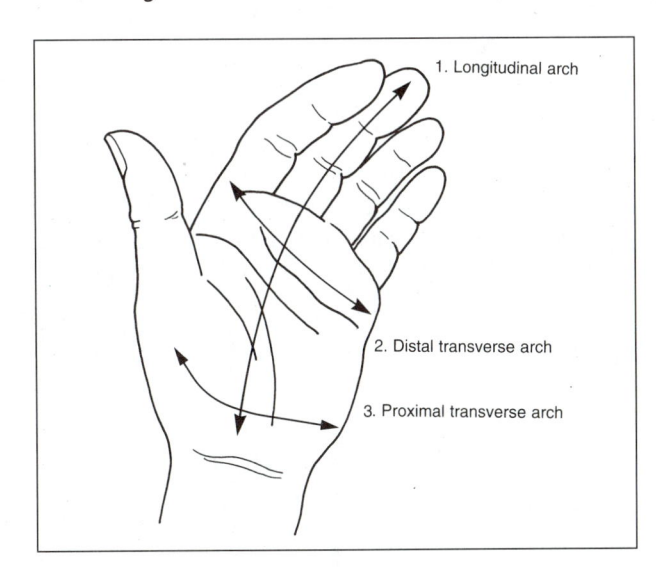

Fig. 15-1 ■ From Coppard BM, Lohman H: *Introduction to splinting: a critical-thinking and problem-solving approach,* St. Louis, 1996, Mosby-Year Book.

2. The proximal palmar crease is an important landmark for splinting. True or False?

The skin on the volar aspect of the hand is thick, tough, and inflexible. These characteristics (especially the inflexibility) account for palmar creases. The distal palmar crease is an important landmark for splinting because it marks the distal edge for splint application. When the splint is positioned proximal to this crease it allows for full metacarpophalangeal joint flexion. Below the distal palmar crease is the proximal palmar crease, which is not a significant landmark for splinting.

Answer: **False**
Coppard, Lohman, p. 23
Malick, p. 16
Refer to Fig. 15-2.

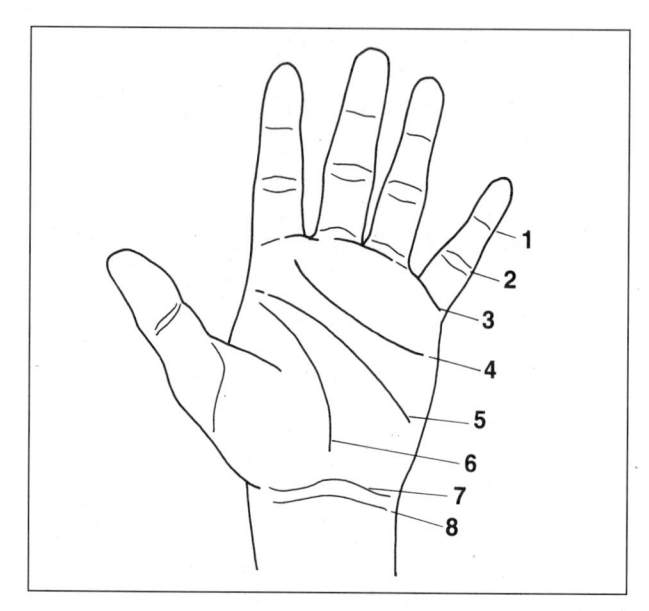

Fig. 15-2 ■ Creases of the hand. **1**, Distal digital crease; **2**, middle digital crease; **3**, proximal digital crease; **4**, distal palmar crease; **5**, proximal palmar crease; **6**, thenar crease; **7**, distal wrist crease; **8**, proximal wrist crease. (From Coppard BM, Lohman H: *Introduction to splinting: a critical-thinking and problem-solving approach,* St. Louis, 1996, Mosby-Year Book.)

3. Open-cell padding is nonabsorbent. True or False?

The two basic types of padding are open-cell and closed-cell foam. Closed-cell foam is nonabsorbent and is easily washed and towel-dried. A therapist can apply closed-cell foam padding to thermoplastic material before molding. This is important to know when planning splint fabrication because padding may cause the splint to be tighter, thus compromising the fit. For example, if one sixteenth-inch padding is added after fabrication, the splint will be one sixteenth of an inch too tight. Open-cell padding absorbs moisture; therefore, it is more difficult to keep clean and can be a breeding ground for bacteria. Open-cell padding usually is softer and more conforming than closed-cell padding.

Answer: **False**
Coppard, Lohman, p. 238

4. Serial splinting for joint contractures depends on the following mechanical phenomenon:

A. Creep
B. Stress relaxation
C. Viscoelasticity
D. Shear fracture

Stress relaxation is the continued decrease in stress **needed** to maintain a given deformation. Stress relaxation occurs over time when tissues are stretched and held at constant length, such as in serial splinting. Because this continued decrease in stress is needed to maintain the new formation of tissue, serial splinting depends on stress relaxation for desirable results.

Creep **results** from stretching tissue under a constant load and is the continued deformation of a material under constant stress. Viscoelasticity is a combination of both viscous and elastic properties and is characterized by hysteresis. Hysteresis occurs when an elastic material immediately springs back to its original shape after stretch or compression. A viscoelastic material returns to its original shape more slowly. Shear fracture occurs when a solid tissue undergoes shear stress sufficient to sustain a fracture.

Answer: **B**
Brand, Hollister, pp. 6, 7, 21, 98, 101-105

5. The length of a splint's forearm trough should be approximately:

A. One fourth the length of the forearm
B. One half the length of the forearm
C. Two thirds the length of the forearm
D. Full length of the forearm

The length of a splint's forearm trough should be approximately two thirds the length of the forearm. This allows full elbow flexion while supporting the musculature. If splint design is too short, pressure points may occur at the proximal end of the splint. The width of the splint trough should be one half the circumference of the forearm.

Answer: **C**
Coppard, Lohman, p. 28

6. All of the following are goals of static splinting, except:

A. Immobilization
B. Preventing deformity
C. Preventing soft-tissue contractures
D. All of the above are goals of static splinting

The goals of static splinting include immobilizing joints to allow them to rest, preventing deformity progression by maintaining an improved position when the splint is applied, and preventing soft-tissue contracture by positioning in a protective fashion. Static splints are used for patients with diagnoses such as rheumatoid arthritis, carpal tunnel syndrome, fractures, and soft-tissue repairs. If they are not contraindicated, static splints should be removed intermittently to perform range-of-motion exercises to decrease stiff joints and associated complications.

Answer: **D**
Coppard, Lohman, p. 14

> **CLINICAL GEM:**
> When securing Velcro, carefully heat the sticky side of the Velcro and/or the splinting material for better adhesion.

> **CLINICAL GEM:**
> Chlorine removes ink marks from splints.

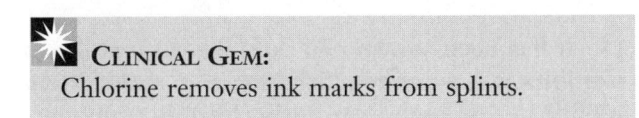

7. Forces between _____ are generally acceptable for dynamic splinting.

A. 50 and 100 grams
B. 100 and 300 grams
C. 300 and 500 grams
D. 600 and 900 grams

When dynamic splints are used to increase the range of motion of stiff joints, the force should be between 100 and 300 grams. It is important to apply a gentle, prolonged force. Too much tension will cause injury to soft tissue structures, resulting in pain, increased inflammation, increased scar formation, and decreased joint mobility. Force can be measured using a Haldex force gauge or spring scale tension gauge. Tension should be monitored regularly to ensure that proper levels of force are consistently applied to the restricted tissues.

Answer: **B**
Hunter, Mackin, Callahan, pp. 166, 1582

8. A dynamic splint is indicated when a joint has a "soft end feel." True or False?

The goals of a dynamic splint are to substitute for loss of motor function, correct existing deformities, provide controlled stress to increase range of motion, and aid in fracture healing. One way a therapist can determine whether a patient is ready for dynamic splinting is to test the "feel" of the joint. If a therapist stretches a joint through its maximum passive range and holds it there, and the tissues feel as if they will continue to respond (the joint feels as if it can go further), the tissues are ready for dynamic splinting. A joint responding in this fashion is said to have a "soft end feel." This usually is noticed in the proliferative stage of wound healing. It is during this stage that dynamic splinting is most effective.

In contrast, when a joint has a "hard end feel," the *most* beneficial splint is a static progressive splint because this splint can be worn for extended periods of time. A stiff joint with an abrupt and firm response is described as a joint with a "hard end feel." The prolonged stress of the static progressive or serial static splint is necessary to effect this type of stiffness. This type of splinting is helpful in the chronic stage of wound healing.

Serial static splinting is useful throughout all stages of wound healing because of its ability to rest the tissue as well as gain motion. The serial static splint is applied with the tissues at their maximum length and is worn for long periods of time to allow the tissues to adapt to the new position. An example of a serial static splint is a serial cast.

Answer: **True**
Hunter, Mackin, Callahan, p. 1155
Refer to Fig. 15-3.

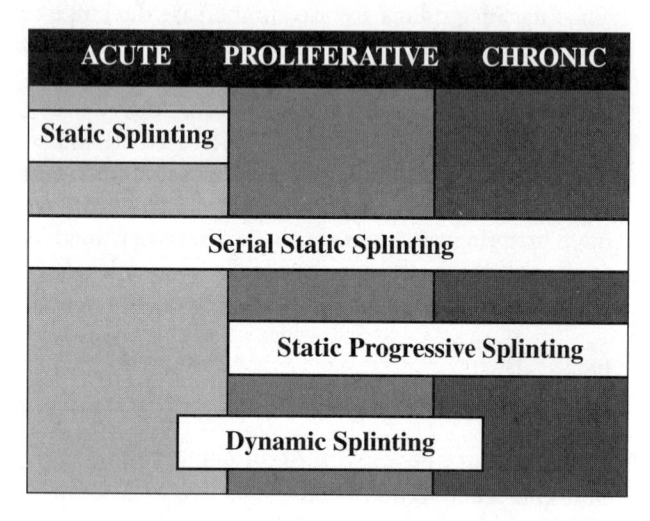

Fig. 15-3 ■ Different types of splints are effective during different stages of healing. (From Hunter JM, Mackin EJ, Callahan AD: *Rehabilitation of the hand: surgery and therapy,* ed 4, St. Louis, 1995, Mosby-Year Book.)

> **CLINICAL GEM:**
> A MERIT component is a helpful device in static progressive splinting using the total end range time concept developed by P. LaStayo and K. Flowers. This device is available through U. E. Tech (see Appendix 3).

9. Low-profile outriggers lose the required 90-degree angle of pull more quickly than high-profile outriggers. True or False?

Although outrigger height does not influence force magnitude for a dynamic-assist splint, it does influence adjustment schedules. Low-profile outriggers lose the required 90-degree angle of pull more quickly than high-profile outriggers. This concept, however, applies only when working with correctional forces. If the purpose of the splint is to substitute for weak muscles and full passive motion is available, the need for sequential adjustments to accommodate range of motion improvement is unnecessary.

Answer: **True**
Fess, Philips, p. 186

10. You are treating a patient with a diagnosis of carpal tunnel syndrome. A wrist support splint is fabricated and applied. The patient returns to the clinic 2 days later with tenderness over the radial styloid. He removes the splint and the area is red. The redness persists for 30 minutes after splint removal and then subsides. What should be done in this situation?

A. Because the redness resolved in 30 minutes, it is acceptable. The splint should not be adjusted.
B. The splint should be padded around the radial styloid.
C. The splint should be flared out around the radial styloid.
D. The splint should be discontinued because it obviously is not working.

If redness persists around a bony prominence for 20 minutes or longer after splint removal, an adjustment is necessary to decrease pain and pressure on the soft tissue and to increase patient compliance. Padding a splint around the radial styloid without increasing the available space may increase pressure. Therefore, in this case, the best option is to flare the splint out around the radial styloid.

Answer: **C**
Coppard, Lohman, p. 42

> **CLINICAL GEM:**
> Following is a quick reference to common pressure areas:
> • Dorsum of the metacarpophalangeal joints
> • Head of the ulna
> • Base of the thenar eminence
> • Radial styloid
> • Proximal end of a splint

11. It has been shown clinically that to mobilize a stiff joint it is most beneficial to apply intermittent applications of high force rather than low amounts of constant force to increase range of motion. True or False?

To mobilize stiff joints, the application of low amounts of constant force has been shown to be more beneficial than intermittent application of high forces. To favorably influence scar tissue and adhesions, splints are designed to gently maintain tension on the restraining tissues for a prolonged period of time. Forceful tension is not recommended.

Answer: **False**
Fess, Philips, p. 59
Refer to Fig. 15-4.

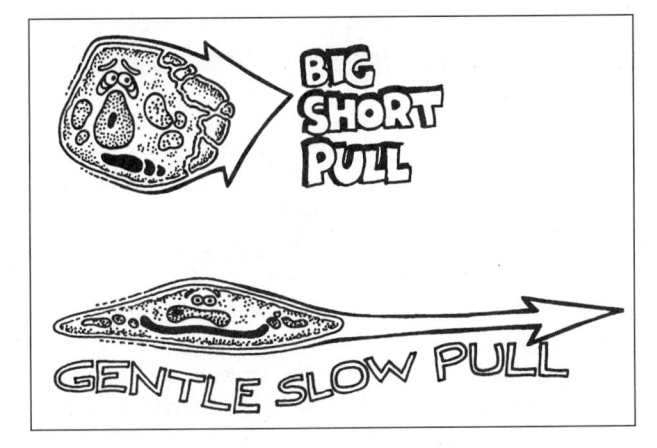

Fig. 15-4 ■ Too much force over a short period of time causes tearing of soft tissues, resulting in an increased inflammatory response and additional scar formation. (From Fess EE, Philips CA: *Hand splinting: principles and methods,* ed 2, St. Louis, 1987, CV Mosby.)

> **CLINICAL GEM:**
> In contrast to the theory of low-load prolonged stress, Bonutti et al report that static progressive splinting can be applied for a short duration with high intensity force to restore range of motion through stress relaxation using the joint active system splint.

Bonutti et al, pp. 128-134

12. You are treating a patient with a proximal interphalangeal joint flexion contracture of 50°. You decide to fabricate a dynamic proximal interphalangeal joint extension splint with a low-profile outrigger. Two weeks later you remeasure the proximal interphalangeal joint and note a 10-degree increase in range. What should you do next?

A. Discard the splint because it already has helped sufficiently
B. Leave the splint alone; it is working fine
C. Modify the outrigger
D. None of the above

Because the patient has shown a 10-degree increase in his range of motion, the splint is no longer pulling at a 90-degree angle and some element of joint compression or distraction may be occurring. The splint should be regularly modified to retain a perpendicular angle (90°) of pull. It is important to know that when the outrigger is at a 90-degree angle of pull, the translational force is zero, resulting in an absence of joint compression or distraction. Splinting should be continued as long as the patient's range of motion is improving.

Answer: **C**
Fess, Philips, p. 136
Refer to Fig. 15-5.

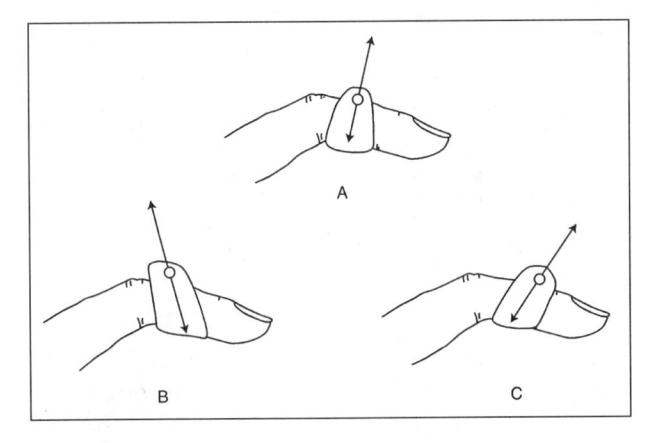

Fig. 15-5 ■ **A,** Angle of approach is 90° to middle phalanx, ensuring that force is not dissipated when proximal interphalangeal joint is pulled into extension. **B,** An angle of approach less than 90° to axis of middle phalanx compresses the joint. **C,** An angle of approach greater than 90° to axis of middle phalanx distracts the joint. (From Pedretti LW: *Occupational therapy: practice skills for physical dysfunction,* ed 4, St. Louis, 1996, Mosby-Year Book.)

13. You are treating a patient who has been provided with a dorsal-based wrist extension splint. The patient complains of pain over the ulnar head. The best way to relieve pressure over this area is to cut a hole in the splint over the ulnar head. True or False?

A common mistake made by therapists is attempting to relieve pressure from a splint by cutting material away and leaving a hole. Cutting holes in splints to relieve pressure can result in greater forces around the circumferential border of the cutout area. This creates a potential for soft-tissue injury. A better way to approach this problem is to **bubble out** the area over the bony prominence and pad the newly bubbled-out area if needed. When this splint was applied, it could have been assumed that the ulnar head area was going to be problematic. The therapist can prevent this problem by adding a pad or piece of putty to the patient's ulnar head, **"bubbling out"** this area during splint fabrication. Once the splint is fabricated, the pad or piece of putty should be removed from the ulnar head and discarded.

Answer: **False**
Fess, Philips, p. 247

> **CLINICAL GEM:**
> A quick reference to decreasing a pressure area follows:
> - Mark the patient's skin over the pressure area with lipstick
> - Apply the splint
> - Remove the splint
> - Look for smudged lipstick on the splint
> - Bubble out the smudged area with a heat gun
> - Reapply the splint
> - Reevaluate the pressure area

14. Which of the following is considered the "safe" position for fingers that have not undergone surgical repair but require immobilization after trauma?

A. Metacarpophalangeal joints at 40° flexion and interphalangeal joints at 0° to 20° flexion
B. Metacarpophalangeal joints at 80° flexion and interphalangeal joints at 30° to 40° flexion
C. Metacarpophalangeal joints at 70° to 90° flexion and interphalangeal joints at 0° to 10° flexion
D. None of the above are safe

Immobilization after trauma of fingers that have not undergone surgical repair should involve protection in the "safe" position splint. The "safe" position is with the metacarpophalangeal joints flexed at 70° to 90° of flexion and the interphalangeal joints at 0° to 10° of flexion. This position considerably decreases the potential for ligamentous contractures, with subsequent limitation of articular motion.

Answer: **C**
Fess, Philips, p. 273

15. The Galveston brace is designed for a metacarpal shaft fracture. True or False?

The Galveston brace (not pictured) is a prefabricated, three-point pressure brace that was introduced and advocated for the treatment of metacarpal shaft fractures. Some reviewers have observed pressure necrosis of the skin on the dorsum of the hand when using the Galveston brace; therefore, the use of this splint has not gained wide popularity. In response to negative feedback regarding the Galveston brace, a custom-molded fracture brace (Fig. 15-6) that widely distributes pressure typically is recommended. Fracture bracing is indicated for stable, isolated, midshaft metacarpal fractures. The splint holds the four metacarpals as a unit, allowing full digital motion. The brace stabilizes the fracture with direct pressure over the bone; the pressure is distributed rather than concentrated, as in the Galveston brace.

Answer: **True**
Hunter, Mackin, Callahan, p. 402

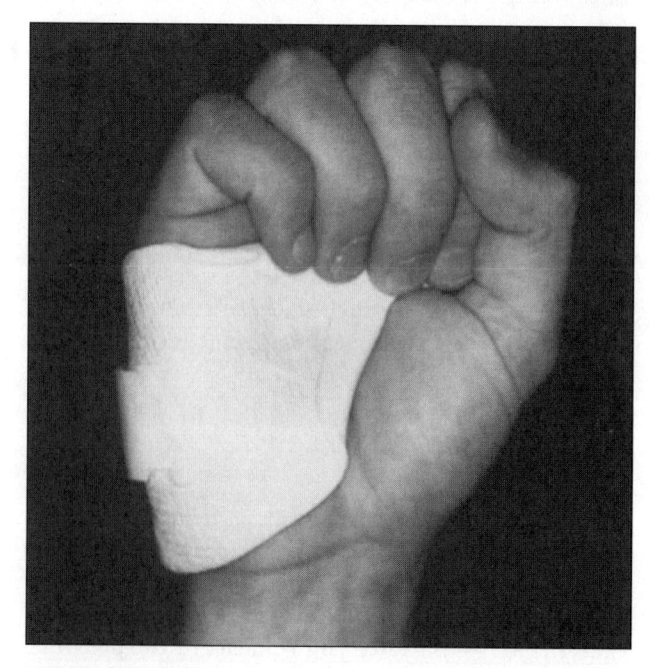

Fig. 15-6 ■ Custom-molded fracture brace. (From Hunter JM, Mackin EJ, Callahan AD: *Rehabilitation of the hand: surgery and therapy*, ed 4, St. Louis, 1995, Mosby-Year Book.)

16. You are treating a patient with a grade-II dorsal dislocation of the proximal interphalangeal joint of the long finger. This patient has been referred to you for a splint. What type of finger splint should be applied?

A. Dorsal splint with proximal interphalangeal joint in 25° of flexion
B. Dorsal splint with proximal interphalangeal joint in 60° of flexion
C. Volar splint with proximal interphalangeal joint at zero
D. Volar splint with proximal interphalangeal joint at 5° to 10° of flexion

Application of the dorsal finger splint with 25° of proximal interphalangeal joint flexion should be sufficient to sustain reduction of a grade-II subluxation. Radiographs should be obtained after application of the splint to confirm reduction. Several weeks of immobilization should be followed by graded range-of-motion exercises (see Fig. 10-6).

Answer: **A**
Hunter, Mackin, Callahan, pp. 378, 383

> **CLINICAL GEM:**
> A quick reference guide to dorsal dislocation grade, description, and splint follows:
>
> | Dorsal Dislocation Grade | Description | Splint |
> |---|---|---|
> | I | Proximal phalanx head damages central attachments distally. Critical corner integrity is maintained (the critical corner is where the volar plate, proper collateral ligament, and accessory collateral ligament merge). Refer to Figure 2-11. | Dorsal finger splint with 25° of flexion for 3 to 10 days; follow-up with buddy taping. |
> | II | Disrupts the critical corner. | Same splint as for grade I; worn for 2 to 4 weeks. |
> | III | Instability occurs volarly and laterally. | Dorsal splint with greater flexion for 6 to 8 weeks. Surgical intervention may be indicated. |

17. You are treating a patient with an acute metacarpophalangeal joint grade-II collateral ligament injury. How should this patient's metacarpophalangeal joint be splinted?

A. Neutrally
B. With 20° flexion
C. With 50° flexion
D. With 90° flexion

Metacarpophalangeal joint collateral ligament injuries occur less frequently than injury to the proximal interphalangeal joint. However, when injury occurs, the metacarpophalangeal joint should be immobilized in 50° of flexion to maintain soft tissue length for 3 weeks. Some authors recommend including adjacent metacarpophalangeal joints. An additional 3 to 6 weeks of buddy taping minimizes stress on the injured ligament.

Answer: **C**
Hunter, Mackin, Callahan, p. 387

18. You are treating a patient with chronic metacarpophalangeal joint extension contractures. Which splinting technique would be most helpful for this patient?

A. Dynamic metacarpophalangeal joint flexion splinting
B. Serial cast with the metacarpophalangeal joints in flexion
C. Static progressive flexion splinting of the metacarpophalangeal joints
D. Splinting would not be helpful for this patient. This patient should be referred for surgery.

Static progressive splinting is especially beneficial for chronic stiffness, such as occurs in metacarpophalangeal joint extension contractures. With this type of splint, the concept of low-load prolonged stress is used. The force of the static progressive splint is lower than with a dynamic splint. A static progressive splint is recommended in this case because it can be worn for longer periods of time. The stress from dynamic splinting is too intermittent and therefore is not the best choice of management for this patient. If there is no progress after several months of static progressive splinting, surgical intervention may be considered.

Answer: **C**
Hunter, Mackin, Callahan, p. 1131

19. The patient in the previous question was treated with static progressive splinting for 4 months and had less than 50° active range of motion at his metacarpophalangeal joints. A capsulectomy was performed. When can splinting be reinitiated to maintain the gains made in surgery?

A. Within 72 hours after surgery
B. 3 to 5 days after surgery
C. 14 days after surgery, when sutures are removed
D. Splinting would not be indicated because the surgeon corrected the restrictions.

This patient was a good candidate for a capsulectomy because he had less than 65° of flexion at the metacarpophalangeal joints. Therapy and splinting should be initiated within 72 hours after surgery. Dynamic splinting should be applied to pull the proximal phalanx into flexion. Dynamic splints can be used during the day as an adjunct to the patient's active exercise program, as well as to protect weakened structures. Static progressive splints often are used at night, placing the metacarpophalangeal joints at near end range of obtainable flexion. The safe position splint is another option for use at night. All splints must be monitored and adjusted frequently. The therapist must pay careful attention to extension lags and if they develop, flexion splinting must be alternated with extension splinting.

Answer: **A**
Hunter, Mackin, Callahan, pp. 1132-1134

20. You are treating a patient after zone-V flexor tendon repair. The patient can fully passively extend his digits only if his wrist is flexed to 30°, and can passively extend the wrist to neutral only with his fingers slightly flexed. Which type of splint is indicated for maximum gains in extension?

A. Dynamic extension of the wrist, with a finger pan to immobilize the fingers in full extension
B. Dynamic wrist extension, with the fingers free
C. Resting pan splint
D. No splint is required. In time, the patient will recover his range of motion.

This patient has extrinsic flexor tightness proximal to the wrist. For specific discussion of extrinsic/intrinsic tightness, refer to Chapter 2, question 5. Because the patient displays a significant change in wrist position with the digits fully extended, it is most beneficial to add a finger pan to a dynamic wrist extension splint (Fig. 15-7). The "pan" immobilizes the fingers in extension in addition to splinting the wrist in extension, which helps to reverse the effects of extrinsic flexor tightness proximal to the wrist.

Answer: **A**
Fess, Philips, p. 265

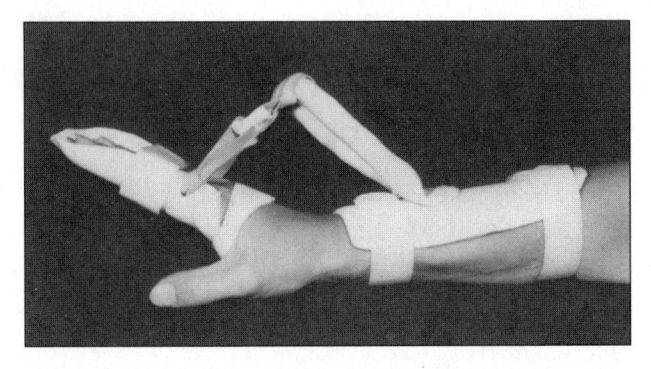

Fig. 15-7 ■ From Fess EE, Philips CA: *Hand splinting: principles and methods,* ed 2, St. Louis, 1987, CV Mosby.

21. A patient is referred to you with a diagnosis of tennis elbow. His physician has recommended a splint. Which splint would you apply?

A. Volar wrist splint with wrist positioned at 10° of dorsiflexion
B. Volar wrist splint with wrist positioned at 45° of dorsiflexion
C. Volar wrist splint with wrist at neutral
D. Volar wrist splint with wrist at 20° of flexion

The purpose of a splint for treatment of lateral epicondylitis is to place the wrist extensor muscles in a position of rest. A volar wrist splint is applied with the wrist in 45° of dorsiflexion. For a very acute lateral epicondylitis, or when a patient experiences pain with elbow flexion or extension, a posterior elbow splint with 90° of elbow flexion and moderate wrist extension can be worn continuously for 2 to 3 weeks to reduce inflammation and pain.

Answer: **B**
Hunter, Mackin, Callahan, p. 1817

22. A patient with rheumatoid arthritis is referred to you for a resting hand splint for night wear. Which splint position is recommended for this patient?

A. Wrist at 10° to 30° extension with the thumb palmarly abducted; metacarpal joints at 15° to 25° of flexion; and digits in slight flexion
B. Wrist at 30° to 50° extension with the thumb radially abducted; metacarpal joints at 30° to 40° of flexion; and digits in slight flexion
C. Wrist at 40° to 50° extension with the thumb palmarly abducted and metacarpal joints at neutral with digits in slight flexion
D. Wrist at slight flexion with thumb radially abducted; metacarpal joints at 10° to 20° of flexion; and digits in slight flexion

In an inflammatory condition such as rheumatoid arthritis, a resting hand splint is recommended. The resting hand splint places the wrist at 10° to 30° extension, with the thumb in palmar abduction, metacarpal joints at 15° to 25° of flexion, and the digits in slight flexion. For patients with severe deformity or exacerbation from rheumatoid arthritis, the resting splint can be modified to position the wrist at neutral or slight extension with slight ulnar deviation. The thumb should be positioned midway between radial and palmar abduction for increased comfort. The recommended thumb position for splinting the rheumatoid hand (at any time) varies among authors.

Answer: **A**
Hunter, Mackin, Callahan, p. 1349
Coppard, Lohman, pp. 97, 98

> **CLINICAL GEM:**
> Too much wrist dorsiflexion may increase the risk of carpal tunnel syndrome.

23. It is important for all patients with radial nerve palsy to receive dynamic splinting regimes to allow for functional use of the hand. True or False?

The most important rationale for splinting a high radial nerve injury is to support the wrist in extension, enhance hand function, and prevent overstretching of the extensors. For many patients, the use of a simple wrist extension splint (not pictured) is sufficient to allow satisfactory hand function because the lumbricals and interossei are able to extend the interphalangeal joints. Extension outriggers for the digits and thumb should be used in situations in which full digital extension is required for successful completion of specific tasks (Fig. 15-8). However, these splints often are considered bulky and excessive and may be discontinued by the patient. Choose patients wisely before fabricating this splint.

Answer: **False**
Fess, Philips, p. 346

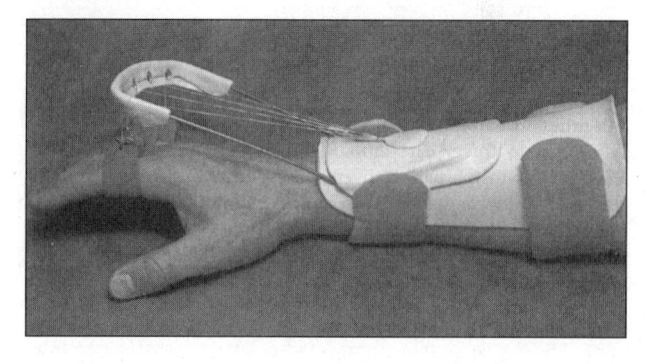

Fig. 15-8 ■ From Coppard BM, Lohman H: *Introduction to splinting: a critical-thinking and problem-solving approach*, St. Louis, 1996, Mosby-Year Book.

24. You are treating a patient with a 6-month-old fixed proximal interphalangeal joint flexion contracture. Which of the following is the best technique for increasing the range of motion of this joint?

A. Dynamic proximal interphalangeal joint extension splint, hand-based
B. Dynamic proximal interphalangeal joint extension splint, forearm-based
C. Serial cast
D. No splint. This is a fixed contracture, which requires surgical intervention.

Casting is one of the most helpful techniques for treating older injuries when remodeling has already taken place. In the case of a fixed contracture, serial casts often are the only form of treatment other than surgical release that provides satisfactory correction. Serial casting often is used preoperatively to improve the chances of successful surgery by reversing the contracture to maximal soft-tissue length. The cast should be changed every other day or a minimum of two times a week to allow exercise and to monitor skin status.

Answer: **C**
Fess, Philips, pp. 453-457
Refer to Fig. 15-9.

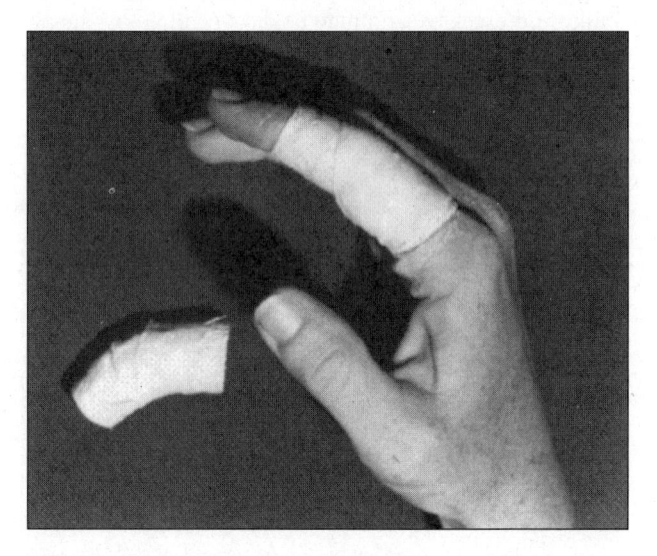

Fig. 15-9 ■ Progressive casting of index interphalangeal joint into extension. (From Hunter JM, Mackin EJ, Callahan AD: *Rehabilitation of the hand: surgery and therapy,* ed 4, St. Louis, 1995, Mosby-Year Book.)

> **CLINICAL GEM:**
> Preconditioning before cast application is achieved with passive exercise, joint mobilization, or other modalities to help bring the tissue to its end-range for several minutes. After preconditioning, cast application should be immediate because the tissues will quickly return to their pre-stretch length.

> **CLINICAL GEM:**
> For serial casting, either plaster of Paris or a low-temperature, thermoplastic material such as Plastofit by Orfit may be used.

25. Golfer's elbow (medial epicondylitis) is treated with which type of splint?

A. Volar wrist splint with wrist at 30° extension
B. Volar wrist splint with wrist at neutral
C. Volar wrist splint with wrist flexed at 20° to 30°
D. No splint will help this condition.

Golfer's elbow is a tendinitis affecting the muscles that originate from the medial epicondyle. During the acute phase, the goal is to reduce inflammation and promote the healing of microscopic tears. A volar wrist splint with the wrist at neutral is applied and worn for 10 to 14 days continuously. After the acute phase, the splint is used for protection or on an as-needed basis for pain.

Answer: **B**
Hunter, Mackin, Callahan, pp. 1811-1812

26. The first web space of the hand often becomes contracted in cases of arthritis, paralysis of the thumb abductors, or scarring. If this contraction occurs, tendon transfers to restore abduction and opposition will fail because they cannot overcome the tension of the tight web. The therapist is given the job of "stretching the web." Splinting is highly effective and is a "low-risk" method of achieving a sustained web stretch. True or False?

Sustained stretch over time is a highly effective method of stretching; however, in the case of the first web space, splinting is not without its risks. In many cases, the therapist incorrectly or inadvertently stresses the metacarpophalangeal joint distally instead of the carpometacarpal joint. The result is that the ulnar collateral ligament at the metacarpophalangeal joint becomes elongated and the thumb web remains shortened and tight. The solution is to apply tension proximally at the head of the metacarpal (watching for pressure ischemia). Surgical correction may be required in severe cases, especially with extensive scarring.

Answer: **False**
Brand, Hollister, pp. 160-162
Refer to Fig. 15-10.

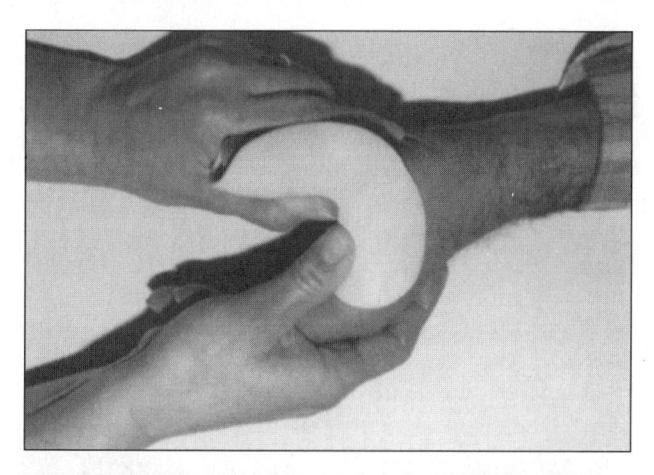

Fig. 15-10 ■ When fabricating a thumb web stretching splint, the therapist should apply the corrective force below the metacarpophalangeal joints of the thumb and index finger to prevent strain on the collateral ligaments. (From Hunter JM, Mackin EJ, Callahan AD: *Rehabilitation of the hand: surgery and therapy,* ed 4, St. Louis, 1995, Mosby-Year Book.)

provocative activities. Therapy for muscle conditioning is not advisable because repetitive finger flexion exercises and sustained grip can increase median nerve compression by increasing pressure in the carpal canal. Although surgery may ultimately be required, conservative treatment for persistent symptoms should include splinting the metacarpophalangeal joints in extension to pull the lumbricals—which take their origin from the flexor digitorum profundi—up out of the carpal tunnel. Studies have shown that the lumbricals lie distal to the carpal tunnel and do not affect intratunnel pressures until finger flexion occurs. Wrist-control splinting alone may not be sufficient to reduce carpal tunnel pressures and digital flexion also may need to be restricted.

Answer: **C**
Evans, pp. 17-18

27. A machinist with "thick, working hands" and well-developed intrinsic muscles was diagnosed with carpal tunnel syndrome. He has been treated for 3 weeks with wrist-control splinting, antiinflammatory medications, oral vitamins, and instructions to avoid provocative wrist positions and repetitive motions. Despite conservative management, his symptoms of low median nerve compression persist. Provocative testing of the cervical spine and proximal upper extremity is negative. The patient is fearful of surgery and resists any suggestion of it. The best method for achieving symptom relief would be:

A. Adding ice massage to treatment and reassessing the patient in 2 weeks
B. Initiating therapy three times a week to improve strength for return to work
C. Incorporating extension of the metacarpophalangeal joints into the wrist extension splint
D. Providing patient education to convince him that surgery is required

Although ice massage is an effective modality for relief of pain and inflammation, this patient has already been taking antiinflammatory medications and has altered

28. You are treating a patient who was referred to you with a humeral shaft fracture. The doctor orders a splint for this patient. Which type of splint would you fabricate?

A. Airplane splint
B. Sarmiento fracture brace
C. Abduction wedge brace
D. Splinting is not indicated for this patient

The humerus is an ideal candidate for functional fracture bracing. A cylinder applied externally to a fractured long bone restrains soft-tissue expansion, directing force equally in all directions during muscle contraction. Sarmiento describes this as a "pseudohydraulic environment." The internal force mechanically stabilizes the fracture. The Sarmiento fracture brace is fastened circumferentially. Active pendulum exercises can be initiated 1 week after humeral shaft fracture, with or without brace application.

Answer: **B**
Hunter, Mackin, Callahan, pp. 396-398
Refer to Fig. 15-11.

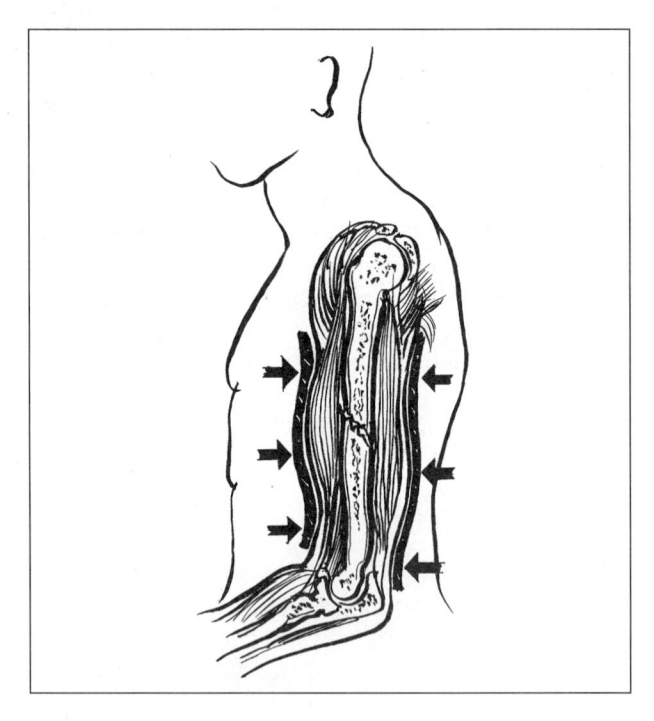

Fig. 15-11 ■ Schematic drawing of a humeral fracture brace (Sarmiento fracture brace) shows how the compressed soft tissue stabilizes a humeral fracture. (Redrawn from Sarmiento A, Latta L: *Closed functional treatment of fractures,* New York, 1981, Springer-Verlag.)

> **CLINICAL GEM:**
> Pendulum or passive exercises are permitted during the first few weeks after humeral shaft fracture. Early active exercise should be avoided until the fracture stabilizes because active exercise can contribute to fracture angulation.

29. A patient with a grade-I skier's thumb injury is treated with a splint for 3 weeks. How should his thumb be positioned in the long opponens splint?

A. Thumb in 30° of palmar abduction, interphalangeal joint free
B. Thumb completely palmarly abducted, interphalangeal joint free
C. Full thumb palmar abduction, interphalangeal joint included
D. Thumb in 30° of palmar abduction, interphalangeal joint included

Ulnar collateral ligament injuries at the thumb metacarpophalangeal joint can be classified as grade I, II, or III. Acute, grade-I injuries (e.g., gamekeeper's or skier's thumb) are most common and are treated with a long opponens splint for 3 weeks, with the thumb in 30° of palmar abduction (Fig. 15-12). The interphalangeal joint is left free to allow for early motion of this joint. Gentle range-of-motion exercises to the metacarpophalangeal joint are initiated 3 weeks after injury. In a grade-II injury, the ligament is partially torn and requires longer immobilization than is needed for a grade-I injury. A grade-III injury is characterized by a complete ligament rupture that requires surgical intervention.

Answer: **A**
Hunter, Mackin, Callahan, p. 1814

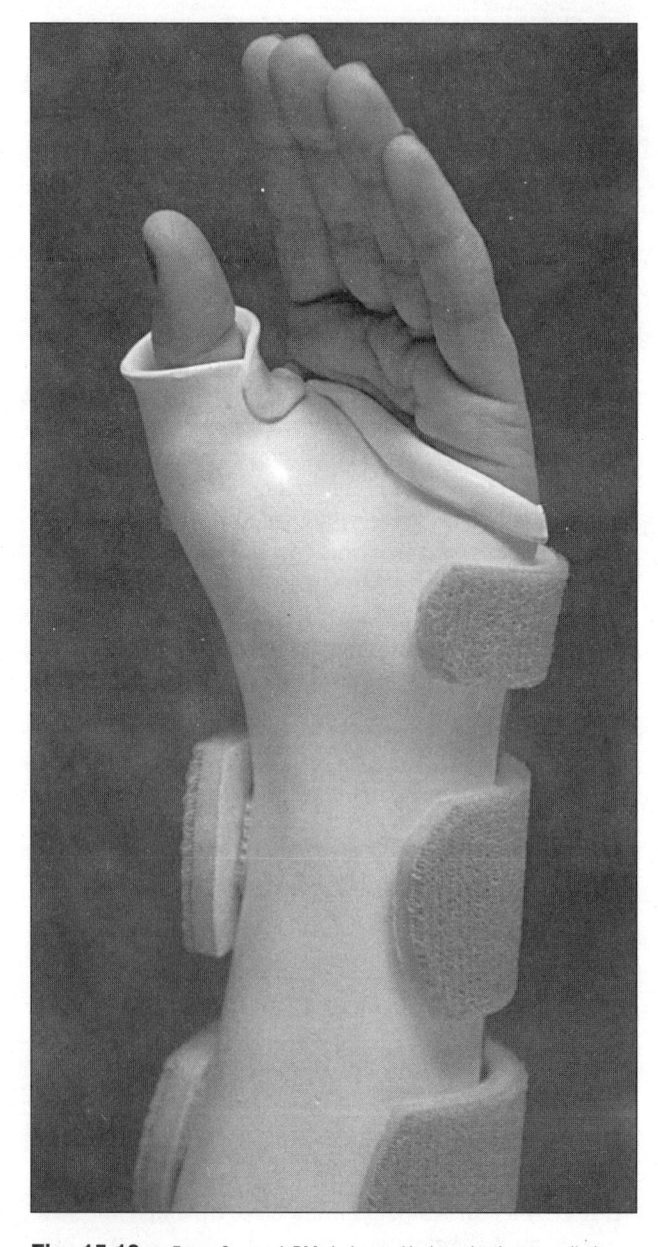

Fig. 15-12 ■ From Coppard BM, Lohman H: *Introduction to splinting: a critical-thinking and problem-solving approach,* St. Louis, 1996, Mosby-Year Book.

> **CLINICAL GEM:**
> Although traditionally managed in a long opponens splint or cast, protection of the healing thumb ulnar collateral ligament can be achieved with a splint that does *not* immobilize the wrist (Fig. 15-13).

The basal joint, or first carpometacarpal joint, often is "worn out" from osteoarthritis. A short opponens splint (Fig. 15-14) can be applied to reduce dorsoradial subluxation of the basal joint. Patients with arthritis in this joint often are greatly relieved by using this small splint during functional activities. The molding must be precise at the base of the first metacarpal to ensure adequate stabilization of the carpometacarpal joint during active use of the thumb.

Answer: **A**
Hunter, Mackin, Callahan, pp. 1164-1165

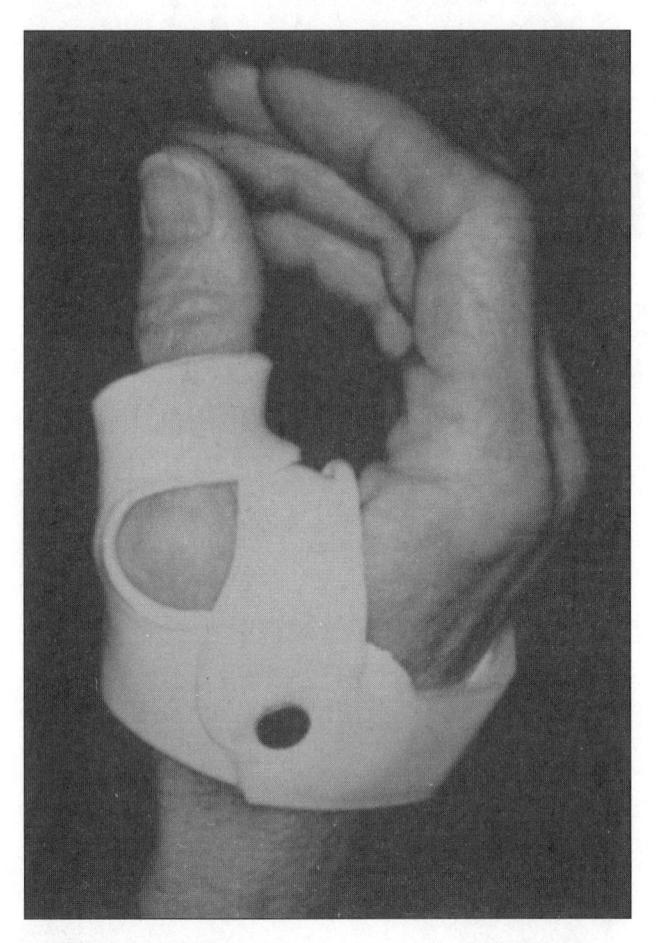

Fig. 15-13 ■ From Hunter JM, Mackin EJ, Callahan AD: *Rehabilitation of the hand: surgery and therapy*, ed 4, St. Louis, 1995, Mosby-Year Book.

30. A patient is referred to you with the diagnosis of mild basal joint arthritis. She reports pain at the base of the thumb with functional task performance. Which type of splint should you fabricate?

A. Short opponens
B. Ulnar gutter
C. Wrist support splint
D. No splint

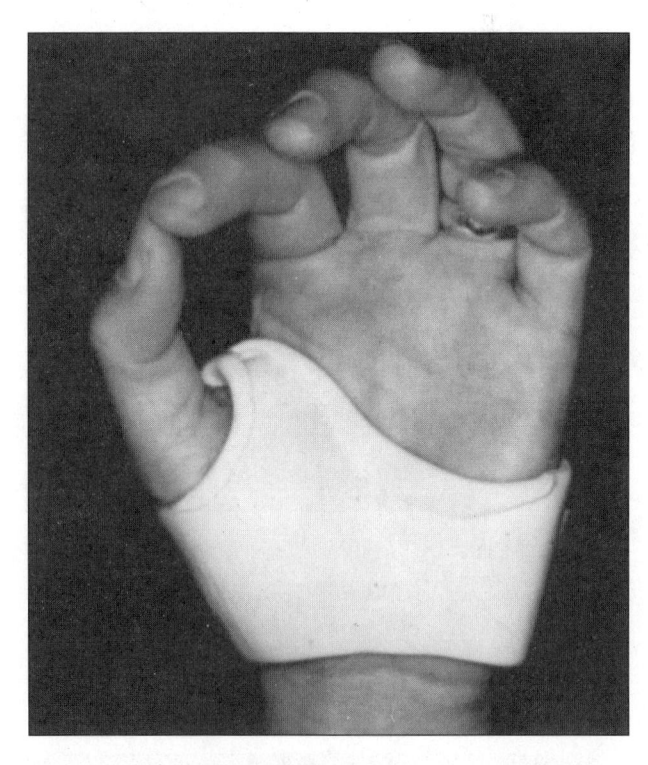

Fig. 15-14 ■ From Hunter JM, Mackin EJ, Callahan AD: *Rehabilitation of the hand: surgery and therapy*, ed 4, St. Louis, 1995, Mosby-Year Book.

> **CLINICAL GEM:**
> If the first carpometacarpal, or basal joint, deformity has progressed to a dislocation and is not manually reducible, a splint is of little value and may increase the patient's pain.

190 CHAPTER 15 Splinting

31. Name the following splints:

Splint

1. _____

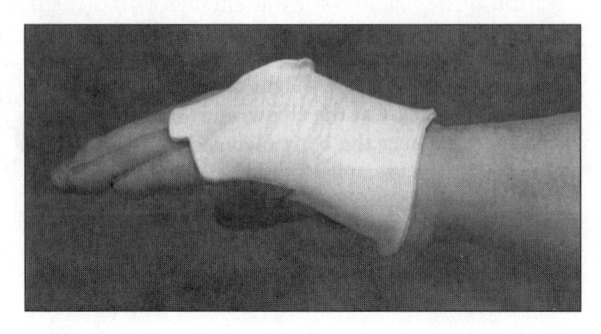

From Coppard BM, Lohman H: *Introduction to splinting: a critical-thinking and problem-solving approach,* St. Louis, 1996, Mosby-Year Book.

2.

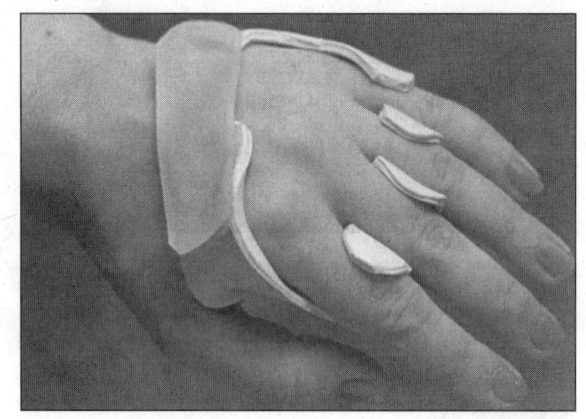

From Coppard BM, Lohman H: *Introduction to splinting: a critical-thinking and problem-solving approach,* St. Louis, 1996, Mosby-Year Book.

3.

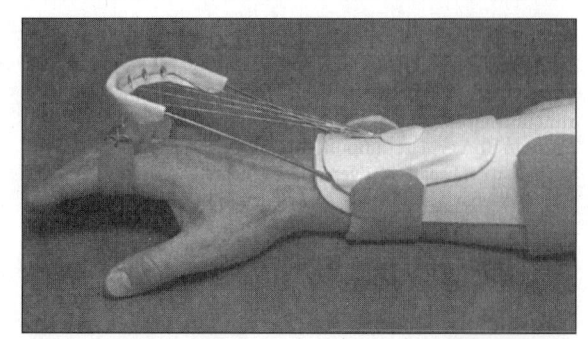

From Coppard BM, Lohman H: *Introduction to splinting: a critical-thinking and problem-solving approach,* St. Louis, 1996, Mosby-Year Book.

4.

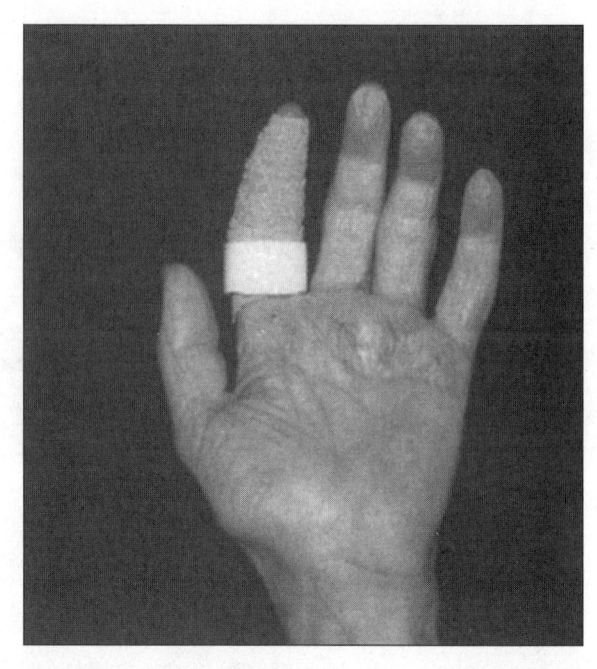

From Hunter JM, Mackin EJ, Callahan AD: *Rehabilitation of the hand: surgery and therapy,* ed 4, St. Louis, 1995, Mosby-Year Book.

5.

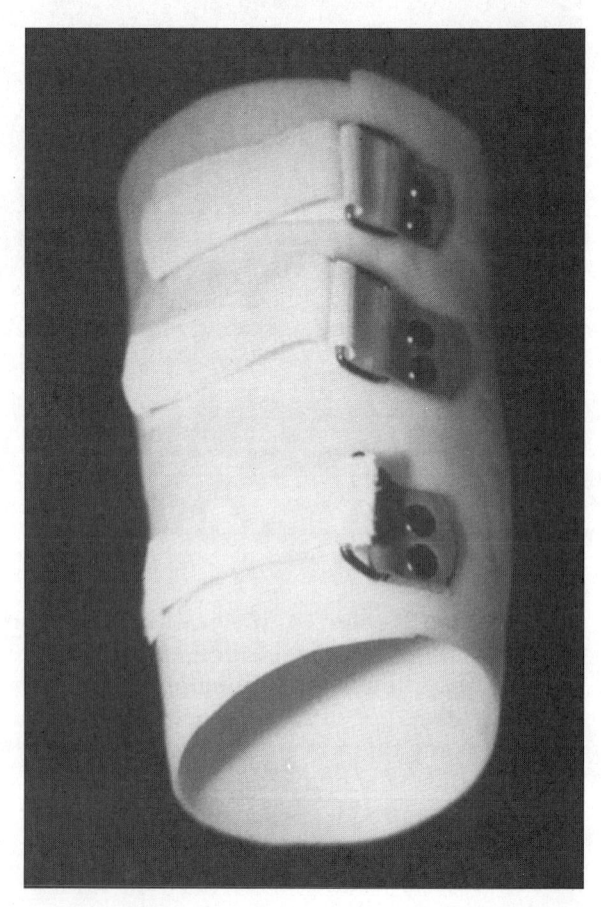

From Hunter JM, Mackin EJ, Callahan AD: *Rehabilitation of the hand: surgery and therapy,* ed 4, St. Louis, 1995, Mosby-Year Book.

CHAPTER 15 Splinting 191

6.

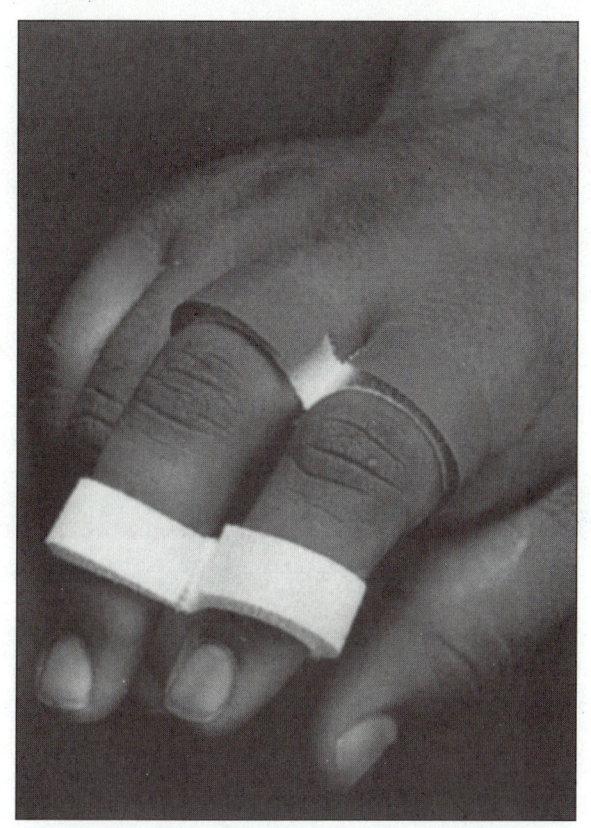

From Hunter JM, Mackin EJ, Callahan AD: *Rehabilitation of the hand: surgery and therapy,* ed 4, St. Louis, 1995, Mosby-Year Book.

Name

A. Pulley ring splint
B. Ulnar nerve injury splint
C. Budding strapping
D. Sarmiento fracture bracing
E. Ulnar deviation splint
F. Radial nerve palsy

Answers: **1. B; 2. E; 3. F; 4. A; 5. D; 6. C**
Hunter, Mackin, Callahan, pp. 318, 399, 470
Coppard, Lohman, pp. 15, 157, 180

Chapter 16

Congenital Anomalies/Amputations/Prosthetics

Topics to be reviewed in random order are:

- Congenital classification system
- Syndactyly/polydactyly
- Madelung's deformity
- Phocomelia
- Clinodactyly
- Kirner's deformity
- Camptodactyly
- Windblown hand
- Hypoplastic thumb
- Desensitization
- Phantom limb
- Early-fit prosthesis
- Prosthesis control mechanism
- Prosthetic types
- Body powered and myoelectric prostheses

1. Match each congenital deformity with the proper classification (pick two deformities for each classification).

Classification

1. Failure of formation (arrest of development)
2. Failure of differentiation (separation)
3. Duplication
4. Overgrowth
5. Undergrowth
6. Congenital constriction band syndrome
7. Generalized skeletal abnormalities

Congenital Deformity

A. Thumb clutched hand
B. Polydactyly
C. Madelung's deformity
D. Transverse deficiencies
E. Maffucci's syndrome
F. Kirner's deformity
G. Macrodactyly
H. Triphalangism
I. Brachydactyly
J. Phocomelia
K. Hypoplasia
L. Gigantism
M. Compression neuropathy
N. Acrosyndactyly

Answers: 1. D and J; 2. A and F; 3. B and H; 4. L and G; 5. I and K; 6. M and N; 7. C and E

Swanson, p. 4
Hunter, Mackin, Callahan, pp. 1428-1433

2. Which of the following means webbed fingers?

A. Polydactyly
B. Ectrodactyly
C. Syndactyly
D. Brachydactyly

Syndactyly means webbed fingers. The incidence of syndactyly and polydactyly is high among infants with congenital anomalies. Syndactyly is most frequently found in the third web space, followed by the fourth web, second web, and first web, respectively.

Answer: **C**
Green, p. 346
Refer to Fig. 16-1.

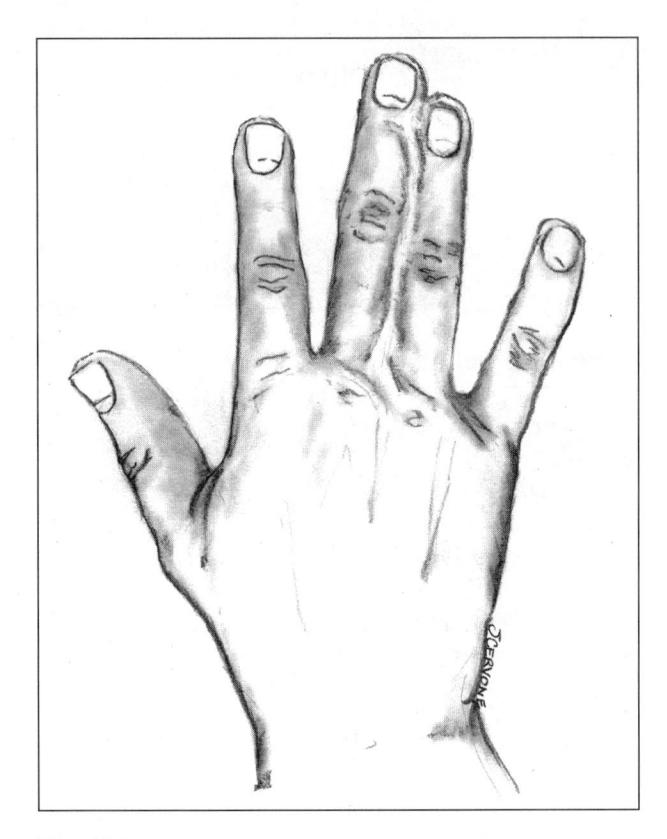

Fig. 16-1

3. Which disorder specifically affects the wrist?

A. Pterygium cubital contracture
B. Kirner's deformity
C. Phocomelia
D. Madelung's deformity

Madelung's deformity is a genetic disorder that does not become obvious until late childhood and is more common in females. The classic deformity is a shortening of the radius at the wrist, resulting in an ulna that is longer than the radius; it appears as a subluxed wrist with a prominent ulnar head. The patient often has limited extension and supination. Madelung's deformity is most frequently seen bilaterally.

Function and appearance are rarely a problem until adolescence. Wrist pain may be noted with vigorous activities. Rest can be used when the pain is exacerbated. Surgical correction can be performed if needed.

Answer: **D**
Green, p. 515
Hunter, Mackin, Callahan, p. 1433

4. Which disorder involves the fifth digit but often is not obvious until the child reaches the age of 12?

A. Kirner's deformity
B. Hyperphalangism
C. Pterygium cubital contracture
D. Arthrogryposis

In 1927, Kirner described a condition of the fifth digit that was characterized by palmar and radial curving of the distal phalanx. This disorder is not considered strictly congenital because it often is not obvious until about age 12. It is more common in females and begins as a painless progressive curving of the distal phalanges of both hands, most commonly in the fifth digit.

Answer: **A**
Green, pp. 353-354
Refer to Fig. 16-2.

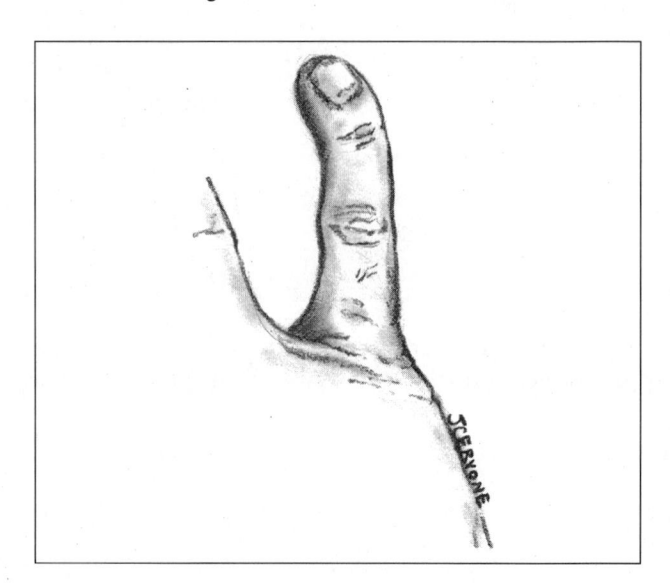

Fig. 16-2

CHAPTER 16 Congenital Anomalies/Amputations/Prosthetics

5. Match each deformity with its definition:

Deformity

1. Pterygium cubital
2. Arthrogryposis
3. Polydactyly
4. Ectrodactyly

Definition

A. Persistent joint contracture
B. Congenital elbow webbing
C. Missing digits
D. Having more than the normal number of fingers and toes

Answers: **1. B; 2. A; 3. D; 4. C**
Green, pp. 304, 363, 370, 480-481

6. Which of the following terms means seal limb?

A. Ectrodactyly
B. Phocomelia
C. Clinodactyly
D. Syndactyly

The term phocomelia means seal limb. Patients with this failure of formation may produce an extreme shortening of the limb. The incidence of phocomelia is approximately 0.8% of all congenital upper limb anomalies. This deformity became notorious in the 1950s and early 1960s when pregnant women took thalidomide. There are few indications for surgery in patients with phocomelia, but prosthetics often are indicated, especially in individuals with bilateral phocomelia.

Answer: **B**
Green, p. 258
Swanson, p. 15
Refer to Fig. 16-3.

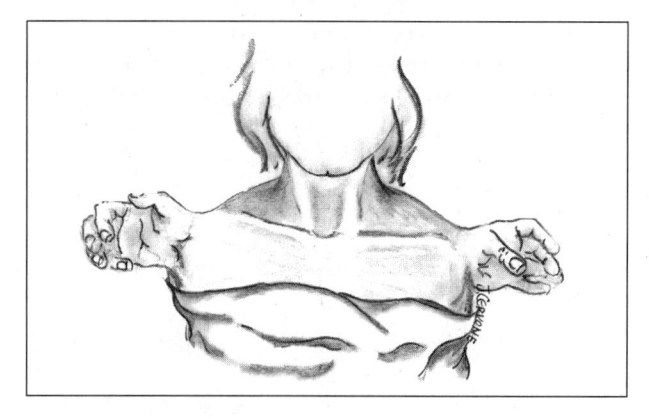

Fig. 16-3

7. Congenital ulnar drift of the fingers and congenital contracture of the digits also are referred to as windblown hand. True or False?

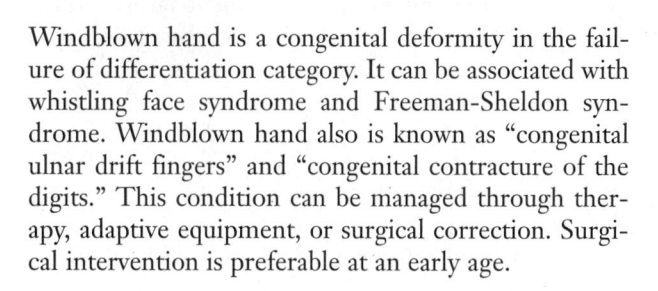

Windblown hand is a congenital deformity in the failure of differentiation category. It can be associated with whistling face syndrome and Freeman-Sheldon syndrome. Windblown hand also is known as "congenital ulnar drift fingers" and "congenital contracture of the digits." This condition can be managed through therapy, adaptive equipment, or surgical correction. Surgical intervention is preferable at an early age.

Answer: **True**
Hunter, Mackin, Callahan, p. 1431
Refer to Fig. 16-4.

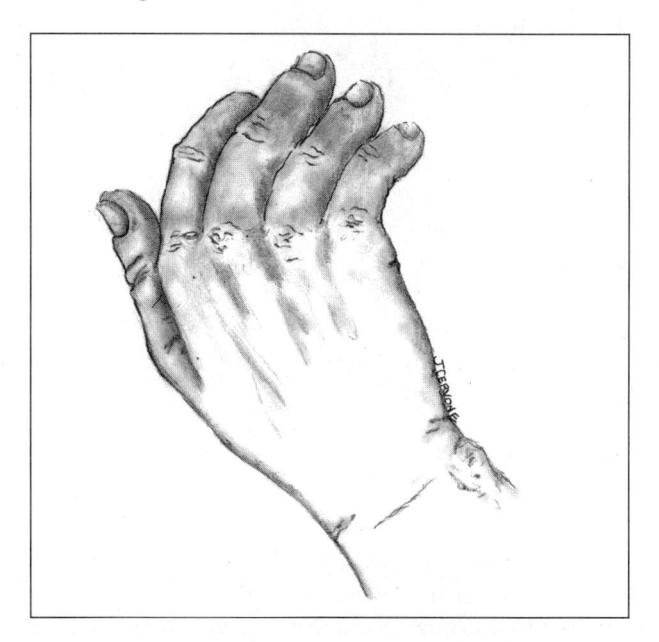

Fig. 16-4

8. Which term is commonly used to refer to a congenital flexion contracture of the proximal interphalangeal joint of the little finger in the sagittal plane?

A. Syndactyly
B. Kirner's deformity
C. Clinodactyly
D. Camptodactyly
E. Trigger digit

Camptodactyly classically presents with a flexion deformity of the proximal interphalangeal joint of the little finger in the sagittal plane (flexion/extension). However, a variety of presentations are noted in the literature. Camptodactyly often is hereditary and may present bilaterally. Frequently, no treatment is necessary, unless it is disabling. Surgical treatment varies because of the multiplicity of structures. Conservative treatment consisting of static, dynamic, or serial casting/splinting has shown favorable results.

Answer: **D**
Swanson, p. 28
Hunter, Mackin, Callahan, p. 1430
Refer to Fig. 16-5.

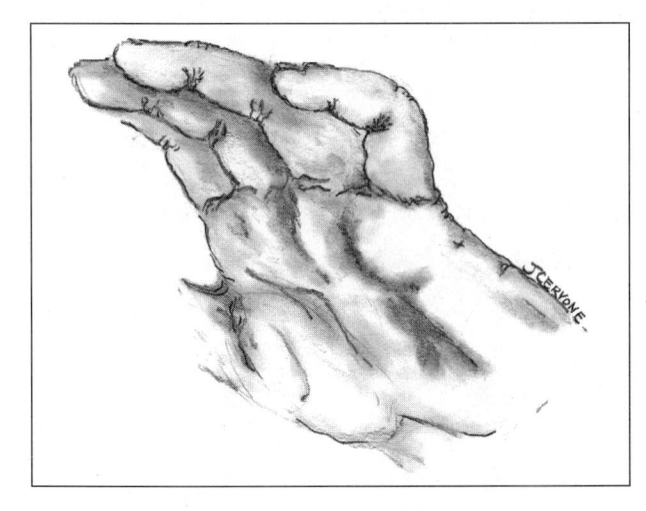

Fig. 16-5

9. An 11-year-old female presents with a bent little finger and has no history of trauma. The patient's complaint is primarily cosmetic. Clinical examination and radiographs reveal middle phalanx involvement with curving in the coronal or radioulnar plane. What would you conclude?

A. Patient has a hypoplastic digit
B. Patient hurt her finger but does not recall injury
C. Patient has Maffucci's syndrome
D. Patient has clinodactyly

The patient's findings are classical indications of clinodactyly, which is a categorization of failure of differentiation. Clinodactyly is similar to camptodactyly; classically, both involve a bent finger in the fifth digit. In clinodactyly, the finger is bent in the coronal or radioulnar plane and most often affects the distal interphalangeal joint; in camptodactyly the finger is bent in the sagittal or extension/flexion plane and most often affects the proximal interphalangeal joint. Often no intervention is needed for clinodactyly. Elective surgery may be indicated for cosmetic purposes.

Answer: **D**
Hunter, Mackin, Callahan, p. 1431
Swanson, p. 28
Green, pp. 411, 423
Refer to Fig. 16-6.

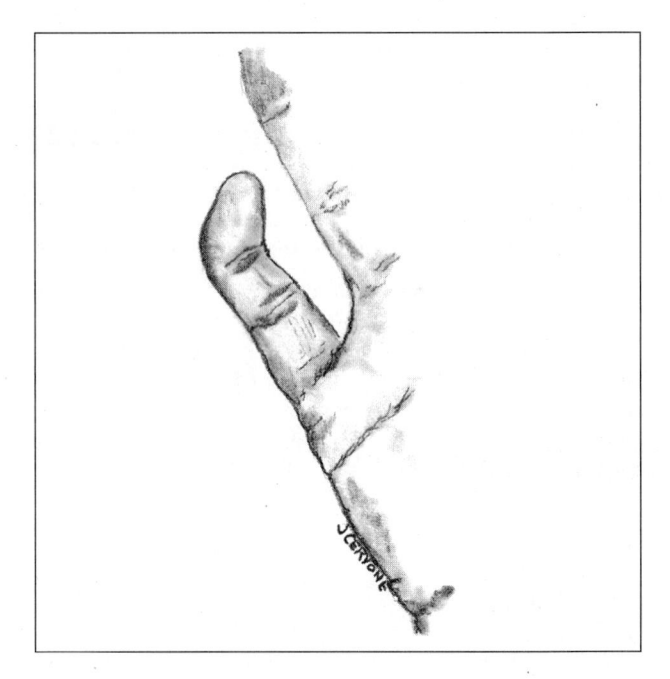

Fig. 16-6

10. Figure 16-7 is an example of:

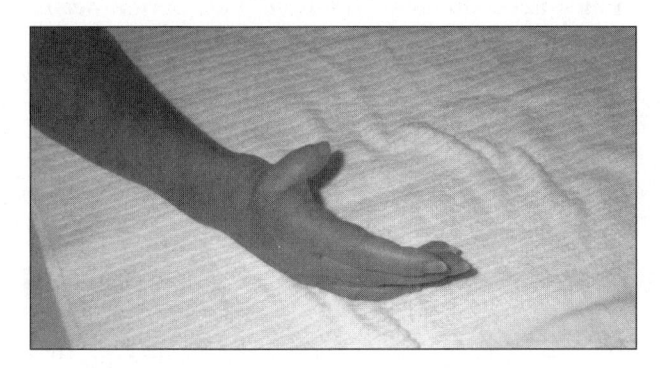

Fig. 16-7

A. Apert's thumb
B. Congenital clasped thumb
C. Retroflexible thumb
D. Hypoplastic thumb

The hypoplastic thumb is a defective digit that is incomplete in its development. The degree of hypoplasia ranges from minimal shortening to complete absence of the thumb. The remaining three answers are specific thumb disorders that are not applicable to the patient shown.

Apert's thumb frequently is short and angulated. The thumb and index webs are deficient, and the thumb must be separated early to allow for function. Congenital clasped thumb is characterized by a thumb that is flexed and adducted; this deformity sometimes is referred to as thumb-clutched hand. The retroflexible thumb is a rare, congenital anomaly; during physical examination, the metacarpophalangeal joint is hyperextended and the distal interphalangeal joint is hyperflexed (resembling a type-III deformity of rheumatoid arthritis).

Answer: **D**
Green, pp. 385-409

11. Amputation at the shoulder level represents which percentage of impairment for the upper extremity?

A. 30%
B. 50%
C. 80%
D. 100%

An amputation of the arm at the shoulder level represents an impairment of 100% of the upper extremity. This corresponds to a 60% impairment of the whole person.

An amputation below the axilla and proximal to the biceps tendon is rated as a 95% to 100% impairment of the upper extremity and a 57% to 60% impairment of the whole person.

An amputation below the elbow and proximal to the metacarpophalangeal joints is rated as a 90% to 95% impairment of the upper extremity and a 54% to 57% impairment of the whole person.

An amputation of the fingers and thumb through the metacarpophalangeal joint is considered a 100% impairment of the hand, a 90% impairment of the upper extremity, and a 54% impairment of the whole person. Digit amputation is rated on a scale that is relative to the entire hand.

Answer: **D**
Hunter, Mackin, Callahan, pp. 1849, 1868

12. Which technique is not appropriate for desensitization of the residual limb?

A. Tapping
B. Vibration
C. Use of graded textures
D. All of the above are appropriate desensitization techniques

---

After the wound has healed, desensitization may be needed for a hypersensitive residual limb. The techniques cited as most appropriate include gentle massage, pressure, tapping, stroking, vibration, and the use of graded textures. Desensitization helps prepare the limb for application of the prosthetic socket.

Answer: **D**
Bowker, Michael, p. 279
Peimer, p. 2461
Hunter, Mackin, Callahan, p. 1229

13. Which of these phenomena is a "normal" response to an amputation that generally does not interfere with function or require any treatment?

A. Phantom limb sensation
B. Phantom limb pain
C. Residual limb pain
D. All of the above

Phantom limb sensation is the ability to perceive cortical images of the lost limb and it occurs in almost every acquired amputee. Phantom limb sensation usually is no more than a minor annoyance and, on occasion, may even be useful during prosthetic training. New amputees should be educated that this is a "normal" phenomenon so that they do not think they are "going crazy" when they still "feel" the areas distal to the amputation. This sensation generally does not interfere with function or require any treatment.

Phantom limb pain can begin in the immediate postamputation phase and should diminish but can become a severe problem and result in chronic pain. If this pain interferes with normal activities of daily living and sleep patterns for more than 6 weeks after the amputation, it must be aggressively treated. Phantom pain is believed to occur because of deafferentation of the peripheral and central pain centers, especially the somatosensory cortex. Pain treatment modalities are used based on their mechanisms in modifying pain messages in these pathways. Many treatment techniques have been employed with varying success. Effective techniques include the use of drugs and conventional occupational/physical therapy modalities.

Residual limb pain is defined as pain in the residual limb that does not descend into the phantom. This pain may be related to neuroma formation or may be caused by physical changes in the residual limb. Another common cause is related to pressure from an ill-fitting prosthesis.

Answer: **A**
Hunter, Mackin, Callahan, p. 1229
Esquenazi, Meier, pp. 5-20
Peimer, p. 2465

CLINICAL GEM:
One way to treat phantom pain is by using a transcutaneous electrical nerve stimulation unit. One technique is electrode placement on the contralateral limb.

14. The "golden period" in prosthetic management denotes the most optimal time for the fitting of an upper-extremity prosthesis in order to promote successful rehabilitation. This period occurs during which time after amputation?

A. The first 6 months
B. The first 60 days
C. The first 30 days
D. The first year

The first immediate-fit prosthesis was reported in 1958 and since then many studies have been conducted to show the effect of early-fit prosthetic fabrication on successful rehabilitation. The study conducted by Malone and others denoted a "golden period" of prosthetic fitting, which appeared to be within the first month after amputation. Early application of a prosthesis promotes the continuation of bilateral activities, better acceptance of the prosthesis, and better healing through edema and pain control. The success rate for patients fit within 1 month of amputation was 93%; the success rate for those fit after 1 month was only 42%.

Answer: **C**
Malone et al, pp. 33-41
Hunter, Mackin, Callahan, p. 1211

CLINICAL GEM:
An early-fit prosthesis may be fabricated within the first 2 weeks after surgery. In fact, an immediate fit can be fabricated in the operating room or shortly thereafter.

15. According to the leading pediatric amputee centers, the most appropriate time to fit a congenital unilateral transverse radioulnar limb-deficient child with his or her first prosthesis is:

A. Before 2 months of age, to aid in visually-guided reaching
B. Birth to 3 months, to help promote incorporation of the prosthesis in the child's body image
C. Around 6 months, when the infant is achieving independent sitting balance
D. When the child is old enough to follow simple two-step commands

The appropriate time to fit a congenital amputee with his or her first prosthesis is probably one of the most controversial topics regarding the limb-deficient child. With recent technical advances and the availability of more types of prostheses, the controversy has become even more complicated because it involves the question of the most appropriate type of prosthesis. Hubbard documents many studies supporting the belief that it is important to fit as a child as early as possible to facilitate the child's ability to become two-handed. She also references many articles that weigh the costs of early fitting against the benefits and questions the cost:benefit ratio. Review of the literature from many of the leading pediatric amputee centers seems to indicate a general agreement that the most appropriate time for fitting a first prosthesis on a congenital unilateral amputee is between 3 and 9 months of age, or at about 6 months, when the child is achieving sitting balance. Support for this follows.

The question of early fit to aid visually-guided reaching was supported in a 1976 article by Fisher. She cited research that supports the belief that the development of visually-guided reaching is dependent on the opportunity to see the limb moving in space. She questioned whether fitting the baby before 3 or 4 months of age would aid visually-guided reaching and thus influence future prosthetic wearing and use patterns.

The Child Amputee Prosthetics Project (CAPP) at the University of California in Los Angeles has long been a proponent of early fitting and bases their criteria on developmental milestones. At The CAPP, the criterion for prescribing the first passive prosthesis for a baby with a below-elbow limb deficiency is the attainment of independent sitting balance. When the baby is sitting securely, has no need to use the arms for support, and has achieved some proficiency in creeping and pulling to a stand, a prosthesis can provide a functional advantage.

Wanner asserts that early fitting at 6 months of age enables the child to incorporate the prosthesis into his body image, which increases the likelihood of long-term prosthetic acceptance. At 6 months of age, most children begin to sit. The prosthesis enables the child to touch down on the limb-deficient side and thereby improves his sitting balance. It also helps the child to do bimanual activities at arm's length.

Hubbard, in her practice with myoprosthetics at the Hugh MacMillan Rehabilitation Center in Canada, also supports this early fit. A passive, cosmetic prosthesis typically is provided to congenital amputees between 3 and 6 months of age to assist them in balance and gross motor activity and to condition them to wearing an artificial limb.

Finally, Jain has outlined in chart form the developmental milestones that are used to guide prescription of various prostheses and their components. He also states that "the initial prosthetic fitting . . . is done at age 3 to 9 months to assist in gross motor development tasks, allowing the use of both limbs for creeping, pulling to stand, and so on. Fitting at a later age (2 to 5 years) has been shown to result in greater rejection of the prosthesis because of the development of compensatory techniques."

Answer: **C**
Hunter, Mackin, Callahan, pp. 1205, 1242, 1246
Bowker, Michael, p. 779
Atkins, Meier, p. 138
Jain, p. 10

16. According to Beasley, which percentage of activities of daily living can be completed with one hand?

A. 30%
B. 50%
C. 70%
D. 90%

According to Beasley, "90 percent of activities of daily living can be accomplished with one normal hand." This fact may account for the large percentage of patients with upper-limb amputations who discard their prostheses.

Answer: **D**
Hunter, Mackin, Callahan, p. 1238
Beasley

17. The Krukenberg procedure initially was indicated for blind, bilateral below-elbow amputees. True or False?

The Krukenberg procedure (Fig. 16-8, *A*) can be considered when treating mutilating upper-extremity injuries. Initially, the Krukenberg procedure was indicated for blind, bilateral below-elbow amputees. This procedure, however, has been used in children with absence of hands and is used in certain countries for unilateral amputees with normal sight. There is concern over the cosmesis of the stump but the amount of function that is possible in these patients is astounding.

There is not much enthusiasm for the Krukenberg procedure in the United States, most likely because of a lack of experience and a poor understanding of both the procedure and how functional (Fig. 16-8, *B*) the patient is afterward.

> *Answer:* **True**
> Hunter, Mackin, Callahan, p. 1055

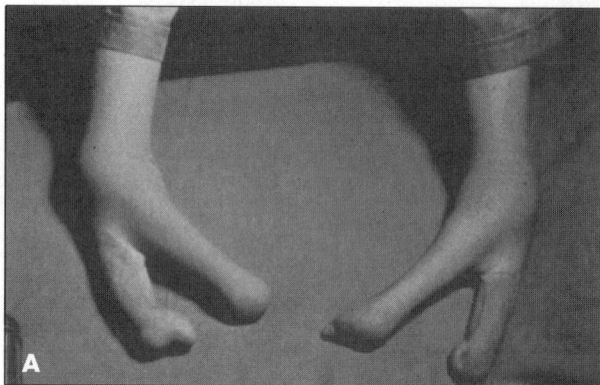

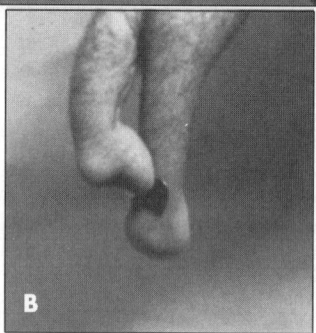

Fig. 16-8 A and B ■ From Hunter JM, Mackin EJ, Callahan AD: *Rehabilitation of the hand: surgery and therapy,* ed 4, St. Louis, 1995, Mosby-Year Book.

18. The control mechanisms needed to lock or unlock a mechanical elbow in a conventional above-elbow prosthesis for a transhumeral amputee are:

A. Chest expansion and scapular abduction of the involved extremity
B. Shoulder depression, shoulder extension, and shoulder abduction of the involved extremity
C. Shoulder depression, shoulder flexion, and internal rotation of the involved extremity
D. Shoulder depression, shoulder extension, and external rotation of the uninvolved extremity

After the prosthesis fit, the first step in training is learning what body movements are needed to control the operation of the prosthetic devices. To operate the elbow lock on a conventional above-elbow prosthesis, the amputee needs **shoulder depression, shoulder extension, and shoulder abduction of the involved extremity.** The therapist must facilitate the full range of motion for these movements before acquisition of the prosthesis and should ensure that the amputee is proficient in these movements for control training before initiating functional use training.

> *Answer:* **B**
> Bowker, Michael, p. 283
> Atkins, Meier, p. 44
> Pedretti, Zoltan, p. 430

19. To power a below-elbow amputee, which motion is used?

A. Humeral flexion
B. Humeral extension
C. Humeral abduction
D. Humeral adduction

A single-control system is used as a power source for a below-elbow amputee to allow for prehension. Humeral flexion is used to operate the terminal device.

Answer: **A**
Hunter, Mackin, Callahan, p. 1234

20. A Muenster socket is necessary for self-suspension when using an above-elbow prosthesis. True or False?

A Muenster socket is necessary for self-suspension in a below-elbow amputee. An above-elbow amputee should have a socket constructed in the shape of a shoulder spica.

> *Answer:* **False**
> Hunter, Mackin, Callahan, pp. 1208, 1227
> *Refer to Fig. 16-9.*

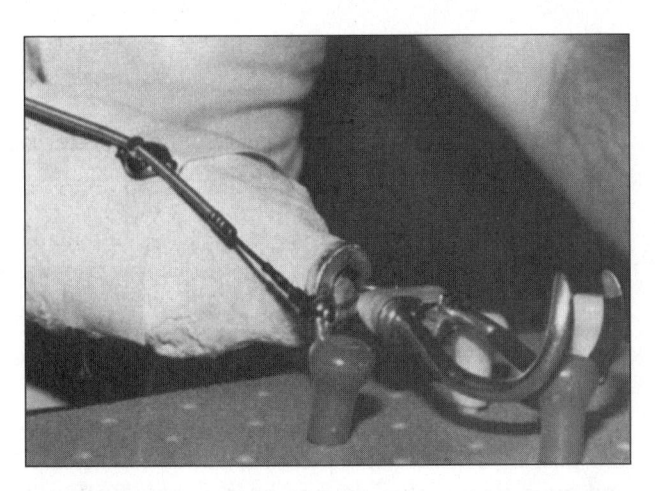

Fig. 16-9 ■ Immediate fit for early training. Cast is applied in the shape of a Muenster below-elbow socket. (From Hunter JM, Mackin EJ, Callahan AD: *Rehabilitation of the hand: surgery and therapy,* ed 4, St. Louis, 1995, Mosby-Year Book.)

21. To what extent should an above-elbow amputee, with a conventional voluntary opening terminal device, be able to open his terminal device when the elbow is fully flexed or extended?

A. At least 50% of maximal available terminal device opening
B. 70% to 100% of maximal available terminal device opening
C. 35% to 55% of maximal available terminal device opening
D. It depends on the level of amputation.

A prosthetic checkout is the key to determining the proper fit, mechanical efficiency, and functioning of the control system. There are many prosthetic evaluation checklists available. Two suggested designs are by New York University and Northwestern University. To evaluate terminal device opening as part of the full evaluation, the above-elbow amputee locks the elbow at 90°. He or she then actively opens the terminal device fully. This opening is measured with a ruler and recorded. The same active opening of the terminal device is next measured with the elbow in full flexion and in full extension. The amputee should be able to open the terminal device at least 50% of the initial measurement when the elbow is at 90°.

A below-elbow amputee should be able to open the terminal device to 70% to 100% of available terminal device opening in full elbow flexion and extension.

Answer: **A**
Hunter, Mackin, Callahan, p. 1233
Trombly, pp. 862-863
Atkins, Meier, p. 42

22. The pediatric "cookie crusher" prosthesis uses which type of control system?

A. One state/two function (hand opening/hand closing)
B. Two state/two muscles
C. Two state/two muscle proportional
D. None of the above

The concept behind myoelectric prosthetics is that the contraction of a muscle can produce a strong enough electric signal that it can be detected at the surface of the skin. This electromyographic signal can be picked up by electrodes that control the flow of myoelectric energy from a battery to a motor. The motor can control a hand, elbow, or even a wrist unit. State control systems function by turning the component either off or on (similar to the operation of a simple light switch). Once the myoelectric system is activated by muscle contraction, the motor will operate at a constant speed until the muscle relaxes and the system is turned off.

Two-state control systems use a contraction of one muscle to activate a motor in one direction, and a second (preferably an antagonistic) muscle to operate the motor in another direction. Therefore, two separate muscles are needed to operate a prosthesis. This two-state/two-muscle control system can operate many commercially available systems and is most commonly used to activate (1) grasp/release in a hand unit using wrist flexors/extensors; and (2) elbow flexion/elbow extension using biceps/triceps. The Otto Block "digital two site" Electric Hand System, the Otto Bock Greifer, and the New York Hosmer-Dorrance electric elbow are all examples of the two-state/two-muscle myoelectric system.

The Utah Artificial Arm System also is a two-state/two-muscle system with the addition of an internal "electronic switch" that is activated by cocontraction of the two muscles, alternating between elbow control and hand control. Spiegel describes the specific control technique in the Utah arm as two-site, five-function myoelectric control.

In proportional control systems, the speed or the prehensile force of the prosthesis is varied with the intensity of the electromyographic signal (similar to the effect of a dimmer switch). The Liberty Mutual Boston Elbow is a proportional two-state/two-muscle system.

In some cases, it is necessary to control a prosthesis with just one muscle site. This may occur when there is only one muscle available (e.g., after brachial plexus injury when only a few muscle sites are available and each is needed to control different movements). In this case, a one-site control system must be used. There are rate-sensitive and level (amplitude)-sensitive control systems. In a rate-sensitive system, the speed at which the muscle is contracted determines the direction of movement. For example, a quick contraction may be used to open the hand and a slow contraction may be used to close it. The hand continues to open or close as long as the muscle remains contracted. In a level-sensitive system, the strength of contraction determines the direction of movement. A hard contraction may be used to open the hand and a gentle contraction may be used to close it. The contractions also must be completed within a specified period of time. The pediatric "cookie crusher" and the University New Brunswick System system are two examples.

Otto Bock's "double channel" Electric Hand System is a one-site, two-function myoswitch controller. So that the Otto Bock Greifer may be completely interchangeable with any of the electric hand systems, it also has the capability to be operated as a one-site/two-function system. Thus, the Greifer can be made to be operated by both one-site or two-state control systems.

Answer: **A**
Hunter, Mackin, Callahan, pp. 1193, 1243
Atkins, Meier, p. 6
Spiegel, p. 62
Esquenazi, Meier, p. 12

23. The most commonly used body-powered terminal device is the:

A. Hosmer-Dorrance voluntary opening hook
B. Otto Bock system hand
C. APRL voluntary closing hand and hook
D. GRIP voluntary closing terminal device

The most distal part of an upper-limb prosthetic is the terminal device (TD). Some authors have stated that this is the most important aspect of the prosthesis, just as the hand is the most important part of the arm. Certainly, a lot of attention has been generated toward the development of various types of TDs.

To date, the most common TD still operates in a gross grasp pattern of function. The mechanical and myoelectric hands function with a "three-jaw-chuck" pinch pattern. Mechanical hooks generally have a stationary post with a movable "finger." All body-powered TDs are operated by a cable in one direction and a spring in the other direction.

Because most upper-limb amputees are unilateral, the residual limb functions as the dominant extremity, with the prosthetic limb operating as a functional assist. This is especially true because the science of prosthetic development has not progressed to isolated finger function in a prosthesis.

A "voluntary opening" indicates that the amputee must use his or her own body power to pull on the cable and **open** the terminal device; the spring automatically closes the device. The Hosmer-Dorrance hook terminal device is the device most commonly prescribed in North America. The pinch force of this TD is determined by the number of rubber bands or springs that are used. Each rubber band on the hook provides approximately 1 to $1\frac{1}{2}$ pounds of pinch force.

Voluntary closing, conversely, uses the pulling action on the cable to **close** the TD. The advantages of the voluntary closing TD are that a greater maximal pinch strength is available and that graded prehension is allowed. The pinch force is as gentle or strong as the force generated by the amputee. Unfortunately, the mechanical complexity of this device makes it both expensive and prone to break down; for this reason, the voluntary closing TD is not popular.

Both voluntary closing and voluntary opening hands have the disadvantages of frictional losses in the mechanics, which are far greater than with either type of hook; restriction of movement by the cosmetic glove; and contours that block visualization of the fingertips. In addition to these disadvantages, some authors suggest that the practice of the hook-type TDs may have a high incidence of prosthetic rejection because psychosocial issues are not addressed.

Answer: **A**
Trombly, p. 854
Bowker, Michael, p. 107
Hunter, Mackin, Callahan, pp. 1193-1196
Esquenazi, Meier, p. 25

> **CLINICAL GEM:**
> Some authors believe that the terminal device is the most important component of the prosthesis; others believe the socket is the most important component.

Hunter, Mackin, Callahan, p. 1232

24. You are treating a patient, after an amputation, who wants a myoelectric prosthesis. Which testing device is used to assess the strength of a potential muscle group?

A. Nerve conduction velocity unit
B. Galvanic stimulation unit
C. Myotester
D. Direct current stimulation device

The myotester is useful in assessing the signal strength of potential muscle groups. A myotester also helps determine the best electrode placement. Visual feedback is provided on the unit with a meter or a light. The test is first performed on the sound side for training and then applied to the side with the amputation.

Answer: **C**
Hunter, Mackin, Callahan, p. 1248
Refer to Fig. 16-10.

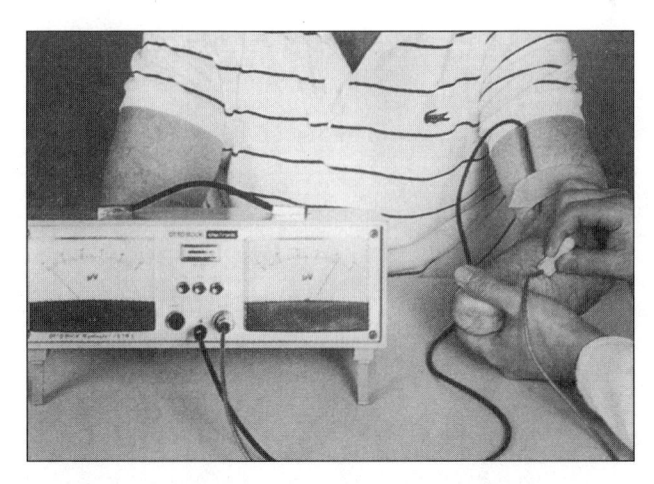

Fig. 16-10 ■ From Pedretti LW: *Occupational therapy: practice skills for physical dysfunction*, ed 4, St. Louis, 1996, Mosby-Year Book.

25. A 36-year-old female sustained a traumatic left transradial amputation. The perfect terminal device for maximizing her functional capabilities would be:

A. A myoelectric hand because of its cosmesis and functional abilities
B. A conventional body-powered voluntary opening hook because of the increased ability to visualize objects during functional use
C. A passive cosmetic hand because her non-dominant extremity was amputated
D. None of the above

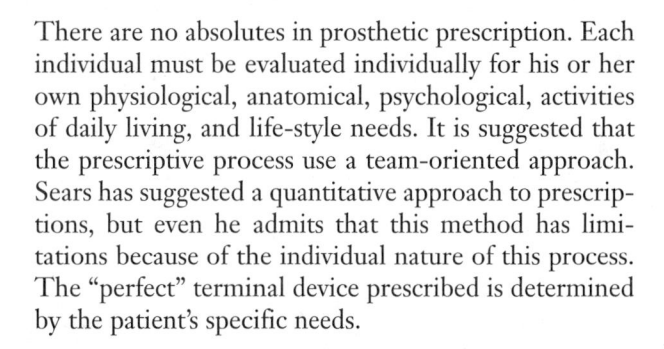

There are no absolutes in prosthetic prescription. Each individual must be evaluated individually for his or her own physiological, anatomical, psychological, activities of daily living, and life-style needs. It is suggested that the prescriptive process use a team-oriented approach. Sears has suggested a quantitative approach to prescriptions, but even he admits that this method has limitations because of the individual nature of this process. The "perfect" terminal device prescribed is determined by the patient's specific needs.

Answer: **D**
Sears, pp. 361-371

> **CLINICAL GEM:**
> Spiegel and Meredith describe the advantages and disadvantages of available components and believe that evaluating the pros and cons are vital to choosing a proper prosthesis.
>
> Meredith, p. 936
> Spiegel, p. 61

26. During functional use training, a unilateral below-elbow amputee is taught to hold dishes with the prosthesis and use the sound extremity to hold the sponge or dishcloth when washing dishes. True or False?

Functional use training usually begins once the amputee has a beginning mastery of the controls. A unilateral amputee will generally find that the prosthesis becomes the non-dominant, gross-assist extremity. Even with recent advances in myoelectrics and hybrid designs, the terminal device still functions in a gross grasp and release. For this reason, during dish washing, the prosthesis is used to grasp the sponge or dishcloth (with care taken to avoid immersing the prosthesis in water) while the sound extremity is used to hold the more fragile dish.

Answer: **False**
Atkins, Meier, p. 46
Bowker, Michael, p. 286

Chapter 17
Modalities

Topics to be reviewed in random order are:

- **Ultrasound treatment indications and precautions**
- **Iontophoresis treatment and techniques**
- **Phonophoresis**
- **Continuous passive motion**
- **Whirlpool treatment indications**
- **Heat treatment indications**
- **Cold therapy treatment indications**
- **Biofeedback treatment indications**
- **Intermittent compression pump treatment indications**
- **Electrical stimulation treatment indications and parameters**
- **Conduction/convection/conversion**
- **Strength duration curve**

1. Which of the following is not an example of conduction?

A. Hot packs
B. Paraffin wax
C. Cold packs
D. Fluidotherapy

Conduction is the process whereby a state of excitation affects successive portions of a tissue or cell so that the disturbance is transmitted to remote points. All of the above, except fluidotherapy, transfer energy by conduction. Fluidotherapy is a form of convection that transfers heat by means of currents in liquids or gases.

Answer: **D**
Michlovitz, pp. 115, 385

2. Match each modality to the correct answer(s). Answers A through E may be used more than once.

Modality

1. Paraffin
2. Ultrasound
3. Fluidotherapy
4. Cold bath
5. Fluori-methane spray
6. Whirlpool
7. Ultrasound, pulsed

Answer

A. Conversion
B. Convection
C. Low, specific heat
D. Conduction
E. Evaporation

Answers: **1. C and D; 2. A; 3. B; 4. D; 5. E; 6. B; 7. A**
Michlovitz, pp. 115, 119
Hunter, Mackin, Callahan, pp. 1505, 1521

CHAPTER 17 Modalities

3. Which process attempts to deliver medicine across the skin into deeper structures?

A. Ultrasound
B. Interferential electrical stimulation
C. Phonophoresis
D. Diathermy

Phonophoresis is a method of introducing medicine to a local area without skin invasion. It is a painfree, safe means of treatment. The increase in cell membrane permeability that occurs with ultrasound most likely is the mechanism that allows the introduction of medicine. No well-controlled clinical trials have provided support for using phonophoresis rather than ultrasound alone.

Answer: **C**
Hayes, p. 43
Hunter, Mackin, Callahan, p. 1526

> **CLINICAL GEM:**
> The drugs most frequently used with phonophoresis are:
>   Hydrocortisone
>   Dexamethasone
>   Lidocaine
>   Trolamine salicylate

4. Intermittent compression pumping should:

A. Be set no higher than 50 mm Hg for the upper extremity
B. Have a ratio of 3:1 of inflation to deflation
C. Not exceed the patient's diastolic blood pressure
D. All of the above

Adhering to all of the above guidelines is important when using the intermittent compression pump.

Answer: **D**
Hayes, p. 71
Refer to Fig. 17-1.

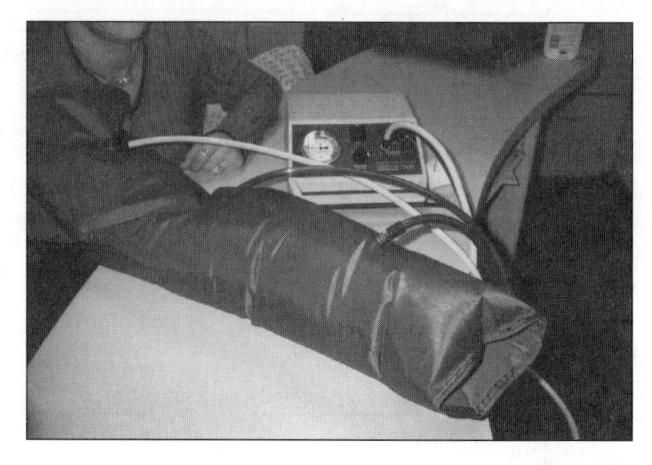

Fig. 17-1

5. Which of the following is false about cold therapy?

A. It is the thermal agent of choice for the first 24 to 48 hours after injury.
B. It decreases inflammation.
C. It decreases pain.
D. All of the above are true.

All of the above are considered accurate. There is controversy in the literature regarding the effects of cold therapy; therefore, further research is warranted.

Answer: **D**
Michlovitz, pp. 84-86

6. Redness of the skin after cold therapy may occur in response to:

A. Highly oxygenated blood
B. Low oxygenation of blood
C. Reactive hyperemia
D. A and C are correct.
E. B and C are correct.

When tissue temperature is lowered, oxygen does not split from hemoglobin in the blood. This saturates the venous system with oxygen and produces redness in the affected area. Reactive hyperemia, which is an increased presence of blood in a particular area, occurs during restoration of blood flow after a decreased supply of blood. It may occur 10 to 15 minutes after the removal of cold.

Answer: **D**
Michlovitz, pp. 98, 392

7. One disadvantage of using fluidotherapy is the risk of patient intolerance to the medium. True or False?

One disadvantage of using fluidotherapy is the risk of patient intolerance to both the medium and the confined space. Advantages of fluidotherapy include the availability of a temperature-control device and the ease of administering active range-of-motion exercises.

Answer: **True**
Michlovitz, p. 124
Refer to Fig. 17-2.

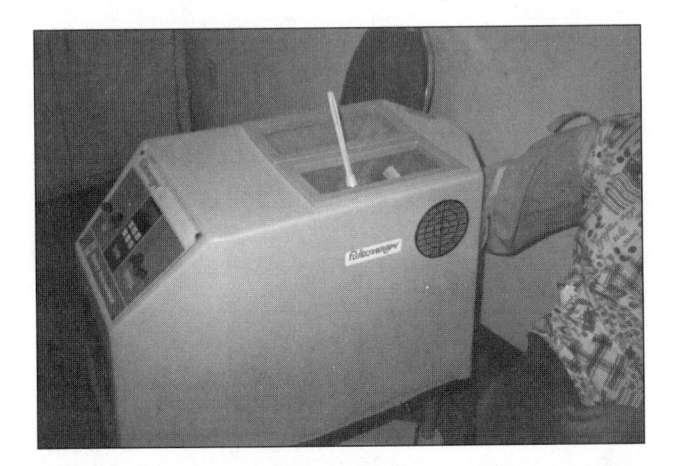

Fig. 17-2

8. Increased tissue temperature is a thermal effect of ultrasound. How does this increased temperature affect the blood flow to the treated area?

A. The tissue has a decrease in blood flow.
B. The tissue has an increase in blood flow.
C. The tissue has no change in blood flow.
D. The tissue initially has a decrease in blood flow, followed by an increase in blood flow.

The principle reason for using ultrasound for thermal effects is elevated tissue temperature. With increased tissue temperature, a normal response is an increase in blood flow.

Answer: **B**
Michlovitz, pp. 177-179

9. Which of the following is not a contraindication when using ultrasound for therapy treatment?

A. Fractured bone
B. Testes
C. Pregnant uterus
D. Malignant tissue

In the past, therapists were advised to avoid ultrasound over unhealed fracture sites. According to Michlovitz, there is no reason to avoid ultrasound over fracture sites unless sensation is impaired or the site is asensate (without sensation). In fact, studies have indicated that pulsed ultrasound may accelerate fracture healing. Pulsed ultrasound also may be used on patients diagnosed with myositis ossificans.

Ultrasound treatment should be avoided over the pregnant uterus because the increase in temperature has been shown to adversely affect the fetus, causing low birth weight, brain size reduction, and orthopedic deformities. Research also has shown that ultrasound should be avoided over malignant tissues because it may increase cellular detachment and cause metastasis. Ultrasound also should be avoided for patients with thrombophlebitis or decreased sensation, for areas with reduced circulation, during active infection, during exacerbations of rheumatoid arthritis, or for individuals with pacemakers. Ultrasound should not be used over the eyes, heart, or testes. Caution should be used when applying ultrasound to epiphyseal areas (growth areas) in children.

Answer: **A**
Michlovitz, p. 205

208 CHAPTER 17 Modalities

10. It is important to heat ultrasound gel for patient comfort and to increase transmission. True or False?

Heating ultrasound gel is inadvisable because it makes the gel runny and decreases viscosity, which leads to runoff. Gel is an excellent coupling agent for transmission. Using gel helps to decrease air bubbles and friction. Heating increases oxygen in gel, thus decreasing the coupling medium effectiveness. Water is an adequate coupling medium; however, increased air bubbles in water will reduce transmission.

Answer: **False**
Michlovitz, p. 199

> **CLINICAL GEM:**
> A quick reference to gel temperature follows:
> less than 66° F = 90% effective
> greater than 66° F = 73% effective

11. When treating supraspinatus tendonitis with ultrasound, which shoulder position is most beneficial?

A. Arm abducted and internally rotated
B. Arm externally rotated and abducted
C. Position of comfort
D. Position that most aggravates pain

When using ultrasound as a treatment modality for supraspinatus tendonitis, the position of choice is arm abducted and internally rotated to expose the supraspinatus tendon from under the acromion process.

Answer: **A**
Michlovitz, p. 203
Refer to Fig. 17-3.

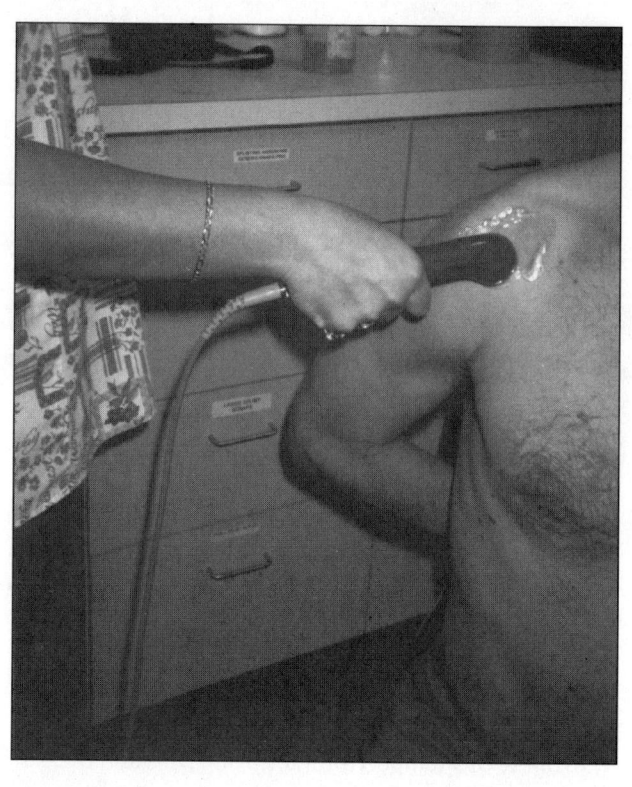

Fig. 17-3

12. You are treating a stiff digit with abundant scar tissue. Which ultrasound frequency would be best for elongating the scar?

A. 1 MHz
B. 3 MHz
C. 1.5 w/cm^2
D. 1.0 w/cm^2

When a depth of penetration of up to 2 cm is desired, the therapist should use 3 MHz ultrasound. Three megahertz is ideal for treating hand and wrist pathologies. Ultrasound has been shown by some authors to be helpful in elongating scar tissue.

A 1 MHz ultrasound treatment is best used to treat deeper tissue when desired penetration is up to 5 cm in depth. One megahertz is ideal for treating the back and lower extremities. Answers C and D are incorrect because they relate to intensity.

Answer: **B**
Hunter, Mackin, Callahan, p. 23

13. Match each modality to the correct temperature application:

Modality

1. Paraffin
2. Hot pack in hydrocollator
3. Fluidotherapy
4. Whirlpool

Temperature Application (° F)

A. 102 - 118
B. 113 - 129
C. 158 - 167
D. 96 - 104

Answers: **1. B; 2. C; 3. A; 4. D**
Michlovitz, pp. 117, 119, 123, 160

14. Intermittent compression pumps may be used with all of the following, except:

A. Postmastectomy lymphedema
B. Venous insufficiency
C. Arterial insufficiency
D. Amputations
E. Traumatic edema

Patients with arterial insufficiency have increased peripheral resistance and compression worsens this condition. Other contraindications include infections, thrombi, cardiac dysfunction, kidney dysfunction, obstructed lymphatic channels, and cancer (see Fig. 17-1).

Answer: **C**
Hayes, p. 71

> **CLINICAL GEM:**
> Sequential pumps with gradient pressure are much more effective than one-chamber intermittent pumps when treating lymphedema.

15. An 80-year-old woman slipped and fell on a wet pavement. She landed on an outstretched arm, which resulted in a Colles' fracture of her right wrist. After 8 weeks in a cast, the patient continues to suffer from severe, chronic edema of the wrist and hand. Her treatment included intermittent pneumatic compression (IPC). Necessary chart information for determining progress when treating this condition with IPC would be:

A. Right wrist muscle strength
B. Pre- and posttreatment measurements of girth of the right forearm and wrist
C. Grip strength
D. Active range of motion of right wrist flexion and extension
E. Right forearm and wrist sensation

The comparison of girth measurements before and after treatment and from treatment to treatment is an important clinical indication of the effectiveness of intermittent pneumatic compression.

Answer: **B**
Hecox, Mehreteab, Weisberg, pp. 424, 427

16. An active tennis player developed a gradual onset of muscular pain in the dorsal aspect of his right wrist and forearm. Trigger points were elicited in the extensor digitorum muscle. The stretch-and-spray method was selected for treatment. Of the following, choose the most suitable sequence for treating this patient:

A. Fully support elbow in extension; extend wrist and fingers; spray the painful muscle in parallel sweeps proximal to distal; follow with a hot pack to the forearm musculature
B. Fully support elbow in extension; fully flex wrist and fingers; spray the painful muscle in parallel sweeps proximal to distal; follow with a hot pack to forearm musculature.
C. Fully support the elbow in flexion; extend the wrist and fingers; spray the painful muscle in perpendicular sweeps proximal to distal; follow with a cold pack to the forearm musculature
D. Fully support the elbow in extension; fully flex wrist and fingers; spray the painful muscle perpendicular to the length of the muscle fibers; follow with a hot pack to the forearm musculature

To treat this tennis player with the stretch-and-spray technique, fully support his elbows in extension and fully flex his wrist and fingers. To fully inactivate trigger points by passive stretching, the muscle must be extended to its full, normal length and then held at a point of tolerable discomfort. Often verbal reinforcement to help the patient relax is beneficial. The jet stream of vapor coolant is directed at an acute angle of 30° and swept over the skin parallel to the affected muscle fibers in a proximal to distal fashion (Fig. 17-4). Any given area should be sprayed two to three times before applying a hot pack. After the skin is warm, stretch and spray can be repeated.

Ethyl chloride and Fluori-methane are common sprays; however, ethyl chloride is not recommended. Fluori-methane is safer to use but can freeze the skin when a stream is directed on one area for 6 seconds or longer; therefore, Fluori-methane should be used with caution.

Answer: **B**
Travell, Simons, pp. 65-74, 503-504

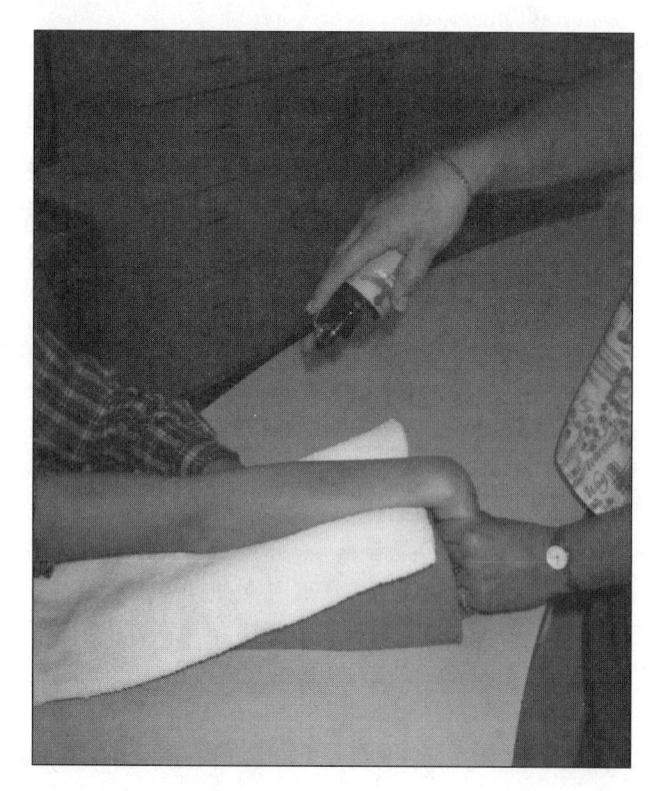

Fig. 17-4

17. The use of the Jobst compression pump is not contraindicated in the presence of:

A. Infection
B. Vascular damage
C. Pain
D. Fractures
E. It is contraindicated for all of the above.

Compression units should not be used when a patient has an active infection, vascular damage, and/or unhealed fractures. If using a compression pump increases the patient's pain level, it should be modified or discontinued; however, pretreatment pain is not a contraindication to the use of a compression unit.

Answer: **C**
Malick, Kasch, p. 98

18. Melzack and Wall theorized that small-diameter fibers of light touch and proprioception can close the gate to pain fibers. True or False?

The gate-control theory proposed by Melzack and Wall in 1965 theorizes that large-diameter fibers (light touch pressure and proprioceptive sense) can "close the gate" to the slower, smaller, nonmyelinated C fibers that conduct pain.

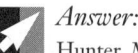

Answer: **False**
Hunter, Mackin, Callahan, p. 1536

19. You have a patient with hypergranulation tissue on his hand wound. You choose to treat this patient with a lukewarm whirlpool for 15 minutes. This is the best method of treatment. True or False?

Hypergranulation tissue, also referred to as "proud flesh," occurs when granulation tissue continues to form over the original wound. The proper way to treat such a wound is with the application of silver nitrate or corticosteroid cream. A therapist also should use semipermeable dressings on the wound and decrease the frequency of wound cleansing and dressing changes.

Answer: **False**
McCulloch, Kloth, Feedar, p. 143

20. Whirlpool is the modality of choice for which of the following?:

A. Débriding loosely adherent necrotic tissue
B. Cleansing dirt from wounds
C. Facilitating softening of eschar from a wound
D. All of the above

All of the above are appropriate uses of a whirlpool bath. Whirlpool is not used as frequently as it once was but it continues to serve an important role in wound care. A limited amount of whirlpool treatments are helpful for cleaning and débriding wounds.

Answer: **D**
McCulloch, Kloth, Feedar, p. 153

21. Which of the following is an incorrect statement?

A. Wounds should be débrided immediately after whirlpool.
B. Therapists use whirlpool primarily for cleansing wounds.
C. Whirlpool is helpful in decreasing moderate vascular occlusion.
D. All of the above are correct.

After whirlpool, a wound should be tended to immediately; otherwise, tissues may desiccate (dry out). Cleansing the wound is the primary goal of whirlpool treatment. Whirlpool is not a good choice if the primary goal is to significantly increase circulation. Surgery is the treatment of choice for moderate to severe vascular occlusion.

Answer: **C**
McCulloch, Kloth, Feedar, pp. 55-56, 153

22. Which of the following patients is a good candidate for contrast baths as a treatment modality?

A. A patient with small vessel disease secondary to diabetes
B. A patient with arthrosclerotic endarteritis
C. A patient with Buerger's disease
D. A patient who received a flexible implant arthroplasty of the metacarpophalangeal joints
E. All of the above patients are poor candidates for contrast baths

A patient with flexible implant arthroplasties of the metacarpophalangeal joints might benefit from the use of contrast baths. All of the answers except D describe patients who cannot use contrast baths as a treatment modality. Caution also should be exercised when using contrast baths for a patient with peripheral vascular disease if the water temperature is set higher than 40° C (104° F).

Contrast baths are used for patients with arthritis of the peripheral joints, joint sprains, muscle strains, and to toughen amputation stumps. Unfortunately, no well-controlled studies are available regarding the efficacy of contrast baths. If a contrast bath is used, the temperature should be between 38° C (104° F) and 44° C (111.2° F) in one basin and 10° C (50° F) to 18° C (64° F) in the other basin. The extremity to be treated should be placed in the warm basin for 10 minutes, then immersed in the cold basin for 1 minute, and returned to the warm basin for 4 minutes. This cycle should be continued for 30 minutes, with the last immersion being in the warm basin.

Answer: **D**
Hunter, Mackin, Callahan, p. 1371
Michlovitz, pp. 161-162

CLINICAL GEM:
For severe edema some authors advocate ending contrast bath treatment in cold water for 1 minute.

23. Continuous passive motion enhances the healing and regeneration of musculoskeletal tissues. True or False?

212 CHAPTER 17 Modalities

Continuous passive motion (CPM) enhances the healing and regeneration of musculoskeletal tissues, including articular cartilage, synovial membranes, joint capsules, ligaments, and tendons. CPM also is used to overcome joint stiffness and pain, and minimizes the effects associated with immobilization.

Answer: **True**
Hunter, Mackin, Callahan, p. 1545
Refer to Fig. 17-5.

24. Continuous passive motion can provide low-load prolonged stress. True or False?

Continuous passive motion is probably effective in preventing or overcoming joint stiffness because of the machine's ability to provide low-load prolonged stress (LLPS) to tissues. The phenomena of LLPS is best

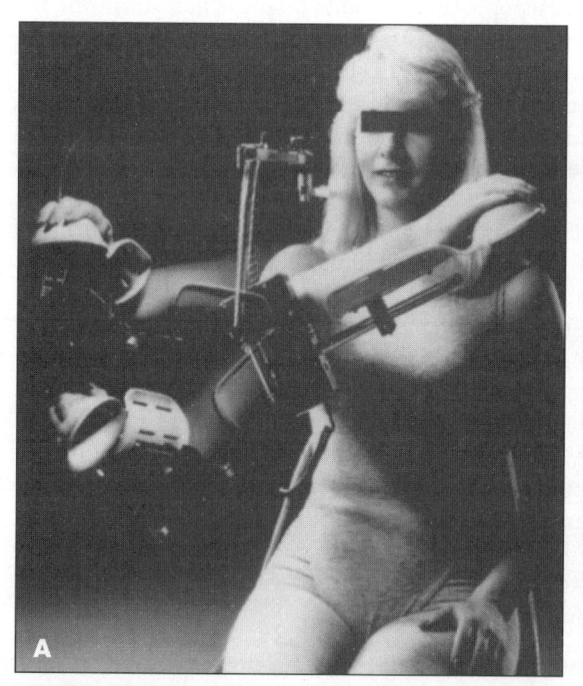

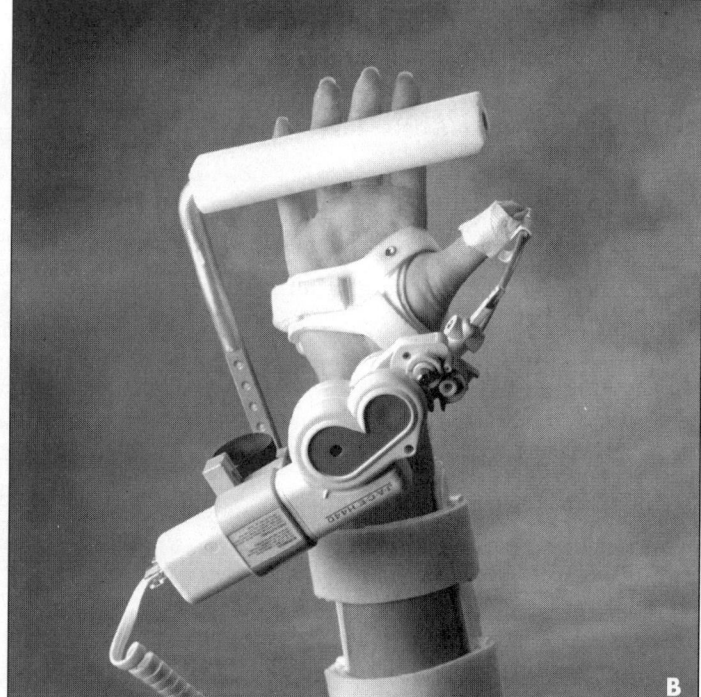

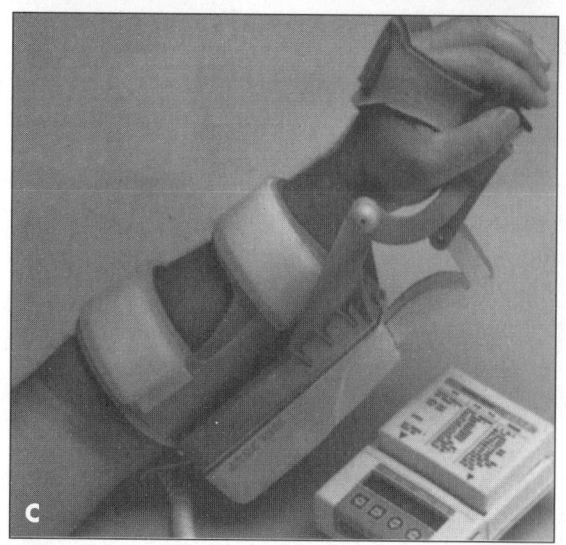

Fig. 17-5 ■ Examples of continous passive motion (CPM) devices used in treating the upper extremity patient. **A,** JACE S600 shoulder chairmount CPM; **B,** JACE H440 hand rehabilitation system; **C,** JACE W550 portable wrist CPM. (Courtesy of Thera-Kinetics Inc., Cherry Hill, NJ.)

explained by Atkinson and others, who state that "the fibroblasts of the fibrous connective tissue matrix apparently respond to physical forces by a homeostatic biofeedback loop to maintain the proper balance of tissue constituents." LLPS addresses structural changes in the tissues after trauma and stiffness after immobilization. The mechanics of LLPS and its effects on connective tissue are still somewhat speculative.

Answer: **True**
Hunter, Mackin, Callahan, p. 1546

25. For which of the following is continuous passive motion contraindicated?

A. Burn patients
B. Capsulotomies
C. Fractures with open reduction internal fixation
D. Unstable fractures

Continuous passive motion (CPM) is indicated for fractures that are stable after open reduction internal fixation. CPM is not indicated for an unstable fracture. It is, however, indicated in surgical release of joints, capsules, tendons, and extraarticular scar adhesions. CPM has some indications for use with surgical repair of tendons or repair of ligaments. Other indications include overcoming joint stiffness, inflammatory conditions, pain, burns, and total joint replacements.

Answer: **D**
Hunter, Mackin, Callahan, pp. 1548-1551

26. When treating lateral epicondylitis, the best form of cold therapy is:

A. Cold pack
B. Ice massage
C. Cold bath
D. Controlled cold-compression units

An ice massage is the best technique for treating a small area, such as in lateral epicondylitis. Ice massage also is helpful when treating a muscle belly, bursa, or trigger point. An area 10 × 15 cm can be covered in 5 to 10 minutes. When ice massage is performed, it is not uncommon for a patient to experience cold followed by burning, then aching, and finally numbness or analgesia.

Answer: **B**
Michlovitz, pp. 99, 100
Refer to Fig. 17-6.

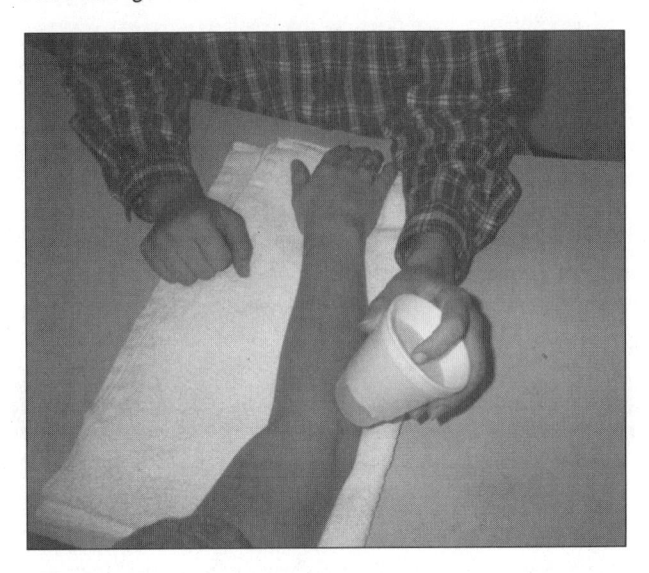

Fig. 17-6

> **CLINICAL GEM:**
> A quick way to remember the order of physiological events during ice massage is to think of "CBAN": C—Cold, B—Burning, A—Aching, N—Numbness.

27. Match each electrical stimulation parameter to the corresponding word(s):

Parameter

1. Amplitude
2. Pulse duration
3. Frequency
4. Rise time
5. On time/off time

Word(s)

A. Rate, pulse/second, Hz
B. Width
C. Duty cycle
D. Intensity
E. Ramp/surge

Answers: **1. D; 2. B; 3. A; 4. E; 5. C**
Hunter, Mackin, Callahan, p. 1512

28. The cathode is the positive electrode. True or False?

The cathode is the negative electrode and the anode is the positive electrode. The negative electrode (cathode), or active electrode, should be placed over the motor point when performing functional electrical stimulation.

Answer: **False**
Hunter, Mackin, Callahan, p. 1513

> **CLINICAL GEM:**
> One way to remember polarity is to recall that A+ (anode +) is a better grade than C− (cathode −).

29. Match each wave form to the corresponding current:

Wave Form

1.

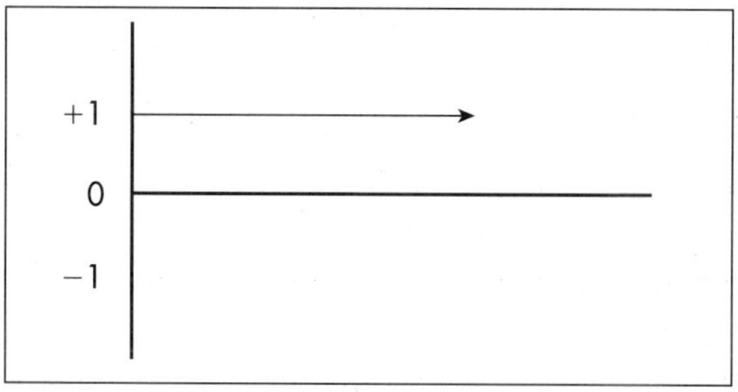

2.

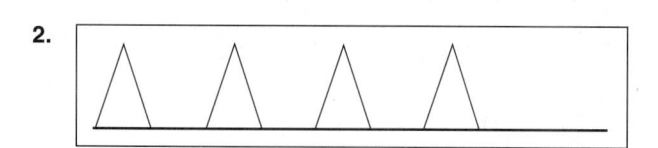

3.

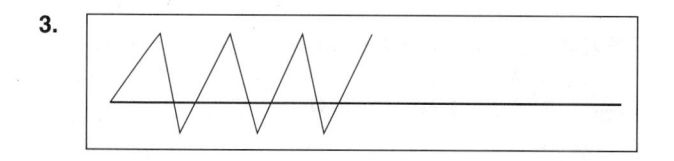

4.

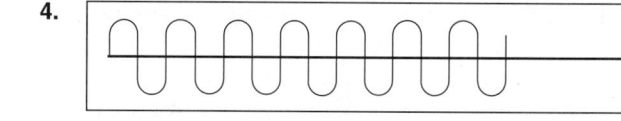

Current

A. Biphasic short duration current
B. Direct current
C. Polyphasic sinusoidal alternating current
D. Monophasic short duration current

Answers: **1. B; 2. D; 3. A; 4. C**
Hunter, Mackin, Callahan, p. 1511

30. You are treating a patient after flexor tendon repair with electrical stimulation to increase the pull-through of his flexor digitorum profundus to the middle finger. You notice with your current electrode placement that you are only getting the flexor digitorum superficialis to fire. One option would be to move the electrodes closer together to result in deeper penetration of current. True or False?

When treating this patient you must take into consideration that the flexor digitorum profundus lies deep to the flexor digitorum superficialis. To obtain a deeper penetration of current, the electrodes should be placed further apart. Other options include changing the electrode size or varying the placement of the electrodes.

Answer: **False**
Malick, Kasch, p. 84
Hunter, Mackin, Callahan, p. 1513

31. Strength-duration tests help determine the excitability of nerve and muscle tissues. Test results are plotted on log paper with the stimulus intensity on the Y axis and duration on the X axis. The relative position of the curve and the rheobase and chronaxie are identified on the graph. Answer true or false to the following statements:

A. Rheobase is the minimum intensity required to elicit a minimally visible contraction when the duration is infinite. True or False?

B. Chronaxie is the duration required for a stimulus with twice the rheobase intensity to elicit a visible contraction. True or False?
C. The strength-duration curve of a denervated muscle requires a lower intensity for a given duration than does an innervated muscle. True or False?
D. Sensory nerve tissue has a higher threshold than muscle tissue. True or False?

Rheobase is the minimum intensity required to elicit a minimally visible contraction when the duration is infinite and the chronaxie is twice the rheobase.

Although it is excitable tissue, denervated muscle requires a stimulus of higher amplitude and longer duration than does a normally innervated muscle.

Sensory nerve tissue responds more quickly than a motor (muscle) nerve and requires a lower intensity and shorter duration than muscle tissue.

Answers: **A. True; B. True; C. False; D. False**

Hecox, Mehreteab, Weisberg, pp. 277, 278
Meyer, pp. 124, 225
Hunter, Mackin, Callahan, p. 1510
Refer to Fig. 17-7.

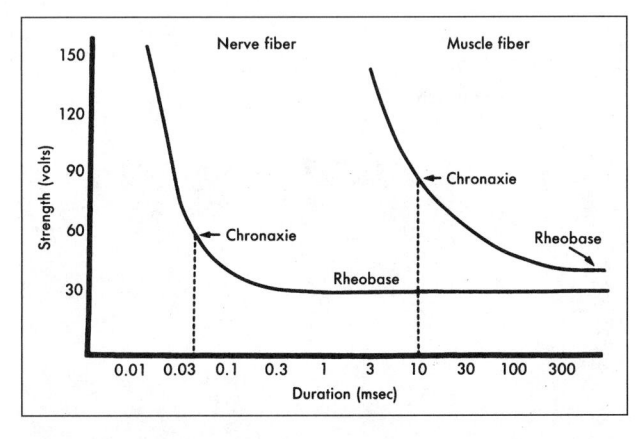

Fig. 17-7 ■ Strength duration curve of nerve and muscle fiber. (From Hunter JM, Mackin EJ, Callahan AD: *Rehabilitation of the hand: surgery and therapy*, ed 4, St. Louis, 1995, Mosby-Year Book.)

32. Which type of current should be used with denervated muscle tissue?

A. Strong, low-rate transcutaneous electrical nerve stimulation
B. Brief, intense transcutaneous electrical nerve stimulation
C. Direct current
D. Alternating current

Direct current typically is used for denervated muscle tissue. It has the capacity for the long pulse duration that is needed to elicit muscle contraction. It is important to know, however, that there is a great deal of thermal buildup with this treatment and that burns can readily occur. Some authors recommend only 10 contractions per session because of thermal effects. Use of this type of treatment is controversial; for every report advocating its use there is another report contraindicating it.

Answer: **C**
Lee, p. 32
Hunter, Mackin, Callahan, p. 1510

33. A 33-year-old, active tennis player developed a gradual onset of extensor tendonitis in the right forearm and is unable to play tennis secondary to severe, sharp pain at the common extensor tendon origin when extending his wrist. Iontophoresis has been indicated as a treatment option. Which solution is the most appropriate choice for this diagnosis?

A. Copper sulfate
B. Saline
C. Lidocaine
D. Dexamethasone

This patient has developed lateral epicondylitis. Dexamethasone is the most appropriate solution to use with iontophoresis. Dexamethasone is an antiinflammatory and is effective for treating arthritis, bursitis, and tendonitis with iontophoresis.

Answer: **D**
Hecox, Mehreteab, Weisberg, p. 297
Hunter, Mackin, Callahan, p. 1517

34. Iontophoresis is chosen to treat edema and pain on the dorsum of a wrist. Which of the following is incorrect with regard to setting up iontophoresis treatment?

A. Clean skin and perform a sensation assessment
B. Use a continuous direct current generator
C. Use an active electrode with the opposite polarity of the ion to be delivered
D. Place a second, larger dispersive electrode on a distant area
E. Electrodes should be buffered by the manufacturer

An active electrode with the **same** polarity as the ion to be delivered is necessary. The ions are delivered to the tissues while they are repelled by an electrode with the same polarity. All of the other answers are correct statements regarding iontophoresis.

Answer: **C**
Hecox, Mehreteab, Weisberg, pp. 296-297
Refer to Fig. 17-8.

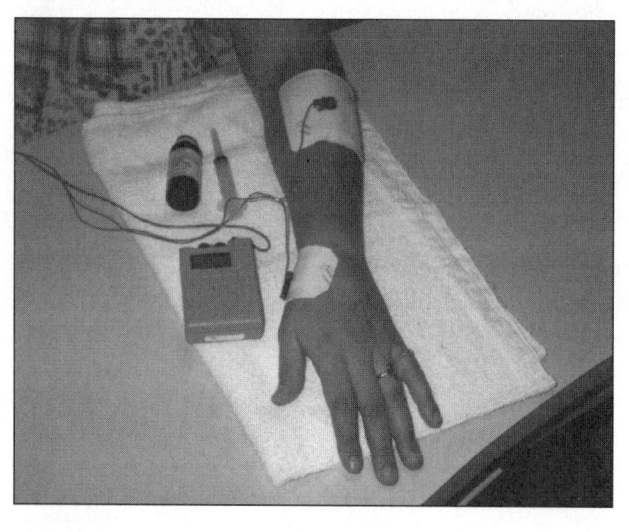

Fig. 17-8

35. A 25-year-old man presents with pain of the left wrist 2 days after playing in a racquetball contest. When using electrical stimulation to treat such an injury, which of the following treatment parameters is most appropriate for decreasing pain?

A. Continuous, high voltage at 50 to 120 Hz for 10 to 30 minutes
B. Surged, Russian stimulation at 2500 Hz for 30 to 60 minutes
C. Interrupted, low voltage at 5 Hz for 20 minutes
D. None of the above are appropriate

To help reduce acute pain, high voltage electrical stimulation typically is used, with a rate of 50 to 120 Hz for 10 to 30 minutes. A continuous mode is most effective because an ongoing, unmodified series of pulses is comfortably tolerated by the patient. This mode allows muscle relaxation and a reduction in pain.

Answer: **A**
Meyer, p. 215
Hecox, Mehreteab, Weisberg, pp. 266-267

36. Which of the following transcutaneous electrical nerve stimulation modes is appropriate when painful procedures (e.g., débridement) are performed on a patient?

A. Conventional
B. Low rate
C. Brief intense
D. All of the above

The brief intense technique involves a brief and intense high-rate (above 100 pulses/second) and high-width (above 200 microseconds) current at an intensity as high as the patient can tolerate. Brief intense transcutaneous electrical nerve stimulation produces a tetanic contraction and results in surface analgesia for 10 to 15 minutes. This is a noxious stimulus and is best used with and before painful procedures such as burn débridement, passive stretching, or minor surgery.

Answer: **C**
Hecox, Mehreteab, Weisberg, p. 302
Refer to Fig. 17-9.

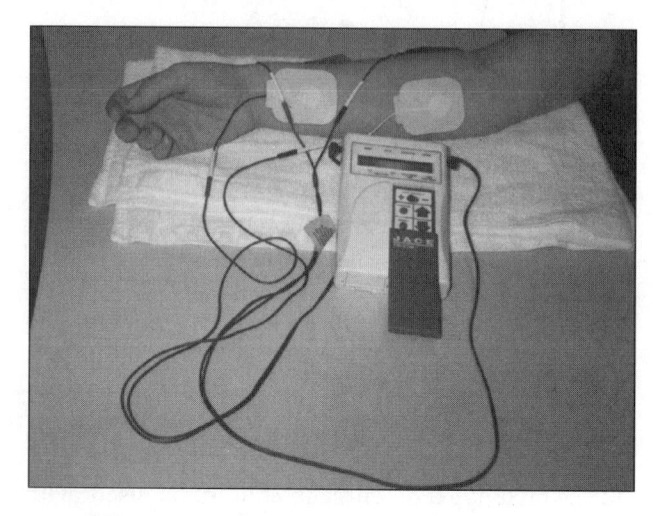

Fig. 17-9

37. High-voltage galvanic stimulation has proved to be a popular modality at wound sites for enhancing and accelerating healing. Answer true or false to the following statements:

A. High-voltage galvanic stimulation with a negative polarity will retard bacterial growth. True or False?
B. High-voltage galvanic stimulation at the positive electrode increases collagen synthesis and accelerates wound epithelialization. True or False?
C. On infected wounds, a positive electrode is used first until the infection is cleared; this is followed by a negative electrode for stimulation of tissue healing. True or False?

Clinicians agree that the negative electrical field has a greater bacterial effect and that the positive electrical field is more effective for tissue healing. The negative electrode is thus used initially to clean an infected wound and is followed by the positive electrode for tissue repair.

Answers: **A. True; B. True; C. False**
Hecox, Mehreteab, Weisberg, pp. 290-291

38. Electrical current is used to stimulate muscle and cause a contraction. The quality of a muscle contraction will change according to the changes in current parameters. A variety of therapeutic gains can be made by stimulating a muscle contraction. Match each muscle effect with the appropriate electrical current parameter:

Muscle Effect

1. Muscle pumping
2. Muscle strengthening
3. Muscle reeducation

Current Parameter

A. High-frequency alternating current; tetanic contraction (50 to 100 pulse/second); surged mode (15 seconds on, 50 seconds off); 10 repetitions
B. Comfortable contraction (30 to 50 PPS); interrupted or surged mode; 15 to 20 minutes
C. High-voltage direct current (20 to 40 PPS); surged mode (5 seconds off, 5 seconds on); 20 to 30 minutes

Answers: **1. C; 2. A; 3. B**
Arnheim, Prentice, pp. 332-333
Refer to Fig. 17-10.

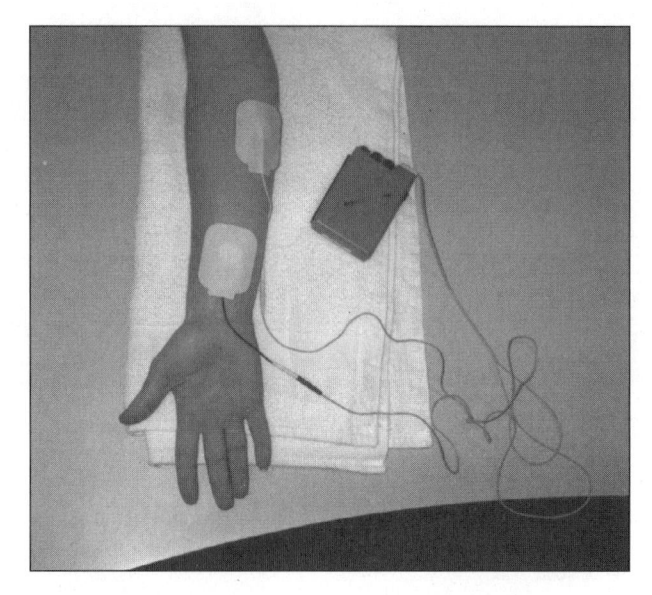

Fig. 17-10

39. A 31-year-old patient with multiple sclerosis is having difficulty drinking from a cup using her left arm because of tremor. Which of the following modalities would be the most appropriate for educating this patient to control her tremor?

A. Electromyogram feedback
B. Russian stimulation
C. Paraffin wax
D. Transcutaneous electrical nerve stimulation
E. Ultrasound

Electromyogram feedback has been used successfully for a variety of neurological conditions, including multiple sclerosis, cerebrovascular accident, cerebral palsy, and spinal cord injuries. It aids the patient in learning muscle control that would be beyond the reach of more traditional treatments. It can help clarify a particular patient's abnormal motor pattern and heighten a patient's awareness regarding proper versus improper movement.

Answer: **A**
Hecox, Mehreteab, Weisberg, p. 373

Chapter 18
Cumulative Trauma

Topics to be reviewed in random order are:

Evaluation and management of the following:

- Radial tunnel syndrome
- Carpal tunnel syndrome
- Cubital tunnel syndrome
- Anterior interosseous nerve and posterior interosseous nerve syndrome
- Wartenberg's disease
- Lateral and medial epicondylitis
- Handlebar palsy
- de Quervain's disease
- Trigger finger
- Intersection syndrome
- Ergonomic problems

The roof of the cubital tunnel is the arcuate ligament or Osborne's band (ligament). It also can be called the humeral ulnar aponeurotic arcade or the triangular ligament. The floor of the tunnel is formed from the medial collateral ligament and the walls are formed by the medial epicondyle and the olecranon.

Answer: **C**
Idler, p. 379
Refer to Fig. 18-1.

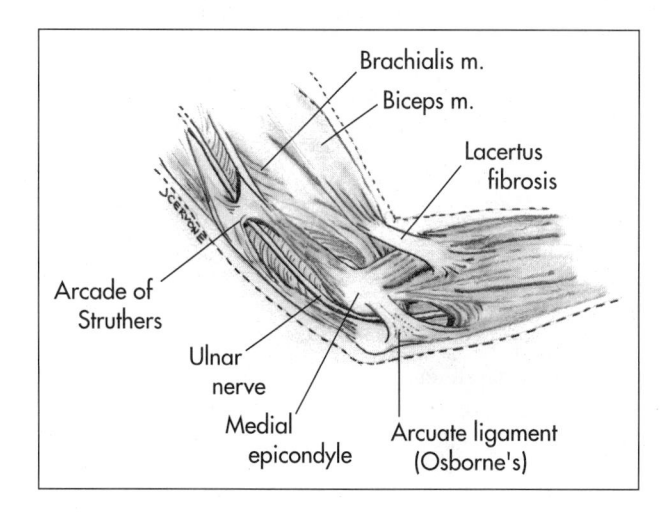

Fig. 18-1

1. Another name for the arcuate ligament is:

   A. Transverse retinacular ligament
   B. Arcade of Frohse
   C. Osborne's band (ligament)
   D. Ligament of Struthers

2. Trigger finger is associated with:

   A. Middle-aged females
   B. Rheumatoid arthritis
   C. Using tools with hard or sharp edges
   D. All of the above

Trigger finger is associated with all of the above. It is caused from stenosis (thickening) at or around the A1 pulley. If the patient has sufficient swelling in this region, the tendon can become locked in flexion and can cause a snap (often painful) as it pulls under the A1 pulley. The most commonly affected digit is the thumb. A thickened pulley and an hourglass enlargement of the tendon are consistent findings with trigger finger. Conservative treatment includes steroid injection and a splinting regime. Operative treatment is performed if conservative management has failed (see Fig. 1-17).

Answer: **D**
Putz-Anderson, p. 16
Hunter, Mackin, Callahan, pp. 1007-1009

> ★ **CLINICAL GEM:**
> Following is a quick reference to trigger-finger rehabilitation:
> • Splint metacarpophalangeal joint in extension, with proximal interphalangeal and distal interphalangeal joints free, for 3 to 6 weeks.
> • Perform passive range of motion to metacarpophalangeal joint to avoid stiffness.
> • Use modalities to reduce pain and inflammation.
> • Use Coban to reduce edema.

3. de Quervain's disease is tenosynovitis of which tendons?

A. Abductor pollicis longus and extensor pollicis brevis
B. Abductor pollicis longus and palmaris brevis
C. Palmaris brevis and extensor pollicis brevis
D. Extensor pollicis longus and abductor pollicis longus
E. Extensor pollicis longus and abductor pollicis brevis

In the 1893 edition of *Gray's Anatomy*, "washerwoman's sprain" was first described. In 1895, Fritz de Quervain further described this condition as a stenosing tenosynovitis. The tendons of the abductor pollicis longus and the extensor pollicis brevis (Fig. 18-2, *A*) are housed in the first of six compartments residing beneath the extensor retinaculum. Pain usually is the predominant symptom, with tenderness and swelling noted proximal to the radial styloid. de Quervain's disease typically is caused from overuse of the hand and wrist, especially when the patient has combined pinch with wrist motion and forearm rotation. Metabolic abnormalities such as diabetes, hypothyroidism, and rheumatoid arthritis may be associated with this disease. Pregnancy also may be associated with de Quervain's disease. A positive Finkelstein test usually is noted with de Quervain's disease (Fig. 18-2, *B*). See the following Clinical Gem for a quick reference to performing this test.

Answer: **A**
Hunter, Mackin, Callahan, pp. 1012-1014

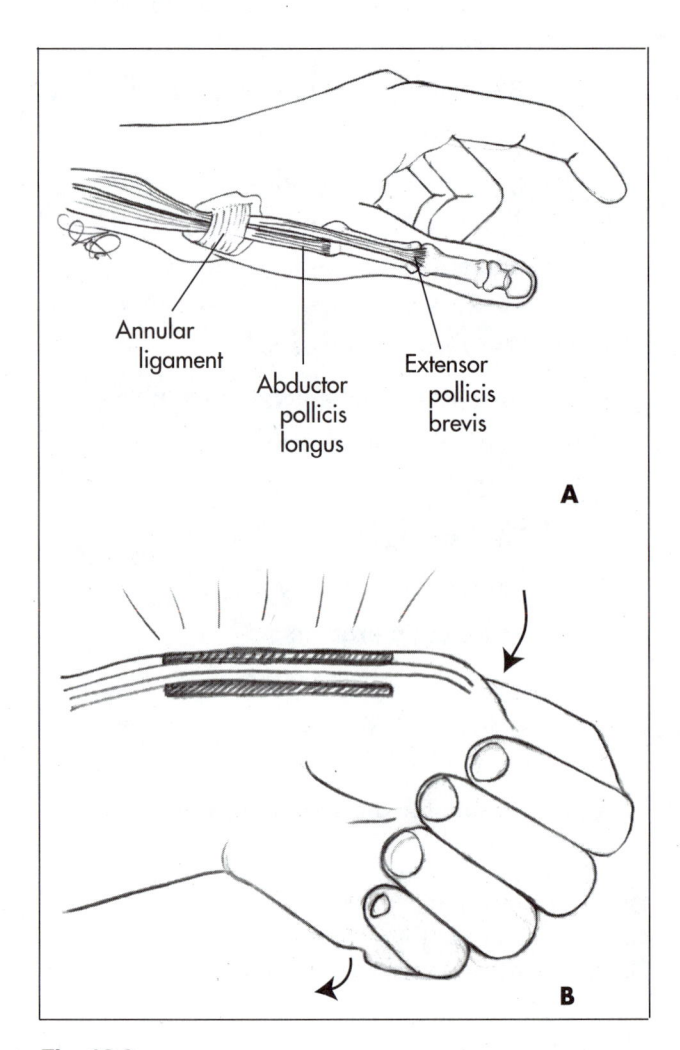

Fig. 18-2

> **CLINICAL GEM:**
> Following is a quick reference to performing a Finkelstein test:
> - Place patient's thumb across his palm
> - Wrap patient's fingers around his thumb
> - Passively move the patient's wrist into ulnar deviation
> - Excruciating pain around the radial styloid indicates a positive test

> **CLINICAL GEM:**
> Did you know that pain elicited with resisted thumb extension at the metacarpophalangeal joint is referred to as a positive "hitchhiker's test"? This test indicates inflammation of the extensor pollicis brevis tendon in the first dorsal compartment.

4. Which of the following should be avoided or modified to reduce the risk of developing cumulative trauma disorder?

A. Tool vibration
B. Extreme or awkward joint postures
C. Repetitive finger action
D. All of the above

All of the above contribute to cumulative trauma disorders (CTDs) and should be decreased when possible. Avoiding or modifying high-contact forces and static loading also reduces the chance of acquiring CTDs.

Answer: **D**
Putz-Anderson, p. 10

5. Gantzer's muscle is an accessory muscle of the:

A. Extensor pollicis longus
B. Abductor pollicis longus
C. Flexor pollicis longus
D. Extensor pollicis brevis
E. Flexor digitorum superficialis

Gantzer's muscle is an accessory slip off the origin of the flexor pollicis longus muscle. It can be a site of compression in anterior interosseous nerve pathology.

Answer: **C**
Spinner, p. 339
Refer to Fig. 18-3.

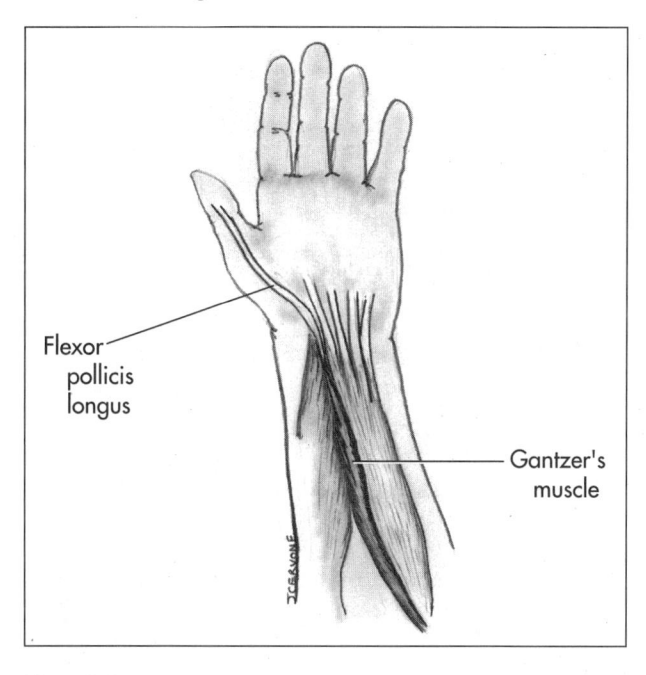

Fig. 18-3

6. What causes nocturnal pain with carpal tunnel syndrome?

A. Sleeping position
B. Vascular stasis
C. Thenar atrophy
D. A and B
E. All of the above

Patients with carpal tunnel syndrome often complain of nocturnal pain that awakens them. They relieve this symptom by shaking their hands. Sleeping posture can cause nocturnal pain because of the flexed position of the wrist that often is assumed during the night. Vascular stasis, which can occur in the canal at night from inactivity, contributes to compression of the median nerve by increasing canal pressure as the blood vessels become full, thus causing pain.

Answer: **D**
Hunter, Mackin, Callahan, pp. 909-910

7. Intersection syndrome involves which dorsal wrist compartments?

A. First and second
B. First and third
C. Third and fifth
D. Fourth and fifth
E. Fifth and sixth

Intersection syndrome is a condition triggered by repetitive use of the wrist or a traumatic incident. This syndrome tends to be more common among weightlifters, people who row or canoe, and writers. Patients complain of pain and tenderness in the distal forearm, where the extensor carpi radialis longus and extensor carpi radialis brevis tendons (second dorsal wrist compartment) cross over the extensor pollicis brevis and abductor pollicis longus tendons (first dorsal wrist compartment). Treatment includes thumb spica splinting, antiinflammatory medications, steroid injections, ice, and avoidance of provocative activities.

Answer: **A**
Hunter, Mackin, Callahan, pp. 1012-1013
Refer to Fig. 18-4.

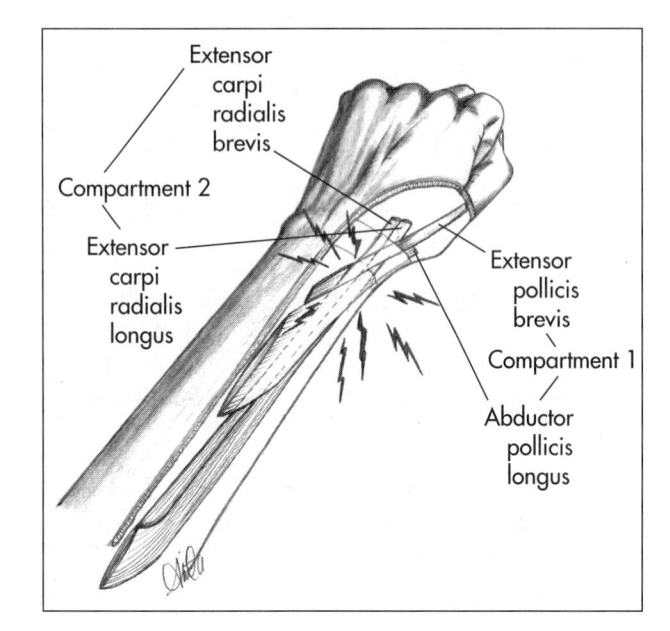

Fig. 18-4

8. Which type of splint should be used on a patient referred to you with de Quervain's disease?

A. Wrist support splint
B. Thumb spica splint with the interphalangeal joint free
C. Thumb spica splint including the interphalangeal joint
D. Elbow extension splint
E. Short opponens splint

A patient with de Quervain's disease is splinted in a thumb spica with the interphalangeal joint free. It is unnecessary to immobilize the interphalangeal joint because the extensor pollicis longus tendon is not an offender in this disorder. Steroid injections commonly are used in conjunction with splinting to reduce inflammation (see Fig. 15-12, question 29).

Answer: **B**
Hunter, Mackin, Callahan, p. 1013

9. Injury of the posterior interosseous nerve presents with all of the following symptoms, except:

A. Weak extensor digitorum muscle
B. Weakness of triceps
C. Weakness of the extensor indicis muscle
D. Weakness of wrist extensor muscles

The triceps is innervated by the radial nerve before it branches into the posterior interosseous nerve (PIN). As the deep branch of the radial nerve exits from the supinator, its name becomes the PIN. PIN syndrome elicits pain in the dorsal forearm, weakness of the metacarpophalangeal joint extensors, and weak wrist extension because of loss of the extensor carpi ulnaris and of the extensor carpi radialis brevis in 50% of cases. **There is no sensory loss.** The PIN is vulnerable for a variety of reasons, whether traumatic or nontraumatic. Some causes of entrapment include: (1) soft-tissue tumors; (2) radial head fractures; and (3) compression at the arcade of Frohse.

Answer: **B**
Prasartritha, Liupolvanish, Rojanakit, p. 107
Refer to Fig. 18-5.

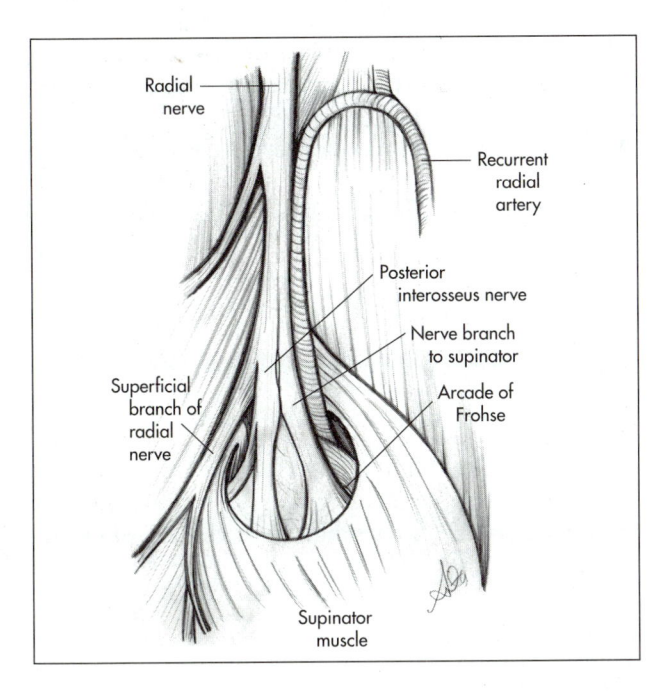

Fig. 18-5

10. Golfer's elbow is another name for medial epicondylitis. True or False?

Medial epicondylitis involves the flexor muscles in the forearm and also is termed golfer's elbow. Patients report aching or burning at the flexor carpi ulnaris and flexor carpi radialis origins (the most frequently involved tendons). Conservative management is similar to that of lateral epicondylitis, except that the wrist is splinted at neutral and the air cast is applied to the flexors rather than the extensors.

Answer: **True**
Hunter, Mackin, Callahan, p. 1812

11. Which tendon is most commonly involved in lateral epicondylitis?

A. Extensor carpi radialis longus
B. Extensor carpi radialis brevis
C. Supinator
D. Extensor carpi ulnaris

The extensor carpi radialis brevis is the extensor tendon most commonly injured in lateral epicondylitis. The supinator and extensor carpi ulnaris also may be involved in lateral epicondylitis. The extensor carpi radialis longus usually is not involved because its origin is proximal to the lateral epicondyle.

Answer: **B**
Stanley, Tribuzi, p. 430
Refer to Fig. 18-6.

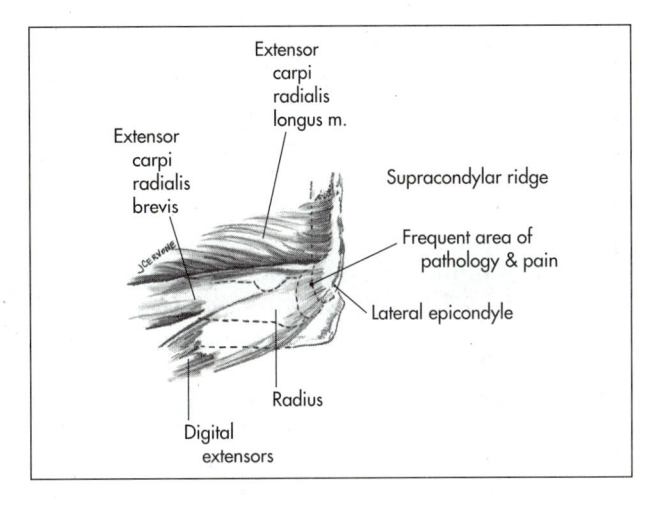

Fig. 18-6

12. A 46-year-old woman is referred to you with a diagnosis of acute lateral epicondylitis. What is the best choice for treatment?

A. Wrist immobilization splint
B. Elbow flexion block splint
C. Strengthening exercises
D. Aggressive stretching of the extensor musculature

Most cases of lateral epicondylitis are treated conservatively. The goals of therapy are to decrease pain and inflammation and restore functional use. This may be accomplished by applying a wrist immobilization splint (20° to 45° of extension), which allows the common extensor muscles to rest. During the acute phase, ice, rest, and education are mandatory. Once the pain and inflammation have decreased, you may begin gentle stretching for both the extensor and flexor muscles of the forearm. At this point, a proximal pneumatic air splint may be worn in conjunction with the wrist immobilization splint. The air cast is proposed to counterforce the loading to the wrist extensors (use of an air cast is controversial). Once the patient's pain is managed and is not exacerbated easily, strengthening exercises can be progressed.

Answer: **A**
Stanley, Tribuzi, p. 431

224 CHAPTER 18 Cumulative Trauma

> **CLINICAL GEM:**
> Air casts used for lateral epicondylitis may cause compression of the posterior interosseous nerve. The therapist must watch for symptoms of posterior interosseous nerve irritation.

13. A 39-year-old woman presents with complaints of chronic ulnar wrist pain. With forearm rotation you notice a snapping on the ulnar side of the wrist. The patient reports increased pain with excessive wrist motion. What might this patient have?

A. Subluxation of the extensor carpi ulnaris
B. Rupture of the extensor digiti quinti
C. Tendinitis of the triangular fibrocartilage complex
D. Tendinitis of the intrinsic muscles

The extensor carpi ulnaris inserts on the fifth metacarpal base and constitutes the sixth dorsal compartment; it also has a separate compartment that is deep to the extensor retinaculum. Traumatic rupture of the extensor carpi ulnaris retinaculum causes subluxation of the extensor carpi ulnaris. Patients also can have a chronic subluxation that becomes symptomatic with excessive wrist range of motion. During physical examination, the therapist can palpate the extensor carpi ulnaris coming out of the ulnar groove while inspecting forearm rotation.

Answer: **A**
Millender, Louis, Simmons, p. 137
Refer to Fig. 18-7.

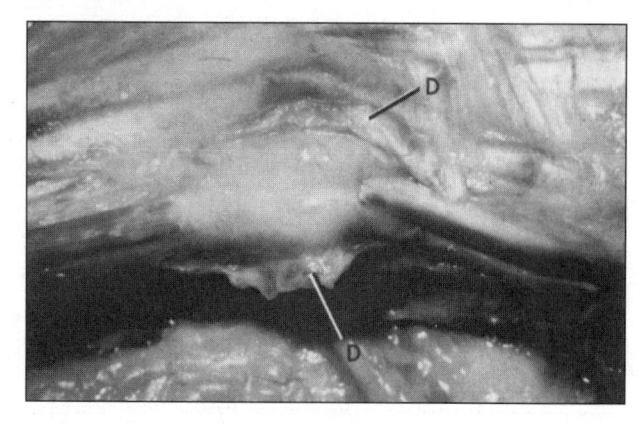

Fig. 18-7 ■ Sixth dorsal compartment. Supratendinous extensor retinaculum is seen reflected. Extensor carpi ulnaris (ECU) tendon is fixed distal to the ulna by synovial-lined tunnel of fascia derived from the infratendinous retinaculum. Angulation of the tendon increases displacement forces during supination. Insertion of the tendon is on the fifth metacarpal to right. *D,* Extensor retinaculum. (From Hunter JM, Mackin EJ, Callahan AD: *Rehabilitation of the hand: surgery and therapy,* ed 4, St. Louis, 1995, Mosby-Year Book.)

14. What would be your first recommendation for treatment of the patient in the previous question?

A. Splint or cast in pronation, with slight dorsiflexion and radial deviation
B. Splint in slight flexion and ulnar deviation
C. Fluidotherapy for desensitization
D. Strengthening

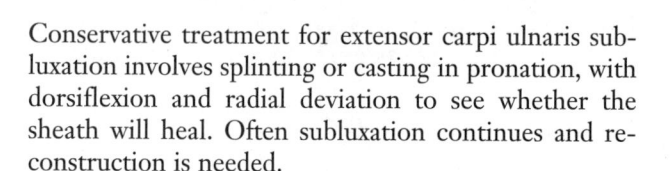

Conservative treatment for extensor carpi ulnaris subluxation involves splinting or casting in pronation, with dorsiflexion and radial deviation to see whether the sheath will heal. Often subluxation continues and reconstruction is needed.

Answer: **A**
Millender, Louis, Simmons, pp. 136-138
Thorson, Szabo, p. 425

> **CLINICAL GEM:**
> A circumferential wrist cuff with padding pressing on the extensor carpi ulnaris may help decrease subluxation and allow for greater function than a long arm cast or splint.

15. In which position should a patient's wrist be splinted for conservative management of carpal tunnel syndrome?

A. Wrist extension (20°)
B. Wrist neutral (0°)
C. Wrist flexion (20°)
D. Wrist flexion (40°)

Carpal tunnel syndrome traditionally was splinted with the wrist in a "cock-up" splint, with moderate amounts of wrist extension. Currently, however, it is recommended that the wrist be at neutral to reduce pressure in the carpal canal (Table 18-1). This gives patients more relief of symptoms than the original protocol of wrist cock-up splinting.

Answer: **B**
Ranney, p. 70
Gilberman, p. 747

Table 18-1

Wrist Position Correlation with Carpal Canal Pressure

Wrist Position	Carpal Canal Pressure
Neutral	18 mm Hg
20° extension	35 mm Hg
20° flexion	27 mm Hg
40° flexion	47 mm Hg

16. Putty is an excellent choice for conservative rehabilitation of carpal tunnel syndrome. True or False?

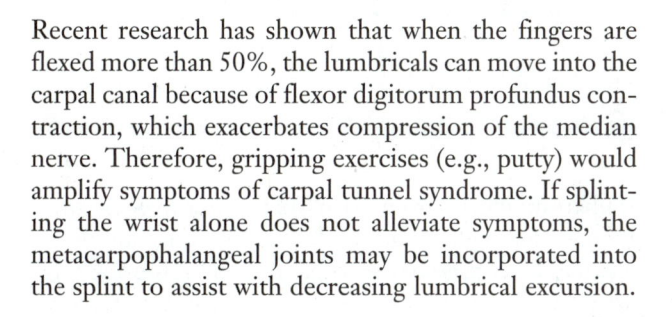

Recent research has shown that when the fingers are flexed more than 50%, the lumbricals can move into the carpal canal because of flexor digitorum profundus contraction, which exacerbates compression of the median nerve. Therefore, gripping exercises (e.g., putty) would amplify symptoms of carpal tunnel syndrome. If splinting the wrist alone does not alleviate symptoms, the metacarpophalangeal joints may be incorporated into the splint to assist with decreasing lumbrical excursion.

Answer: **False**
Evans, p. 17

17. The radial nerve enters the forearm between the two heads of which muscle?

A. Flexor carpi ulnaris
B. Pronator teres
C. Supinator
D. Brachioradialis

The radial nerve arises from the posterior cord of the brachial plexus and winds posterior to the humerus. The radial nerve **subdivides** at the elbow into the superficial sensory branch and a deep motor branch termed the posterior interosseous nerve. The latter dives between the two heads of the supinator as it enters the forearm.

Answer: **C**
Hunter, Mackin, Callahan, p. 70-73
Refer to Fig. 18-8.

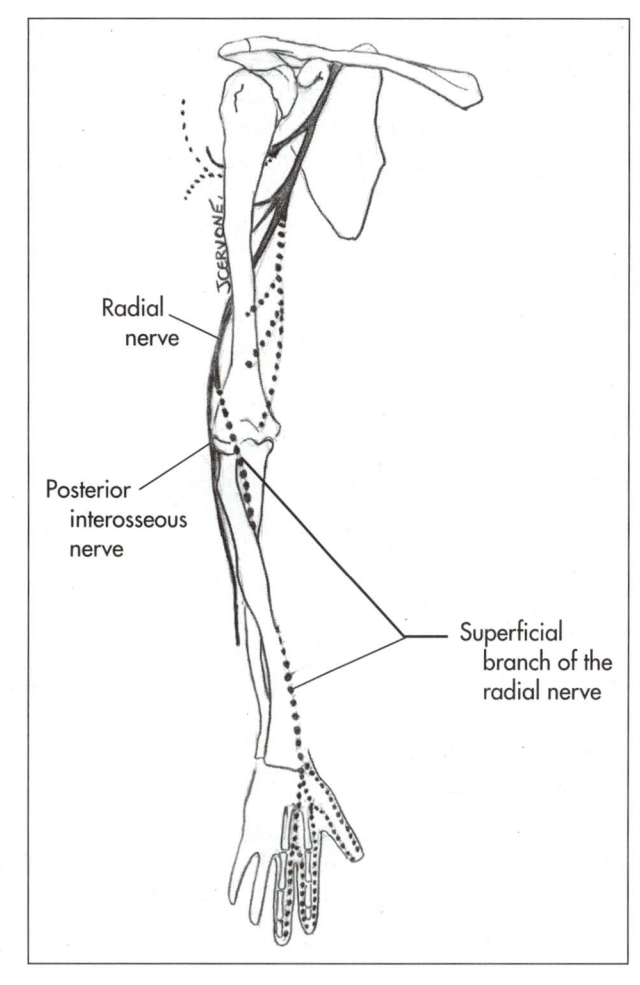

Fig. 18-8

18. Which nerve emerges between the brachioradialis and the extensor carpi radialis longus tendons in the forearm and may become irritated after de Quervain's release?

A. Posterior interosseous nerve
B. Superficial branch of the radial nerve
C. Recurrent branch of the median nerve
D. Ulnar nerve

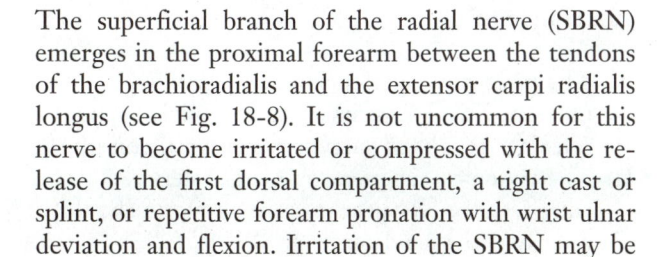

The superficial branch of the radial nerve (SBRN) emerges in the proximal forearm between the tendons of the brachioradialis and the extensor carpi radialis longus (see Fig. 18-8). It is not uncommon for this nerve to become irritated or compressed with the release of the first dorsal compartment, a tight cast or splint, or repetitive forearm pronation with wrist ulnar deviation and flexion. Irritation of the SBRN may be misdiagnosed as de Quervain's tenosynovitis. Dellon and Mackin suggest testing with the patient's elbow in extension, forearm in hyperpronation, and wrist in ulnar flexion for 1 minute. A positive test for the SBRN results in numbness and tingling over the dorsoradial aspect of the hand. A positive Tinel's sign over the course of the nerve also may be present.

Answer: **B**
Ranney, p. 187

19. Wartenberg's disease is:

A. Compression of the ulnar nerve
B. Compression of the superficial branch of the radial nerve
C. Compression of the digital nerve to the thumb
D. Intrinsic weakness
E. Intrinsic muscle wasting

Wartenberg's disease also is known as radial sensory nerve entrapment. Patients complain of hypersensitivity, dorsal hand and radial wrist pain, and possibly dysesthesia of the dorsal thumb/index fingers on the dorsum of the hand. A positive Tinel's sign around the radial styloid often is present. See question 18 for causes and evaluation techniques.

Answer: **B**
Ranney, p. 187

20. A 29-year-old female is referred to you from her primary care physician with a diagnosis of dorsal hand and wrist pain. She complains of decreased sensation in the dorsal thumb and index. Evaluation revealed point tenderness at the distal forearm on the radial side, an inconsistent positive Tinel's sign at the site of pain, mild edema along the distal radial forearm, and a 4.31 reading with the Semmes-Weinstein monofilament for the dorsal thumb. The patient's job requires repetitive forearm pronation with wrist flexion and ulnar deviation. Her primary care physician issued a prefabricated wrist support splint, which increased her symptoms. What might you conclude?

A. The patient is experiencing de Quervain's tenosynovitis. Her primary care physician should refer her to a hand surgeon for surgical consult.
B. The patient is experiencing median nerve compression. Her primary care physician should refer her to a hand surgeon.
C. The patient is experiencing Wartenberg's disease. The appropriate splint should be applied.
D. Current splint protocol should be continued. The patient needs time to adjust to the brace.

This patient has Wartenberg's disease. Her splint increased her symptoms because the splint did not protect the thumb. This patient needs a long thumb spica splint to protect from excessive thumb and wrist range of motion.

Answer: **C**
Ranney, p. 187

21. Radial tunnel syndrome presents with symptoms of muscle paralysis in the wrist extensors. True or False?

Radial tunnel syndrome (RTS) is a controversial topic because some physicians and therapists question its existence. RTS presents with pain in the posterior forearm (Fig. 18-9) without associated muscle paralysis. It can occur with unresolved chronic lateral epicondylitis and/or repetitive forearm and wrist motion.

Clinical tests include the resisted wrist extension test, the resisted supination test, and the resisted middle-finger extension test. These provocative tests also may be used to determine lateral epicondylitis and are positive if pain is reproduced during the examination. The key to differentiation between lateral epicondylitis and RTS is point tenderness. There is pain and tenderness with palpation over the supinator with RTS; with lateral epicondylitis, the pain usually is over the extensor carpi radialis brevis origin, radial head, and lateral epicondyle.

Common sites of compression in RTS include: (1) the radial nerve against the capitellum by the extensor carpi radialis brevis (see Fig. 18-9); (2) arcade of Frohse (see Fig. 18-9); (3) leash of Henry (fan-shaped vessels); and (4) fibrous bands anterior to the radial head. Treatment for RTS is similar to treatment for lateral epicondylitis and includes decreasing wrist motion, splinting (wrist support), modification of activity, modalities, and a balance between activity and rest.

Answer: **False**
Ranney, p. 183
Hunter, Mackin, Callahan, p. 1816
Refer to Fig. 18-9.

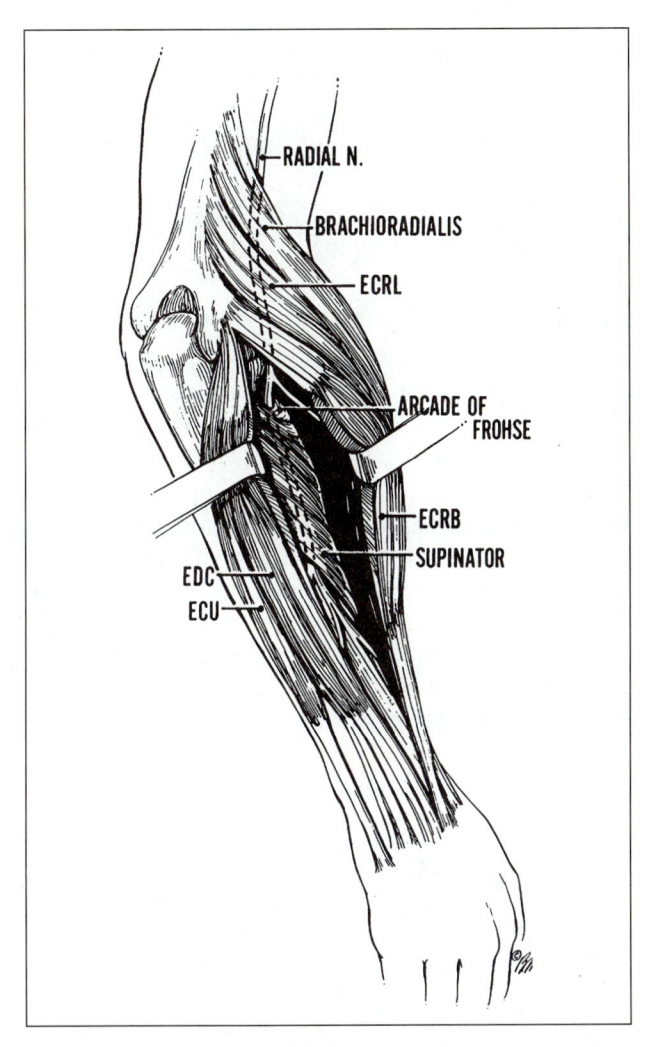

Fig. 18-9 ■ Copyright, Elizabeth Roselius, 1993. From Eversmann C: *Entrapment and compression neuropathies.* In Green DP, editor: *Operative hand surgery,* New York, 1993, Churchill Livingstone, with permission.

22. When testing for acute lateral epicondylitis, grip strength will be increased with the elbow extended. True or False?

Lateral epicondylitis, also known as tennis elbow, occurs from excessive loading to the extensor mass and/or a rapid grasp. One way to test lateral epicondylitis is to test grip strength with the elbow flexed and then with the elbow extended. If grip strength is significantly diminished with the elbow extended, the test for lateral epicondylitis is positive. This extended position puts increased tension on the extensor tendons.

Answer: **False**
Hunter, Mackin, Callahan, p. 1816

23. John H. is a patient referred to you with complaints of hand weakness and numbness in the ring and small fingers. Your sensory tests reveal diminished sensation of digits four and five, both volarly and dorsally. This patient might have nerve compression at:

A. Guyon's canal
B. The cubital tunnel
C. The carpal tunnel
D. The arcade of Frohse

This patient has ulnar nerve symptoms that narrow your choices to either Guyon canal or the cubital tunnel. You can rule out Guyon canal because of the dorsal numbness. The dorsal cutaneous branch of the ulnar nerve comes off proximal to Guyon canal. Therefore, dorsal sensory involvement of these digits would indicate a problem proximal to the wrist, such as in the cubital tunnel. See Figure 18-1 for compression at the cubital tunnel.

Answer: **B**
Reiner, Lohman, pp. 11-13

24. Handlebar palsy compresses which nerve?

A. Anterior interosseous nerve
B. Median nerve
C. Ulnar nerve
D. Posterior interosseous nerve

Clinical manifestation of handlebar palsy (a compression of the ulnar nerve at Guyon canal) can present with sensory deficits, intrinsic weakness, or both. The patient describes decreased pinch and grip and pain over the volar wrist and fifth digit. There is a classification system with three types of lesions. Type I involves both motor and sensory branches proximal to the wrist. Type II involves the motor branch at the hook of the hamate and at the distal part of the canal. Type III involves the superficial sensory branch. This palsy does not include the dorsal sensory branch because it branches off proximal to the wrist. Treatment includes rest, splinting, modifying the patient-bicycle fit, padding the handlebars, wearing gloves, and varying hand position while riding.

Answer: **C**
Hunter, Mackin, Callahan, pp. 1825-1826

228 CHAPTER 18 Cumulative Trauma

25. A patient is diagnosed with cubital tunnel syndrome and receives orders for night splinting. The patient's elbow should be splinted in which position?

A. 0° of flexion
B. 30° of flexion
C. 50° of flexion
D. 90° of flexion

The cubital tunnel has the least amount of nerve tension with the elbow fully extended, but this position would be intolerable for most patients. Therefore the recommended position is between 30° to 45° of flexion. It is helpful to include the wrist in the splint, not only for patient comfort but to relax the flexor carpi ulnaris tendon. Other treatments that might be helpful include antiinflammatories prescribed by the physician, modalities, and/or a nerve-gliding program. Patient education is important because the patient must fully understand the pathology in order to modify work, play, and rest.

Answer: **B**
Hunter, Mackin, Callahan, p. 670
Refer to Fig. 18-10.

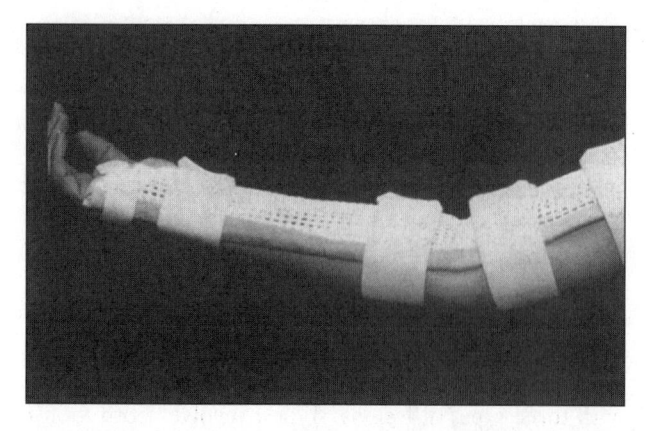

Fig. 18-10 ■ From Hunter JM, Mackin EJ, Callahan AD: *Rehabilitation of the hand: surgery and therapy,* ed 4, St. Louis, 1995, Mosby-Year Book.

CLINICAL GEM:
Conservative treatment for cubital tunnel syndrome, including nighttime splinting and activity modification, should result in a decrease of symptoms within 3 weeks.

26. Therapy after cubital tunnel release with epicondylectomy should be started at which time?

A. Immediately (same day of surgery)
B. 14 days after surgery
C. 21 days after surgery
D. Therapy is not indicated for this procedure.

The literature does not have clear guidelines as to when therapy should be initiated after cubital tunnel release. According to Warwick and Seradge, if range of motion is started at day 3, patients will have full range of motion and minimal chance of flexion contracture. It is not unusual, however, to see a patient immobilized for 14 days before being sent to therapy. According to Sailer, therapy should be initiated at 7 to 10 days after surgery, with end-range stretching started at 4 weeks. According to Hunter, Mackin, and Callahan, range of motion generally is started postoperatively at day 11. Range of motion would not begin on the same day as surgery (answer A) and should not be delayed until day 21 (answer C).

Answer: **B**
Warwick, Seradge, p. 245
Sailer, p. 239
Hunter, Mackin, Callahan, p. 671

CLINICAL GEM:
For a quick reference chart on rehabilitation after cubital tunnel release, refer to the chart provided by Hunter, Mackin, and Callahan in *Rehabilitation of the hand: surgery and therapy,* ed 4.

27. Anterior interosseous nerve syndrome is a motor syndrome. True or False?

The anterior interosseous nerve (AIN) is a branch of the median nerve that innervates the flexor pollicis longus, the flexor digitorum profundus to the index and long fingers, and the pronator quadratus. The AIN syndrome is characterized by an inability to make an "O," which requires thumb interphalangeal joint flexion and index finger distal interphalangeal joint flexion (Fig. 18-11). Patients assume an abnormal pinch. In addition to paralysis, some patients report pain in the proximal forearm. No sensory loss is reported. Treatment includes rest and splinting. If unresolved within 90 days, surgery is indicated.

Answer: **True**
Hunter, Mackin, Callahan, pp. 632-633

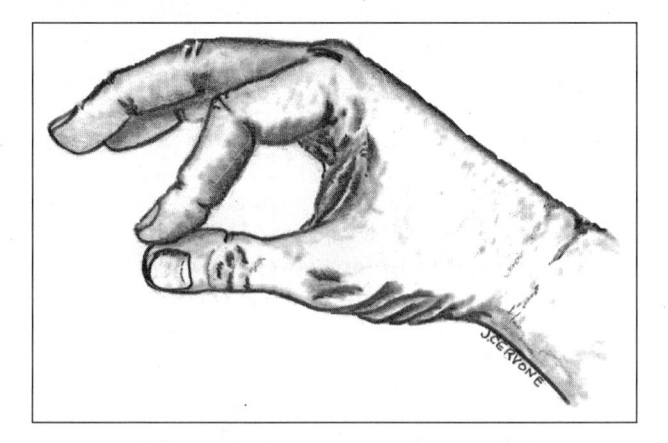

Fig. 18-11

28. You are going to perform a job-site analysis on a patient with a cumulative trauma disorder in the upper extremity. You have a job description from the patient's employer. Which of the following will give you specific information to assist with performing an on-site analysis?

A. Occupational Safety and Health Administration guidelines
B. Local library
C. Dictionary of Occupational Titles
D. None of the above

The Dictionary of Occupational Titles, first published in 1939, is an excellent source to assist with performing a job-site analysis. It was developed to serve as a source for standardized occupational information. The information is divided into seven parts to present data regarding jobs in a systematic manner. These parts include: (1) occupational code number; (2) occupational title; (3) industry designation; (4) alternate titles; (5) the body of the definition; (6) undefined related titles; and (7) definition trailer.

Answer: **C**
Dictionary of Titles, 4th edition

29. With respect to proper work surface heights and positioning, a general rule is to keep elbows close to the body and avoid full elbow extension. True or False?

Anthropometry (measurements of body size) is used as a basis for designing tools, equipment, and work and living places to reduce the incidence of cumulative trauma disorders. It is recommended that elbows be positioned close to the body. Work should be kept within arm's reach and full elbow extension should be avoided. The general work surface should be 5 to 10 cm (2 to 4 inches) below the elbows. For precision work, higher surfaces will decrease overstrain; for heavier work, lower surfaces are recommended.

Answer: **True**
Falkenberg, Schultz, pp. 263-270
Refer to Fig. 18-12.

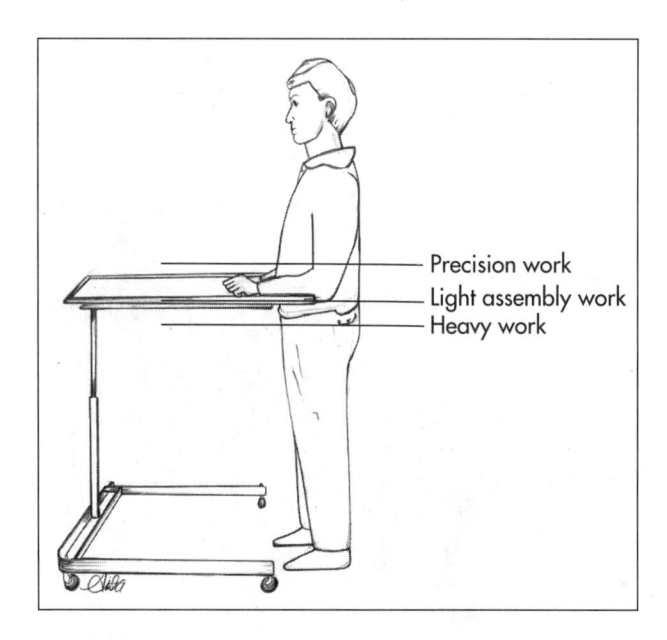

Fig. 18-12

30. Temperature is not a risk factor in the development of cumulative trauma disorders. True or False?

Temperature extremes increase vulnerability to developing cumulative trauma disorders. Cold affects dexterity and coordination, and heat increases fatigue. According to the National Institute of Safety and Health, favorable working temperatures are 68° to 78° F with 20% to 60% humidity.

Answer: **False**
Falkenberg, Schultz, pp. 263-270

31. When designing an ergonomic tool, the handle should be at least 9 cm in length. True or False?

A tool handle should distribute the force over the thenar and hypothenar eminences and digits two through five. If the handle is too short (Fig. 18-13), it may compress the median or ulnar nerve at the palm or the digital neurovascular structures. The tool length should accommodate the average hand width (9 to 12 cm, or 4 to 5 inches), allowing for evenly distributed forces to help reduce exposure to cumulative trauma disorders.

Answer: **True**
Johnson, pp. 299-310

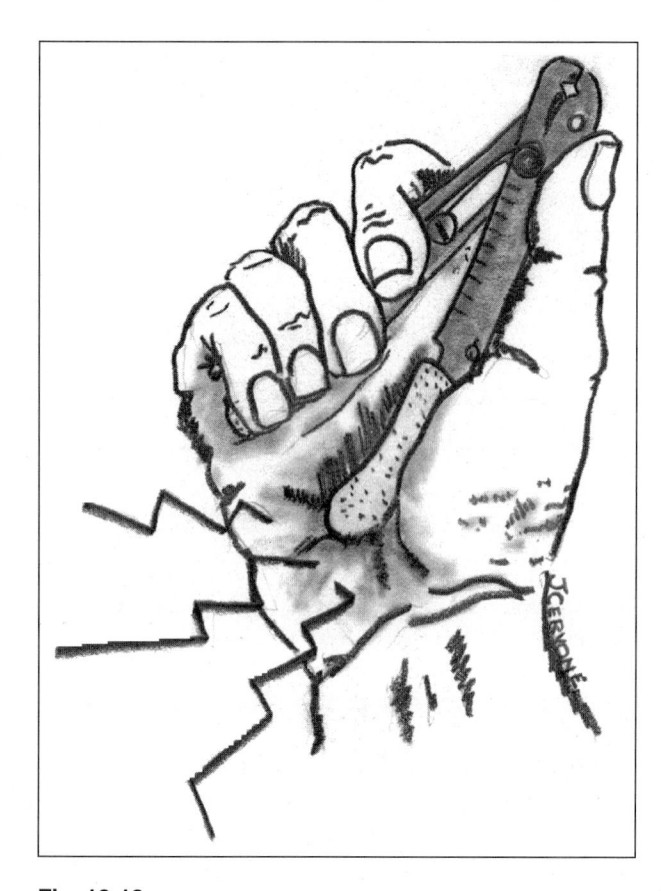

Fig. 18-13

32. The Occupational Safety and Health Administration has an ergonomic minimum standard program that recently has been implemented. True or False?

The Occupational Safety and Health Administration (OSHA) does have a proposed ergonomic standard program; however, it has not been adopted at this time. Currently, OSHA cites facilities under the general duty clause (Section 5a), which states that "each employer shall furnish a place of employment which is free from recognized hazards that are causing or are likely to cause death or serious physical harm to his employees." Ergonomics program management guidelines for meat-packing plants, which are advisory in nature, are currently available. There are no established ergonomic guidelines to cover all professions at this time.

Answer: **False**
Westra

33. Which tool might be used during a job-site analysis to measure the amount of force required to push and pull?

A. Dynamometer
B. Pedometer
C. Chatillon gauge
D. Ergonomic dynamometer

The Chatillon gauge is a valuable tool for performing a job-site analysis to measure the forces required to push or pull certain objects.

Answer: **C**
Hunter, Mackin, Callahan, pp. 1788-1789
Refer to Fig. 18-14.

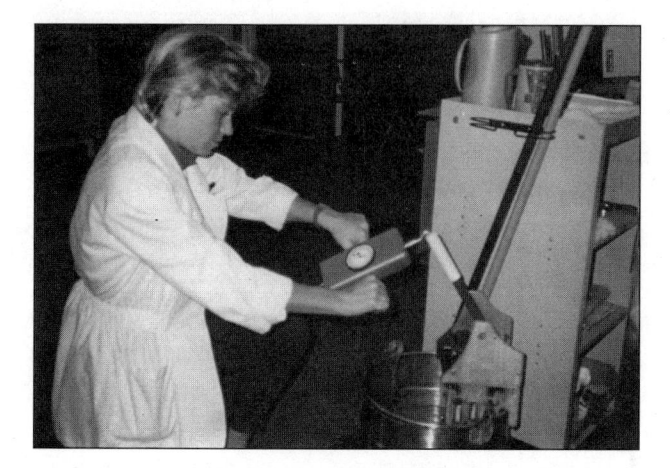

Fig. 18-14 ■ From Hunter JM, Mackin EJ, Callahan AD: *Rehabilitation of the hand: surgery and therapy,* ed 4, St. Louis, 1995, Mosby-Year Book.

34. All of the following are important for healthy computer use, except:

A. Maintaining the wrist in neutral position
B. Taking frequent breaks
C. Always using a wrist rest
D. Stretching frequently

All of the above are good rules to follow, except answer C. A common mistake people make is to rest the wrist while typing. This can cause direct pressure on the carpal canal and can put undue stress on the flexor tendons. Wrist rests are better termed wrist guides. One should only "rest" the wrist on the support when not typing.

Answer: **C**
Pascarelli, Quilter, pp. 178-181

> **CLINICAL GEM:**
> An excellent device to issue for median nerve protection is the soft flex splint. This splint keeps pressure off the median nerve, aids in edema management, and allows full digital motion. This splint can be ordered from durable medical equipment distributors such as AliMed and Northcoast, or directly through Softflex.

35. A 42-year-old woman is referred for therapy with a diagnosis of "wrist pain." After obtaining her history, you learn that she has recently started a new job requiring repetitive wrist flexion. During the evaluation, you note that the patient has volar ulnar wrist pain and tenderness over the ulnar carpus, specifically the pisiform, as well as pain along the ulnar forearm. Increased pain with resisted wrist flexion and passive wrist extension also is noted. You might conclude that she has which of the following?

A. Extensor carpi ulnaris tendinitis
B. Flexor carpi ulnaris tendinitis
C. Radial nerve entrapment
D. Lunate fracture

Flexor carpi ulnaris tendinitis, whether acute or chronic, presents with ulnar wrist pain. It is not uncommon to see this condition when individuals begin a new job requiring frequent wrist flexion or lifting of heavy objects. The pain is over the flexor carpi ulnaris tendon, especially at the pisiform, where it inserts. Conservative treatment usually is successful, with no recurrence of symptoms. If a wrist splint is used, the wrist should be positioned at neutral to 25° flexion with slight ulnar deviation. Job modification also may be beneficial. The physician may prescribe nonsteroidal antiinflammatory drugs or give an injection to reduce inflammation. In some cases surgery is indicated.

Answer: **B**
Millender, Louis, Simmons, p. 131
Thorson, Szabo, p. 425

36. Pain over the thenar and hypothenar eminences after carpal tunnel release is referred to as pillar pain. True or False?

Pillar pain is a well-recognized complication after carpal tunnel release. However, a clear definition of pillar pain has yet to be established. It is variously described as:

- Pain in the thenar **and** hypothenar eminences
- Pain in the thenar **or** hypothenar eminences
- Discomfort in the area of the surgical incision
- Radial and ulnar tenderness

Treatment includes soft-tissue mobilization, vibration, modalities, desensitization, and/or splinting.

Answer: **True**
Hunter, Schneider, Mackin, p. 150
Ludlow, Cox, Hurst, pp. 277-281

> **CLINICAL GEM:**
> It is not uncommon for pillar pain to persist for as long as 6 months. Reassure your patients that the pain will subside.

37. All of the following are potential compression sites for pronator syndrome, except:

A. Lacertus fibrosis
B. Ligament of Struthers
C. Pronator teres
D. Tendinous origin of flexor digitorum superficialis
E. Arcade of Struthers

There are several sites near the elbow where the median nerve is vulnerable to compression. These sites include: (1) between the supracondylar process and the ligament of Struthers; (2) at the lacertus fibrosis, which crosses over the median nerve at the elbow; (3) within the pronator teres muscle; and (4) at the tendinous origin of the flexor digitorum superficialis. The majority of cases are from compression of the median nerve as it passes between the two heads of the pronator teres muscle.

Patients complain of pain in the volar proximal forearm and decreased sensation to the median-nerve innervated digits. Sensory disturbances also may be present in the thenar eminence. Often patients report an occupational onset from repetitive use of the arm, especially resisted pronation. Treatment may include splinting, cessation of the provocative activity, and rest. Steroid injections have not been proven to be effective because minimal synovitis is present. Surgical intervention often is not required. A differential diagnosis from carpal tunnel syndrome is made when there are negative Phalen's and Tinel's signs at the wrist and **no** complaints of nocturnal pain. Answer E, the Arcade of Struthers, is involved with ulnar nerve entrapment.

Answer: **E**
Blair, pp. 754-763

38. **The cause of white finger is:**

A. Vibration
B. C8 nerve compression
C. Peripheral neuritis
D. Diabetes

White finger is a vascular problem caused by industrial overuse of vibratory tools. With the use of vibratory tools, grip force often is doubled because of distortion of position sense. This disorder causes muscle fatigue, pain, numbness, and blanching of the affected fingers and may cause vascular insufficiencies.

Answer: **A**
Ranney, pp. 187-188

CLINICAL GEM:
Interestingly, 50% of people in occupations using vibration tools, such as jackhammers, report symptoms of Raynaud's phenomenon.

Chapter 19
Joint Mobilization/Other Treatment Techniques

Topics to be reviewed in random order are:
- Joint mobilization principles
- Concave-convex rule
- Joint mobilization case studies
- Shoulder taping
- Soft-tissue mobilization
- Trigger-point treatment
- Isotonic/isokinetic/isometric exercises
- Joint protection techniques
- Scar-management techniques

1. When a concave surface is mobilized on a convex surface, the concave joint surface is glided in the same direction that the bone is moving. True or False?

The convex-concave rule denotes the mechanical relationship of the joint surfaces and is the basis for determining the direction of the mobilizing force when joint mobilization gliding techniques are used. When a concave surface is mobilized on a convex surface, the concave joint surface is glided in the same direction that the bone is moving (Fig. 19-1, *A*). If the convex surface is mobilized on a concave surface, bone movement and glide are in the opposite direction (Fig. 19-1, *B*).

Answer: **True**
Kisner, Colby, p. 153
Murphy, p. 2

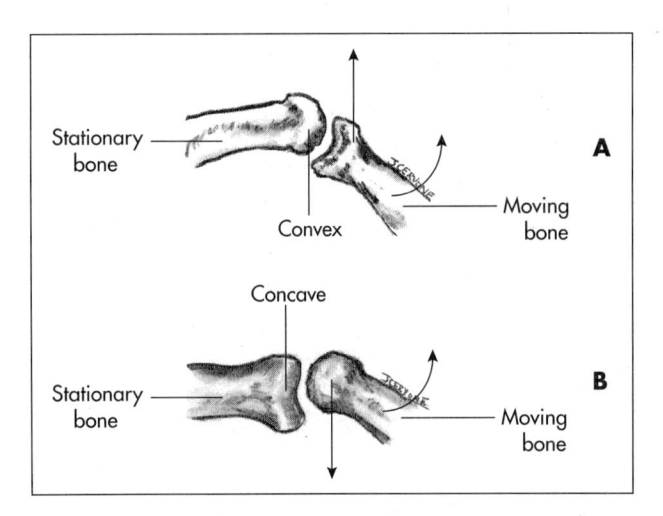

Fig. 19-1 ■ **A**, Moving bone is mobilized in the same direction as desired motion. **B**, Moving bone is mobilized in the direction opposite that of desired motion.

2. Rolling, gliding, and spinning are terms associated with the physiological movements of joint mobilization. True or False?

The techniques used in joint mobilization may be performed with physiological or accessory movements. Physiological movements are performed voluntarily by the patient (e.g., flexion, abduction, and rotation). Accessory movements are those movements within the joint and surrounding tissues necessary for normal joint range of motion that the patient cannot perform voluntarily (e.g., distraction, gliding, compression, rolling, and spinning).

Answer: **False**
Kisner, Colby, p. 158

3. Which of the following is not a contraindication or precaution for joint mobilization?

A. Malignancy
B. Joint replacement arthroplasties
C. Pain
D. Infection

The reference sources cited give overlapping contraindications and precautions. It is important for the therapist to appropriately evaluate the patient and determine whether joint mobilization can be an effective adjunct to treatment. Grade I distraction and grade I oscillatory movements that do not stress or stretch the capsule help block the transmission of pain stimuli. Therefore, pain is not a precaution or contraindication but may be a reason why joint mobilization is used. See the following Clinical Gem for precautions and contraindications to joint mobilization.

Answer: **C**
Kisner, Colby, pp. 156-158
Murphy, p. 1

> **CLINICAL GEM:**
> Following is a list of precautions and contraindications for joint mobilization:
> **Precautions:** Osteoporosis; hypermobility; inability of patient to relax; and presence of protective muscle spasm.
> **Contraindications:** Joint replacement arthroplasty; unhealed fractures; acute arthritis; bone disease; infection; malignancy; and rheumatoid arthritis.

4. Which of the following are benefits of joint mobilization?

A. Increased joint lubrication
B. Increased proprioceptive input
C. Decreased joint stiffness
D. Increased joint nutrition
E. All of the above

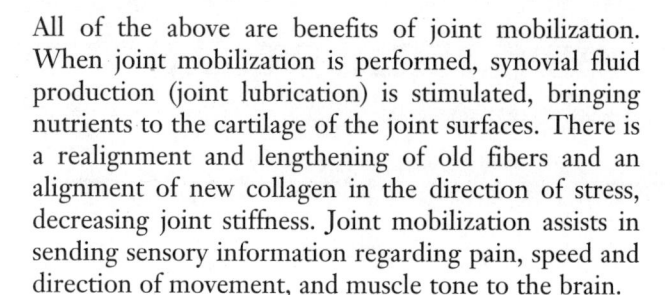

All of the above are benefits of joint mobilization. When joint mobilization is performed, synovial fluid production (joint lubrication) is stimulated, bringing nutrients to the cartilage of the joint surfaces. There is a realignment and lengthening of old fibers and an alignment of new collagen in the direction of stress, decreasing joint stiffness. Joint mobilization assists in sending sensory information regarding pain, speed and direction of movement, and muscle tone to the brain.

Answer: **E**
Kisner, Colby, p. 156
Duda-Huys, p. 7-2

5. According to Kaltenborn, joint play testing and mobilization must be done with the joint in a resting position. True or False?

Kaltenborn refers to bone and joint positions in terms of the maximum loose-packed position (MLPP—the resting position) and the close-packed position. In the MLPP, the greatest amount of joint play is possible; thus the assessment of joint play and treatment are performed in this position. In the close-packed position, there is maximum contact between the concave and convex articular surfaces and therefore the least amount of joint play is available.

Answer: **True**
Duda-Huys, pp. 7-8

6. According to Maitland, a grade-IV joint mobilization movement is a large amplitude movement at end range. True or False?

Maitland's treatment technique involves passive oscillatory movements and sustained stretches. He has defined four basic grades of movement (Fig. 19-2).

Answer: **False**
Kisner, Colby, p. 160
Duda-Huys, p. 7-14

Chapter 19 Joint Mobilization/Other Treatment Techniques

```
                                    Grade IV
                                  _____
                       Grade III
                      _____
         Grade II
        _____
  Grade I
  _____
  A                                          B

  A = Beginning of range
  B = End of range
```

Grade I:	Small amplitude movement at the beginning of range.
Grade II:	Large amplitude movement within the range, but not reaching the limit of range.
Grade III:	Large amplitude movement, performed up to the limit of range.
Grade IV:	Small amplitude movement, performed at the limit of range.

Fig. 19-2

7. Match each practitioner with the associated treatment techniques:

Practitioner

1. Mennel
2. Maitland
3. Kaltenborn
4. Cyriax

Techniques

A. Steroid injection; passive stretch; physiological movement in direction of limitation; deep friction massage
B. Glides; traction; "taking up the slack"
C. Quick thrust; mobilization followed by exercise to maintain range
D. Passive oscillatory movements; anteroposterior and posteroanterior glides; sustained stretch

Answers: **1. C; 2. D; 3. B; 4. A**
Duda-Huys, p. 5-16

8. Which of the following mobilization techniques may be beneficial for increasing shoulder external rotation?

A. Anterior glide
B. Posterior glide
C. Lateral glide
D. Inferior glide

The correct answer is A. External rotation of the humerus stresses the anterior aspect of the capsule, thus allowing further external rotation to occur. With mobilization, the head of the humerus moves anteriorly, helping to stretch the anterior portion of the shoulder capsule. The convex-concave rule should be followed.

Answer: **A**
Donatelli, p. 247

9. A 28-year-old basketball player is referred to therapy 12 weeks after dorsal dislocation of the fifth proximal interphalangeal joint. The patient presents with a 25-degree flexion contracture. One of your treatment techniques is joint mobilization. To increase proximal interphalangeal joint extension, a _____ glide is used.

A. Dorsal
B. Volar
C. Radial
D. Ulnar

According to the convex-concave rule, the digits are mobilized in the same direction as the desired motion. Hence, a dorsal glide is performed to achieve proximal interphalangeal joint extension.

Answer: **A**
Malone, McPoil, Nitz, p. 373

> **CLINICAL GEM:**
> It often is helpful to distract a joint before mobilizing it.

10. To gain dorsiflexion in a hypomobile wrist, you would perform which of the following?

A. Dorsal glide
B. Volar glide
C. Radial glide
D. Ulnar glide

A radiocarpal volar glide increases wrist dorsiflexion according to the concave-convex rule. However, some authors propose that a volar glide at the midcarpal joint will increase flexion. Controversy surrounds the percentage of motion that occurs at the radial carpal versus the mid-carpal joints.

Answer: **B**
Kisner, Colby, pp. 185-186
Refer to Fig. 19-3.

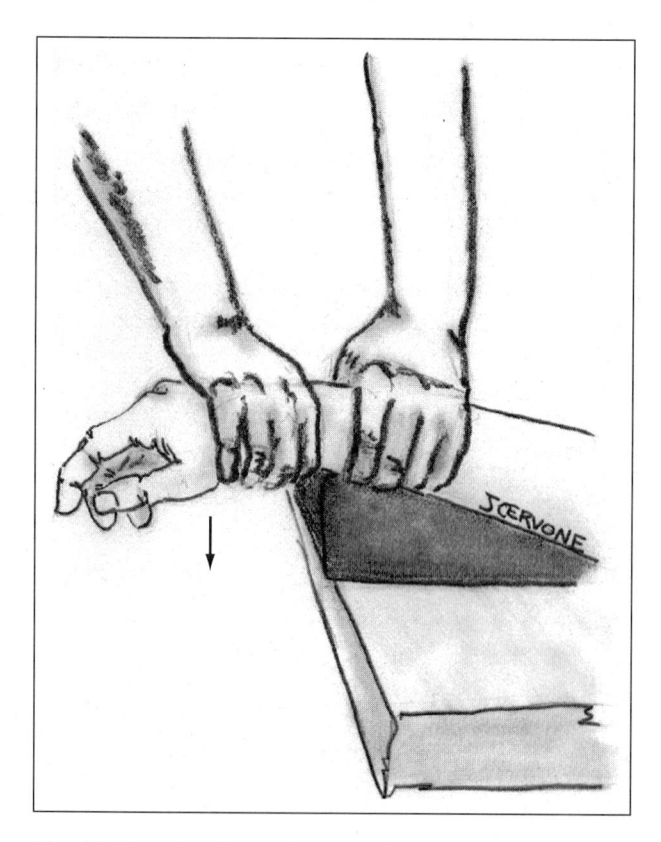

Fig. 19-3 ■ Volar glide at radial carpal joint.

11. According to Cyriax, a "springy" end-feel is significant during evaluation of which condition?

A. Arthritis
B. Fracture
C. Internal derangement of the joint
D. Acute bursitis

According to Cyriax, different sensations can be felt by the examiner's hands at the extreme of the possible range of motion when testing passive movement of a joint. These sensations include bone-to-bone, spasm, capsular, springy block, tissue approximation, and empty. Each of these sensations has an associated condition, which is important to determine so that proper treatment techniques can be administered (Table 19-1). A "springy" end-feel, according to Cyriax, indicates internal derangement of the joint.

Answer: **C**
Cyriax, p. 53
Duda-Huys, p. 7-6

Table 19-1

Cyriax's Description of End-Feel

End-Feel	Description	Significance in Evaluation
Bone-bone	Two hard surfacest meet—abrupt	Anatomic limit of joint
Spasm	Hardish feel Muscles reflexly stop movement	Acute and subacute arthritis Fracture
Capsular	Hardish feel Some give	Arthritis
Spring back	Rebound at end of movement	Internal derangement of joint
Tissue approximation	Soft-arrest movement	No mechanical block
Empty	Pain some distance from anatomic limit	Suspect acute bursitis, abscess, neoplasm

12. All of the following are goals of shoulder taping except:

A. Repositioning the humerus
B. Inhibiting the upper trapezius
C. Decreasing the patient's pain
D. Shortening the lower trapezius
E. All of the above are goals

McConnell reports that shoulder taping repositions the humerus, inhibits activity of the upper trapezius, shortens the lower trapezius, and secondarily decreases pain. McConnell uses taping of the shoulder to treat impingement, simple tendonitis, anterior subluxation, frozen shoulder, and multidirectional instability.

Answer: **E**
Brecker, pp. 10-11

13. Soft-tissue mobilization and myofascial release are both used to treat superficial tissues. True or False?

Soft-tissue mobilization is a gentle technique designed to break up superficial cross restrictions of fascia. Myofascial release is used to release the deeper layer of fascia.

Answer: **False**
Barnes, pp. 5-15

14. According to Barnes, when performing myofascial release the therapist should hold the stretch for a minimum of 30 seconds when a barrier is reached. True or False?

According to Barnes, once a barrier is reached during stretching, the therapist should hold the stretch for a minimum of 90 to 120 seconds. As the barrier releases, the therapist will feel motion under his or her hands and pressure should continue as long as motion persists.

Answer: **False**
Barnes, pp. 5-15

15. A hyperirritable spot in a muscle or its fascia that is painful on compression and can give rise to referred pain might be a:

A. Jump sign
B. Spasm
C. Bruxism
D. Trigger-point

A trigger-point is an area of hyperirritability in a tissue or muscle that, when compressed, is tender and hypersensitive and can give rise to referred pain. Types of trigger-points include myofascial, cutaneous, fascial, ligamentous, and periosteal.

Answer: **D**
Travell, Simons, p. 4

16. Pressure to a trigger-point can result in pilomotor activity. True or False?

Pilomotor activity (gooseflesh) can appear spontaneously with pressure application to active trigger-points (see Fig. 4-10, question 40).

Answer: **True**
Travell, Simons, p. 42

17. Which of the following is not helpful when treating a trigger-point?

A. Light digital pressure
B. Deep stripping massage
C. Stretch and spray
D. Kneading massage

All of the above are useful in helping to inactivate trigger-points, except light pressure.

Answer: **A**
Travell, Simons, p. 25

18. According to Travell, what is the "workhorse" of myofascial therapy?

A. Manual pressure techniques
B. Moist heat treatment
C. Stretch and spray
D. Injection and stretch

Travell reports that stretch and spray is the "workhorse" of myofascial therapy because it quickly inactivates myofascial trigger-points with less discomfort than with injection or ischemic compression (see Fig. 17-4, question 16).

Answer: **C**
Travell, Simons, p. 63

CHAPTER 19 Joint Mobilization/Other Treatment Techniques

19. You are preparing a patient for discharge who sustained a distal tip amputation of his dominant index finger. What would be the most useful tool to help this patient return to his factory job?

A. Valpar work component number eight simulated assembly
B. McCarron-Dial System
C. Baltimore Therapeutic Equipment tool number 162
D. Rolling putty in the clinic

Valpar work samples are used to help return industrial injured workers to gainful employment. Valpar number eight simulates assembly line work and would be useful to assist this patient in training to work on the assembly line at the factory. Valpar work samples are used for evaluation as well as treatment and are easy to administer and score.

The McCarron-Dial vocational rehabilitation system is used for the mentally-challenged population. The use of Baltimore Therapeutic Equipment (BTE) tool number 162 exclusively is not sufficient to return an employee to the assembly line. However, the BTE or Primus are excellent modalities for evaluation, conditioning, functional capacity evaluations, and rehabilitation.

Answer: **A**
Hopkins, Smith, pp. 287-289

20. A concentric contraction is a form of isotonic exercise. True or False?

Isotonic exercise is a dynamic exercise that uses force with movement. An isotonic muscle contraction occurs when tension is developed in a muscle, usually with a constant resistive force. The muscle length decreases or is lengthened during the performance of work or exercise. All of the following are types of isotonic exercise: concentric contraction, eccentric contraction, constant loading, variable loading, and plyometric loading.

Answer: **True**
Hunter, Mackin, Callahan, p. 1733
Taber's

21. Match each isotonic exercise with the correct definition.

Isotonic Exercise

1. Concentric contraction
2. Eccentric contraction
3. Constant loading
4. Variable loading
5. Plyometric loading

Definition

A. Occurs when muscles are loaded suddenly and forced to stretch before they can contract and elicit movement
B. Loading that remains the same
C. Contraction of muscle that results in shortening of muscle fibers
D. Imposing an increasing load throughout range of motion so that a more constant stress is placed on muscles
E. Muscle contraction in a lengthened state

Answers: **1. C; 2. E; 3. B; 4. D; 5. A**
Hunter, Mackin, Callahan, p. 1733

22. A 58-year-old woman complains of pain bilaterally in her basal joints. The patient does not want surgical intervention. She has difficulty peeling vegetables and is seeking your help to ensure success in meal preparation. What can you do for this patient?

A. Refer her to durable medical equipment companies
B. Teach her pinching and grasping strengthening programs
C. Adapt or construct a peeling board
D. Fabricate a short opponens splint
E. C and D are correct

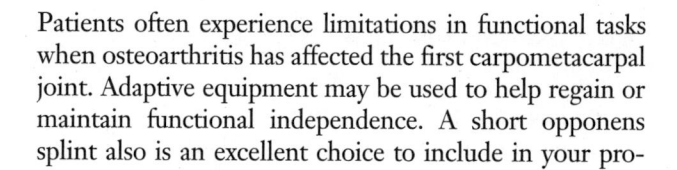

Patients often experience limitations in functional tasks when osteoarthritis has affected the first carpometacarpal joint. Adaptive equipment may be used to help regain or maintain functional independence. A short opponens splint also is an excellent choice to include in your program. Splinting may help decrease inflammation, provide rest and support, position the joint, and minimize joint deformity. Splinting and adaptive equipment are excellent adjuncts that the skilled therapist can implement in a program to manage arthritis.

Answer: **E**
Hunter, Mackin, Callahan, p. 1348

23. A 62-year-old woman with a type-I thumb deformity from rheumatoid arthritis is referred to you for evaluation and treatment. What is the best choice for intervention?

A. Refer her to a surgeon. There is nothing you can do.
B. Fabricate a dynamic interphalangeal joint extension splint
C. Educate your patient in joint protection and adaptive equipment principles
D. Begin an aggressive strengthening program

A type-I thumb deformity (see Fig. 11-1), which is similar to a boutonniere deformity, results in hyperextension of the interphalangeal joint secondary to flexion of the metacarpophalangeal joint. Treatment goals are to decrease pain, decrease edema, maintain joint mobility, and prevent or minimize deformity. Teaching your patient joint protection techniques and using adaptive equipment helps to minimize stress on the thumb.

Answer: **C**
Hunter, Mackin, Callahan, p. 1348

24. You are pushing a full cart of groceries from the store to your car. Which form of exercise are you performing?

A. Isokinetic exercise
B. Stretching
C. Closed-chain kinematics
D. Open-chain kinematics

Pushing a cart is an example of a closed-chain exercise. Closed-chain kinematics are load-bearing exercises used for stability. Closed-chain exercise transfers forces across more than one joint. Open-chain kinematics are exercises performed for mobility in which one joint or muscle group is isolated (e.g., isolated elbow flexion and extension).

Answer: **C**
Hunter, Mackin, Callahan, p. 1734

25. Isokinetic assessment is most often used to measure maximal strength. True or False?

Isokinetic assessment is infrequently used to measure maximal strength. Isokinetic exercise is contraction of a muscle whereby speed is controlled and maximum exertion occurs through the full range of motion. Isometric exercise is a static form of exercise that occurs when a muscle contracts against an immovable object. Isometric assessment is most often used for measuring maximal strength.

Answer: **False**
Hunter, Mackin, Callahan, p. 1733
Taber's

26. Continuous pressure over a scar does all of the following, except:

A. Make it softer
B. Increase elasticity
C. Improve cosmesis
D. Break up scar tissue

Scar-management techniques such as continuous pressure soften tissues, increase elasticity, and improve cosmesis. Scar-management techniques do not break up scar tissue but are used to increase pliability and assist in tissue elongation.

Answer: **D**
Hunter, Mackin, Callahan, p. 1062

27. You are treating a patient after carpal tunnel release. A Silicone gel sheet and Tubigrip are applied 2 days after suture removal to soften scar tissue and decrease edema. During the patient's next visit, she reports increased numbness in the median nerve distribution and hypersensitivity over the incision. Which of the following would you do?

A. Continue Silicone gel sheet and Tubigrip because hypersensitivity will decrease in a few days
B. Refer back to the physician to assess for infection
C. Remove Silicone gel sheet and Tubigrip and reassess
D. Discontinue Silicone gel sheet and commence ultrasound for scar management

Pressure application for scar management can result in skin maceration, allergies to products, decreased circulation, and nerve compression. This patient may have had an allergic reaction to the Silicone gel sheet and/or the Tubigrip may have caused her hypersensitivity. The therapist should consider other scar-management techniques (e.g., otoform or elastomer). This patient's paresthesia may be related to a tight Tubigrip. The current Tubigrip should be removed and a larger size should be applied.

Answer: **C**
Hunter, Mackin, Callahan, p. 1286

> **CLINICAL GEM:**
> Some physicians allow application of otoform while sutures are intact. Others believe that application of otoform or other scar remodeling techniques should be employed after suture removal.

28. A patient is referred to you with bilateral symptoms of pain on the radial side of the forearm and hand. No objective sensory loss is noted. What is a possible diagnosis?

A. de Quervain's tenosynovitis (disease)
B. Intersection syndrome
C. Scalene trigger-points
D. All of the above

If a patient experiences pain on the radial side of the forearm and hand without objective sensory loss, the patient could have a multitude of different diagnoses. Some of the diagnoses may include: intersection syndrome, de Quervain's tenosynovitis, or scalene trigger-points. The therapist must remember to look proximally when treating distal hand problems. It is easy to overlook proximal trigger-points when treating hand patients; however, such oversight may lead to treating an incorrect diagnosis.

Answer: **D**
Travell, Simons, p. 350

Chapter 20

Occupational Safety and Health Administration

Topics to be reviewed in random order are:

- Occupational Safety and Health Administration guidelines
- Personal protection equipment
- Biomedical waste
- Sharps disposal
- Transmittable diseases
- Exposure regulations

1. Personal protection equipment is specialized clothing or equipment worn by an employee for protection against hazards. True or False?

General work clothes, uniforms, pants, and shirts or blouses are not intended to function as protection against hazards. Personal protective equipment includes gloves, masks, eye protection, and gowns and must be provided by the employer.

Answer: **True**
Federal Register

2. When prescription eyeglasses are used for eye protection, they must be equipped with _____ .

A. Tint
B. Adjustable lenses
C. Protective side shields
D. All of the above

To be in compliance with Occupational Safety and Health Administration standards, protective side shields must be used when wearing eyeglasses as personal protective equipment.

Answer: **C**
Florida Administrative Code

3. Occupational Safety and Health Administration mandates the wearing of masks, eye wear, or face shields when one is exposed to:

A. Splashes
B. Spray
C. Droplets
D. Aerosols
E. All of the above

Occupational Safety and Health Administration mandates the use of personal protective equipment whenever an employee is at risk for exposure to any of the above.

Answer: **E**
Florida Administrative Code

242 CHAPTER 20 Occupational Safety and Health Administration

4. **Universal Precautions is the "thread" throughout the Blood-Borne Exposure Plan. This implies:**

A. Treating those 18 to 65 years old as if they were infected with a blood-borne infection.
B. Defining certain patients as "high" risk.
C. Using precautions for all body fluids.
D. Using precautions with selective body fluids and patients.

According to Universal Precautions, all body fluids should be considered possibly infectious regardless of age or "high" risk categorization.

Answer: **C**
Florida Administrative Code

5. **Biomedical waste precautions are specific to:**

A. Occupational Safety and Health Administration standards
B. State law
C. Joint Commission on Accreditation of Healthcare Organizations standards
D. Hospital policy

Although Occupational Safety and Health Administration standards state that biomedical waste precautions must be in place, types and methods of disposal are determined according to state law.

Answer: **B**
Florida Administrative Code

6. **All contaminated dressings are considered biomedical waste.**

A. True
B. False
C. Maybe
D. Depends on state law

Contaminated dressings and gloves may be considered biomedical waste, depending on state law. For example, in Florida, dressings are biomedical waste only if they are supersaturated, with the potential to drip or splash body fluid. Gloves are considered biomedical waste if they are contaminated with blood or body fluid.

Answer: **D**
Federal Registry
Florida Administrative Code

7. **When disposing of biomedical fluids in a rimmed clinical service sink, which type of personal protection should be used?**

A. Gloves
B. Face shield
C. Both A and B
D. None of the above

Splashing from a clinical service sink can be of concern. A face shield and gloves should be used as minimum protection against body fluid splashing into the eyes, mouth, or hands.

Answer: **C**
Florida Administrative Code

8. **Body excretions such as feces, nasal discharges, saliva, sputum, sweat, tears, urine, and vomitus must be treated as biomedical waste. True or False?**

If there is no blood contamination, these body fluids are not considered biomedical waste.

Answer: **False**
Federal Register

9. **Sharps should be packaged in impermeable red polyethylene or polyethylene plastic bags. True or False?**

Sharps should not be packaged in red bags. They must be disposed of in a designated sharps container.

Answer: **False**
Federal Register

10. **Surfaces contaminated with spilled or leaked biomedical waste should be cleaned with an approved disinfectant. True or False?**

Any surface with visible soil must be disinfected with a chemical germicide that is registered by the Environmental Protection Agency.

Answer: **True**
Federal Register

11. At least 20 different pathogens have been transmitted by percutaneous exposure to blood. Which blood-borne diseases are of greatest concern in the healthcare setting?

A. Syphilis; Rocky Mountain spotted fever; malaria
B. Human immunodeficiency virus; hepatitis B; hepatitis C
C. *Staphylococcus aureus*; tuberculosis; *Streptococcus*
D. *Pseudomonas aeruginosa, Escherichia coli, Neisseria meningitidis*

The transmission of all organisms listed above is possible through blood exposure. However, the transmission of most of them is extremely rare compared with the transmission of human immunodeficiency virus, hepatitis B, and hepatitis C, which are the most common concerns of healthcare workers.

Answer: **B**
Centers for Disease Control

12. A client has skin tears on the hands and arms. Which type of personal protection should you use?

A. Gloves
B. Gown
C. Face shield
D. Hair covering
E. All of the above

Personal protection should be selected according to the anticipated body fluid route of exposure. A skin tear could potentially bleed, causing contamination through contact; therefore, in this case, gloves are the protection of choice.

Answer: **A**
Florida Administrative Code

13. A client vomits in your work area. What should you do?

A. Clean the area with alcohol
B. Wear gloves to clean the area
C. Use a hospital approved disinfectant to clean the area
D. B and C
E. A and B

According to the Standard Precautions, body fluids should be cleaned wearing gloves and using a hospital approved disinfectant. Alcohol is not an approved disinfectant. The disinfectant should be tuberculocidal for proper cleaning.

Answer: **D**
Florida Administrative Code

14. An individual receiving the hepatitis B vaccine cannot donate blood. True or False?

The hepatitis B vaccine should be offered to any healthcare worker, free of charge, who potentially could be exposed to the hepatitis B virus. The vaccine boosts the immune system to produce antibodies that will kill the virus if the vaccinated individual is exposed. Because this is a chemical vaccine and not from serum, the vaccinated individual's blood is considered safe for donating.

Answer: **False**
Centers for Disease Control

15. A therapist has been exposed to blood. A contaminated syringe with a needle was left in the patient area and the therapist was stuck. According to Occupational Safety and Health Administration standards:

A. The therapist can report the exposure within 14 days
B. The exposure must be reported immediately
C. The therapist must report on the status of the exposure, in writing, within 6 months of exposure
D. The therapist should ignore the exposure unless the patient is "high" risk

It is necessary to report the incident immediately so that post-exposure follow-up can occur promptly.

Answer: **B**
Federal Registry

16. A therapist's clothing has been saturated with body fluid. The employer must provide:

A. Shower facilities
B. Change of clothing
C. Laundering of the personal clothing
D. All of the above

The Standard Precautions clearly states the provisions that are required for contaminated personal clothing. The skin must be decontaminated by flushing with water, personal clothing must be laundered, and a change of apparel must be provided.

Answer: **D**
Florida Administrative Code

Chapter 21
Research and Statistics

Topics to be reviewed in random order are:

- **Null hypothesis**
- **Scales of measurement**
- **Measures of central tendency**
- **The gaussian distribution**
- **Standard deviation**
- **Reliability and validity**
- **Dependent and independent variables**
- **Type-I and type-II errors**

1. Match the following columns of data in Table 21-1 with the correct scales of measurement (choices A through D).

Table 21-1

Data Column #1	Data Column #2	Data Column #3	Data Column #4
1. Marital Status	2. Satisfaction	3. Time in Treatment	4. Weight (Pounds)
Married	Very satisfied	1 week	40
Single	Somewhat satisfied	2 weeks	50
Divorced	Somewhat dissatisfied	3 weeks	80
Widowed	Very dissatisfied	4 weeks	100

A. Interval
B. Nominal
C. Ordinal
D. Ratio

Nominal: This is a variable such as marital status, in which the only distinction among "married," "single," "divorced," and "widowed" is that they are different categories (Data column #1).

Ordinal: There is a definite order to the measurements in column 2 because they can be ranked in terms of level of satisfaction. However, the distance between "very satisfied" and "somewhat satisfied" cannot be quantified (e.g., "very satisfied" is not a fixed amount better than "somewhat satisfied") (Data column #2).

Interval: Not only is there order to the measurements in column 3, but the distance between any two numbers on the scale is fixed and consistent (e.g., "4 weeks" minus "2 weeks" is the same as "3 weeks" minus "1 week") (Data column #3).

Ratio: The ratio scale is the same as the interval scale, except that it has a true zero, whether real or implied. Weight measurements in column 4 follow a ratio scale because there is a true zero (0 pounds) (Data column #4).

Answers: **1. B; 2. C; 3. A; 4. D**
Knapp, pp. 7-9
Portney, Watkins, pp. 44-48

246 CHAPTER 21 Research and Statistics

> **CLINICAL GEM:**
> Here is a way to remember the differences among nominal, ordinal, and interval scales of measurement. **Nom**inal means that the measurements are *names,* such as the names of categories (e.g., male/female or White/Black/Hispanic/Asian). **Ord**inal means that the measurements can be *ordered* (e.g., high/medium/low or excellent/good/average/poor). Inter**val** means that the measurements are *values* on a well-defined scale, such as degrees Fahrenheit or degrees Centigrade.

2. A histogram is a visual representation of data in which the data values are grouped into intervals and the relative frequency of values in each interval is plotted. True or False?

Individual data values collected in a study may be uninformative by themselves, but by organizing like values together, it may be possible to see trends. For example, the measured calcium values (mg/dL) for a group of 10 patients might be 8.6, 9.2, 8.0, 7.8, 9.7, 8.5, 10.4, 8.5, 9.3, and 10.1. By grouping these values into four intervals of equal width, the raw data can be summarized as follows:

Interval	Count (Frequency)	Relative Frequency
7.0-7.9	1	0.1
8.0-8.9	4	0.4
9.0-9.9	3	0.3
10.0-10.9	2	0.2
Total	10	1.0

Created by Doug Shier.

The last column of this table (the relative frequencies) can be plotted with the intervals on the horizontal axis and the relative frequency on the vertical axis, as in Figure 21-1.

Answer: **True**
Knapp, pp. 28-30

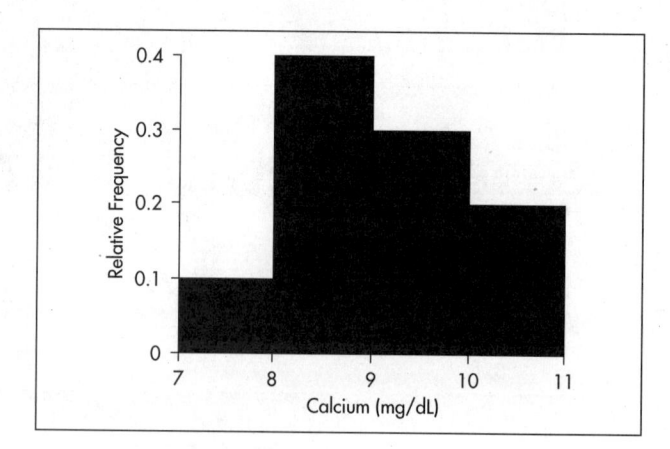

Fig. 21-1 ■ Created by Doug Shier.

3. Match each measure of central tendency with the correct definition.

Measure of Central Tendency

1. Mean
2. Median
3. Mode

Definition

A. The most frequent score in a distribution.
B. The average score in a distribution.
C. The score at the midpoint of the distribution.

Answers: **1. B; 2. C; 3. A**
Portney, Watkins, p. 323
Refer to Fig. 21-2.

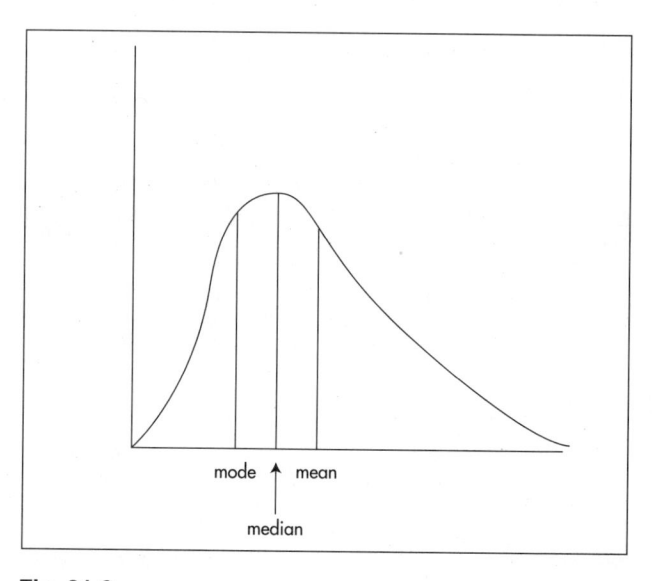

Fig. 21-2

4. What do you call a distribution in which the mean, mode, and median scores are all the same?

A. Gaussian distribution
B. Normal distribution
C. Bell curve
D. All of the above

In a bell curve, which also is known as a gaussian distribution or normal distribution, the mean, mode, and median scores are all the same.

Answer: **D**
Portney, Watkins, p. 323
Refer to Fig. 21-3.

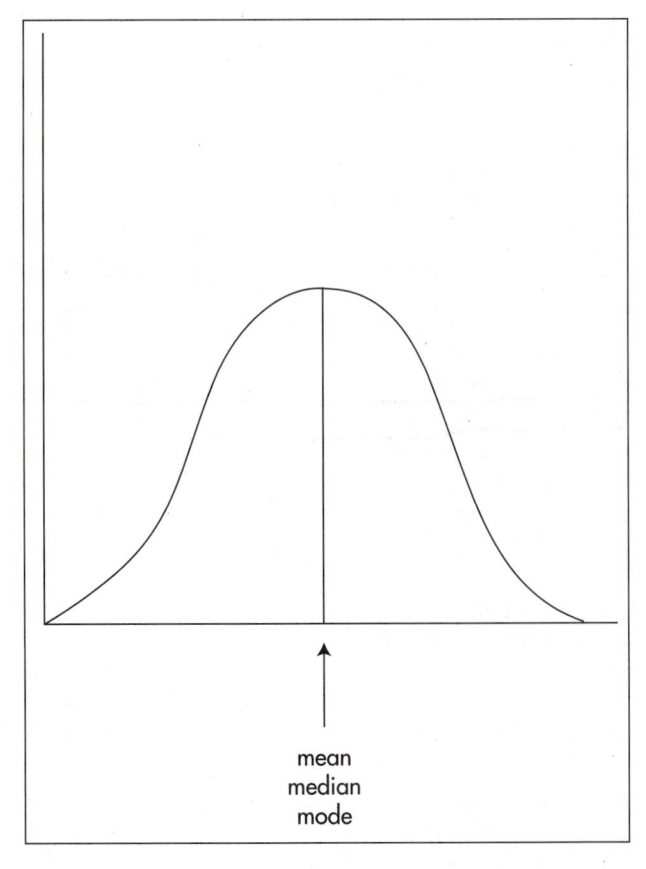

Fig. 21-3

5. The range, by itself (high score minus low score), is a useful measure of variability. True or False?

The range is the difference between the highest and lowest value in a set of variables. A few deviant scores would mislead an observer as to the variability in a distribution. The range by itself is not useful, but in combination with some means of central tendency it can be useful.

Answer: **False**
Portney, Watkins, p. 323

6. The standard deviation is the square root of the variance in a distribution. True or False?

Variance is a measure of variability in a distribution and is equal to the square of the standard deviation. The standard deviation is a descriptive statistic reflecting the variability or dispersion of scores around the mean. The standard deviation is often used as a basis for comparing samples.

Answer: **True**
Knapp, pp. 44-56
Portney, Watkins, pp. 326-327

7. In a screening program for hypertension, the average systolic blood pressure for males in a certain population is 140 mm Hg and the standard deviation is 8 mm Hg. One particular individual has a reading of 165 mm Hg. Does this person have significantly elevated blood pressure? Yes or No?

It is reasonable to assume that this population of individuals has systolic blood pressure values that are normally distributed. In a normal distribution, approximately 68% of the observations fall within (plus or minus) one standard deviation of the mean; 95% fall within two standard deviations of the mean; and 99% fall within three standard deviations of the mean. The individual reading of 165 is 25 units (= 165-140) greater than the mean, and this translates into 3.125 (25/8 = 3.125) standard deviations greater than the mean. This puts the individual over three standard deviations from the mean. Therefore, a blood pressure as high as this occurs in less than 1% of the population. This individual has a blood pressure reading that is statistically significant.

Answer: **Yes**
Knapp, pp. 62-66

248 CHAPTER 21 Research and Statistics

8. The correlation coefficient indicates the degrees of a linear relationship between two measurements. True or False?

When two measurements, such as Scholastic Aptitude Testing scores or grade point averages, covary systematically, the relationship can be graphed as points in a two-dimensional scatter plot, which create a (more or less) straight line. In a significant correlation, the scores may be related **directly** (i.e., as one increases so does the other) or **inversely** (i.e., as one increases the other decreases). Figure 21-4, *A* shows a direct relationship.

Figure 21-4, *B* illustrates an inverse relationship between age and joint flexibility. This relationship shows that as age increases, flexibility decreases.

The degree of linear relationship ranges from −1 (exact inverse relation) to +1 (direct relationship). A correlation of coefficient of zero indicates no linear relationship between the variables.

Answer: **True**
Knapp, pp. 217-218

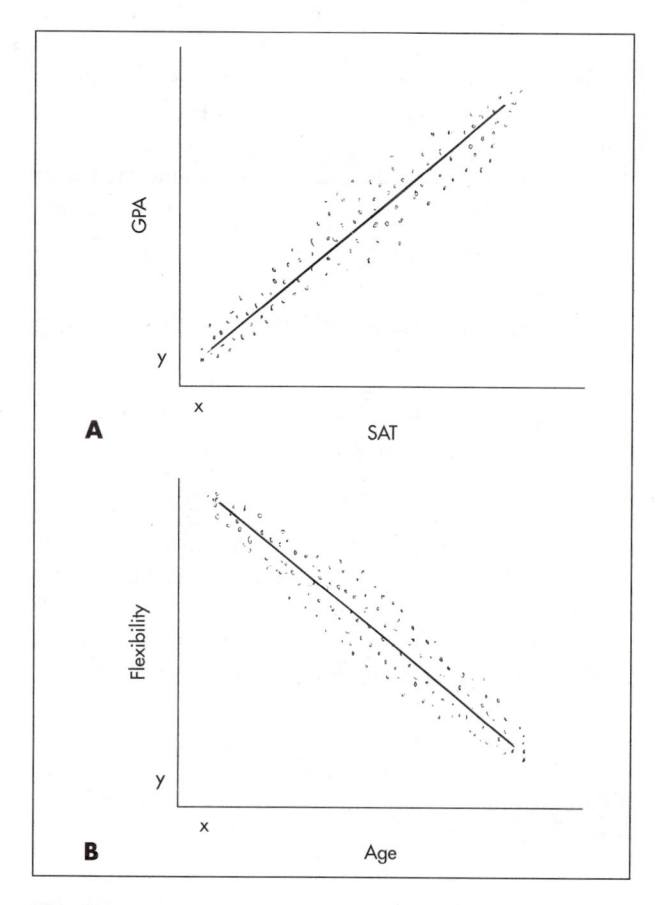

Fig. 21-4

9. In Figure 21-4, grade point averages and flexibility are the dependent variables and Scholastic Aptitude Testing scores and age are the independent variables. True or False?

Grade point average (GPA) and flexibility are dependent variables. Scholastic Aptitude Testing (SAT) scores and age are independent variables. Dependent variables are outcomes or results. Independent variables are presumed to cause or determine outcomes; often these variables are manipulated or controlled by the researcher, who sets their "values" or levels. It should be noted, however, that correlations do not indicate cause and effect. Age, per se, does not cause loss of flexibility. SAT scores do not cause GPAs, although they are clearly a predictor.

Answer: **True**
Portney, Watkins, pp. 90-93, 684
Knapp, pp. 6-7

10. Dependent variables tend to be placed on the Y axis of a graph. True or False?

Researchers tend to place independent variables along the horizontal axis of a graph, which is called the X axis. The results, or dependent variables, appear on the vertical, or ordinate axis (Y axis). In Figure 21-4, *A*, the independent variable, Scholastic Aptitude Testing, is plotted along the horizontal (X) axis and the dependent variable, grade point average, is plotted along the vertical axis (Y).

Answer: **True**
Portney, Watkins, pp. 90-94

11. Which of the following statements describes the difference between statistics and parameters?

A. Statistics are used only in research; parameters can be used in real life.
B. Parameters always are expressed in whole numbers; statistics are expressed in decimals.
C. A statistic is a descriptive measure based on a sample. When an entire population is measured, it is called a parameter.
D. All of the above are true.

This question has to do with how researchers can look at a segment of a population and make inferences about the whole population. This process is called sampling. The researcher determines the population, which is the entire set of individuals or units to which data will be generalized. However, if the researcher samples randomly from that population and measures that sample, the results can be generalized to the entire population. A sample is a subset of a population chosen for study. The results obtained from the sample are called statistics.

Answer: **C**
Portney, Watkins, pp. 111-124

> **CLINICAL GEM:**
> To remember the concept "populations," think of a large group of individuals, such as those who comprise the U. S. population. In contrast, a "sample" consists of a small group of individuals, such as 100 patients participating in clinical research. Samples are the basis for making inferences about an entire population.

12. The null hypothesis states that the differences found among samples are caused by an experimental intervention. True or False?

The statement above characterizes the experimental (alternative) hypothesis, not the null hypothesis. The null hypothesis states that differences found among samples are caused by sampling error. Typically, the null hypothesis is a hypothesis of no difference. Experiments can never prove or disprove either hypothesis; rather, they report the probability that one or the other is true.

Answer: **False**
Portney, Watkins, p. 346
Knapp, pp. 108-109

13. Match each statistical term with the correct definition.

Statistical Term

1. T test
2. β level
3. Parameter
4. Type-II error
5. $p < .01$
6. Independent variable
7. α level
8. Type-I error

Definition

A. The probability that the observed difference is caused by sampling error
B. A parametric test for comparing two means
C. The percent set by the experimenter at which she/he will reject the null hypothesis when it is true
D. An incorrect decision to reject the null hypothesis
E. An incorrect decision to accept the null hypothesis
F. A descriptive measurement of a population
G. The characteristic of experimental units that is expected to influence an outcome
H. The percent set by the experimenter at which she/he will accept the null hypothesis when it is false

Answers: **1. B; 2. H; 3. F; 4. E; 5. A; 6. G; 7. C; 8. D**
Portney, Watkins, pp. 677-694

> **CLINICAL GEM:**
> Here is a way to remember type-I and type-II errors. In the western justice system, a person is presumed innocent until proven guilty beyond a reasonable doubt. In this case, the null hypothesis is that the defendant is innocent (the presumption), and the experimental hypothesis is that the defendant is guilty. A type-I error is rejecting the null hypothesis when it is true (i.e., convicting an innocent person). Use the mnemonic **ONE: O**ne is **N**eedlessly **E**xecuted. A type-II error is not rejecting the null hypothesis when it is false (i.e., letting a guilty person go free). Use the mnemonic **TWO: T**he **W**icked get **O**ut.

14. Clinical services continue to be offered without an established base of experimental data. True or False?

With increasing economic challenges in healthcare, practitioners must justify clinical decisions with an identified body of knowledge. Unfortunately, many health professionals share the dilemma that clinical services continue to be offered without a base of experimental data. A scientific rationale does exist for practice, but often it comes from other disciplines such as anatomy, physiology, or psychology. Healthcare professionals must establish their own special professional knowledge base to effectively change or develop practice techniques.

Answer: **True**
Portney, Watkins, p. 3

15. Intrarater reliability refers to the variation between two or more raters who measure the same group of subjects. True or False?

Intrarater reliability refers to the stability of data recorded by one individual across two or more trials. In contrast, **interrater** reliability concerns variation between two or more raters who measure the same group of subjects. Often researchers decide to use one rater in a study to avoid the necessity of establishing **interrater** reliability. This is useful for ensuring consistency within the study but it does not strengthen the generalizability of the research outcomes.

Answer: **False**
Portney, Watkins, pp. 60, 61

16. Validity is the degree of consistency with which an instrument or rater measures a variable. True or False?

Reliability is the degree of consistency with which an instrument or rater measures a variable. Validity is the degree to which an instrument measures what it is intended to measure.

Answer: **False**
Portney, Watkins, pp. 690, 694

17. The goal of the researcher is to reject the null hypothesis. True or False?

The null hypothesis, H_0, states that any observed differences between the means are caused by chance. The goal always is to statistically test the null hypothesis, usually with the intent of rejecting it. This concept is similar to a legal assumption that a person is innocent until proven guilty. The null hypothesis suggests we assume that no relationship exists between variables until significant evidence is accumulated to convince us otherwise. The goal is not to "prove" the null hypothesis but to give the data a chance to disprove the null hypothesis.

The alternative hypothesis, H_1, is what the researcher hopes the data will support; the alternative hypothesis indicates that the observed difference is "real."

Answer: **True**
Portney, Watkins, p. 346

18. While establishing a research study, you decide that the level of significance in your study will be .05. To improve your confidence level, what would you do to the "P" value?

A. Lower it to .025
B. Increase it to .10
C. Increase it to .50
D. None of the above

The traditional designation of .05 is an arbitrary standard. When this standard is used, it means that we are willing to accept a 5% chance of incorrectly rejecting the null hypothesis. To improve our confidence level, we can minimize the risk of statistical error by lowering the level of significance in the study to .025 or .01.

Answer: **A**
Portney, Watkins, p. 349

Appendix 1

Drugs Commonly Encountered in Hand Therapy

Jodi Jones Knauf, OTR, PA-C

One of the areas of upper extremity rehabilitation seldom addressed in the occupational and physical therapy literature is prescription and nonprescription drugs and their effects on wound care, healing, and rehabilitation. The goal of this appendix is to introduce the hand therapist to some of the most common medications prescribed by hand surgeons and frequently encountered in a rehabilitation setting. Commonly used or abused nonprescription drugs such as nicotine, alcohol, and caffeine also are presented. Finally, an alphabetical list of the drugs discussed in this appendix and the classification of each is provided for your quick reference. It is beyond the scope of this appendix to address all classes of medications and their indications, side effects, and interactions. Please refer to the Physicians' Desk Reference and other pharmacology reference books for such information.

Common Medications Prescribed by Hand Surgeons

Narcotic Analgesics

Narcotic pain medicines are among the most common drugs encountered on a daily basis by hand therapists. They are most often prescribed to reduce pain after surgery or trauma. Narcotics may be useful, especially in the early postoperative period, in allowing the patient to comply with the treatment regimen without undue discomfort so that therapeutic progression may be achieved. Narcotics, however, can be associated with a number of common side effects that may interfere with treatment sessions and compliance with exercises at home. These include sedation, drowsiness, and other symptoms associated with central nervous system (CNS) depression (see alcohol); nausea and vomiting; rash; and pruritis (itching). Narcotics also have the potential to be abused. If you believe that your patient exhibits any of these symptoms, it is important to notify the referring physician, who may change the patient's medication or place the patient on a structured pain medication protocol. Remember that because therapists typically spend more one-on-one time with patients than do physicians, therapists often are in a better position to identify these problems; physicians generally appreciate such observations and input.

Common narcotic analgesics (or drugs containing a narcotic analgesic) include: Codeine, Darvocet-N, propoxyphene (Darvon), meperidine (Demerol), hydromorphone (Dilaudid), Hydrocodone, Lorcet, Lortab, dolophine (Methadone), MS Contin, nalbuphine (Nubain), Oxycodone, Percocet, Percodan, morphine (Roxanol), butorphanol (Stadol), pentazocine (Talwin), Tylox, and Vicodin. Another drug that is commonly prescribed for pain and related to the opiates but not considered a narcotic is tramadol (Ultram). This drug acts on the CNS and should not be given in conjunction with narcotics or given to patients who are addicted to narcotics.

Nonsteroidal Antiinflammatory Drugs

Nonsteroidal antiinflammatory drugs (NSAIDs) are an expanding class of drugs that are useful in the treatment of arthritis, musculoskeletal disorders and injuries, and postoperative patients because of their analgesic, antipyretic, and antiinflammatory properties. Their mechanism of action is the inhibition of prostaglandin synthesis. Prostaglandins cause pain, redness, fever, and edema in various musculoskeletal conditions including osteoarthritis, rheumatoid arthritis, and related disorders. NSAIDs do not produce the CNS side effects associated with narcotics or the many adverse reactions associated with steroids; however, they commonly cause gastrointestinal (GI) side effects that may be serious. These include abdominal pain, indigestion, nausea, diarrhea, constipation, and possibly even GI bleeding (typically causing dark tarry stools) from gastritis or peptic ulcer disease. NSAIDs that have a salicylate (aspirin) component may cause oozing, bleeding, and bruising postoperatively because of their anticoagulant (blood thinning) properties. Other common side effects of NSAIDs include rash, pruritis, headache, and dizziness. Commonly prescribed and over-the-counter NSAIDs include: ibuprofen (Advil), naproxen (Aleve), naproxen sodium (Anaprox), flurbiprofen (Ansaid), aspirin products, sulindac (Clinoril), oxaprozin (Daypro), diflunisal (Dolobid), piroxicam (Feldene), Ibuprofen, indomethacin (Indocin), etodolac (Lodine), ibuprofen (Motrin), fenoprofen (Nalfon), naproxen (Naprosyn), ibuprofen (Nuprin), ketoprofen (Orudis), nabumetone (Relafen), ketorolac (Toradol), and diclofenac (Voltaren).

Corticosteroids

Corticosteroid drugs are used principally as antiinflammatory agents for most patients encountered in a hand therapy setting. Oral steroids are used to treat medical conditions such as asthma, chronic obstructive pulmonary disease, dermatologic conditions, and rheumatic or autoimmune disorders, but in hand surgery they are used primarily to decrease edema and inflammation. Side effects of oral steroids may be serious in conditions requiring high doses and/or prolonged treatment and may include gastrointestinal ulcers, osteoporosis, hip necrosis, hyperglycemia or diabetes, insomnia, irritability, weight gain, cushingoid features, impaired wound healing, and susceptibility to infections. In hand conditions, however, steroids are more commonly used in an injectable form that allows a localization of their effect and causes fewer systemic side effects. Depending on the condition being treated and its location, the steroid may be combined with a local anesthetic such as lidocaine (Xylocaine) or bupivacaine (Marcaine). Injections should not be given in a previously infected or unstable joint because they can interfere with the body's ability to fight infection and wound healing responsiveness. Local injections, especially if repeated, can cause thinning of overlying skin, a discolored and shiny appearance, and atrophy of subcutaneous tissues. Oral corticosteroid preparations include: Cortisone, dexamethasone (Decadron), prednisone (Deltasone), and Medrol and methylprednisolone (Medrol Dosepak). Injectable steroids include: triamcinolone (Aristocort), betamethasone (Celestone), dexamethasone (Decadron), methylprednisolone (Depo-Medrol), and triamcinolone (Kenalog).

Antibiotics and Antimicrobial Drugs

Antimicrobial drugs commonly are employed postoperatively in hand surgery patients, topically or orally, and for severe infections, intramuscularly or intravenously. Depending on the type of surgery, conditions of the injury, and preference of the surgeon, oral antibiotics may be given prophylactically in the early postoperative period. However, because of the increasing emergence of resistant strains of bacteria, these medications should not be given casually for "possible" infection, and ideally a culture should be taken before treatment is initiated. Once a patient has started to take an antibiotic, the full prescription should be completed, even if the infection appears to have been resolved. The most common side effects of these medications are gastrointestinal and may present as abdominal pain, indigestion, nausea, vomiting, diarrhea, or constipation. Rash, pruritis, photosensitivity, headache, and dizziness also are common. Antibiotics that are likely to be encountered in a hand setting include: cefazolin IM/IV (Ancef), amoxicillin/clavulanate (Augmentin), clarithromycin (Biaxin), cefaclor (Ceclor), cefotetan IM/IV (Cefotan), cefuroxime (Ceftin), cefprozil (Cefzil), ciprofloxacin (Cipro), cefotaxime IM/IV (Claforan), clindamycin (Cleocin), cefadroxil (Duricef), erythromycin (E-mycin), erythromycin (E.E.S.), metronidazole (Flagyl), ofloxacin (Floxin), ceftazidime IM/IV (Fortaz), cephalexin (Keflex), cefazolin IM/IV (Kefzol), penicillin V (Pen-Vee K), ceftriaxone IM/IV (Rocephin), ampicillin/sulbactam IM/IV (Unasyn), nafcillin (Unipen), doxycycline (Vibramycin), and azithromycin (Zithromax).

Anticoagulants and Antithrombotics

Patients who undergo microvascular surgery or are predisposed to thromboembolic complications (including patients with a history of deep venous thrombosis, pulmonary embolism, peripheral vascular disease, stroke, cardiac arrhythmias, or other cardiac diseases) often are placed on blood-thinning or anticoagulant medications. In hand surgery these drugs are used to prevent arterial (and venous) occlusions, especially after soft-tissue flaps are inserted or replants. Arterial thrombosis or embolism may otherwise lead to necrosis or death of a flap, digit, or entire extremity. In some cases, hand surgeons may use medicinal leeches to decrease venous engorgement of skin flaps postoperatively; the leeches suck out the blood and fall off when they are full. Bleeding is, of course, the most common complication of anticoagulant therapy, and patients on these medications typically have repeated blood testing to maintain the equilibrium between the desired effect and frank bleeding. While on these drugs patients typically will have more oozing and drainage and prolonged wound healing times. Many prescription and over-the-counter medications may affect the blood levels of these drugs or intensify the anticoagulant effect; therefore, if your patient is experiencing increased or continued problems with bleeding, you should have the patient make a list of all current medications and contact the referring physician. As patients progress postoperatively, physicians may substitute aspirin products such as Bayer, Bufferin, or Ecotrin (Aspirin) for more potent anticoagulants. Some of the more potent anticoagulant drugs include: warfarin (Coumadin), heparin, enoxaparin (Lovenox), ardeparin (Normiflo), danaparoid (Orgaran), dipyridamole (Persantine), and ticlopidine (Ticlid).

Sympatholytic or Antiadrenergic Drugs

These medications work by interfering with the sympathetic nervous system's constriction of peripheral blood vessels in the skin and subcutaneous tissues of the upper extremity in conditions such as Raynaud's syndrome and reflex sympathetic dystrophy (RSD). They do not significantly increase skeletal muscle blood flow, and therefore are not very useful in the treatment of other types of peripheral vascular disease; however, they can cause dilation of blood vessels in the superficial tissues and skin. The most common side effect of these agents is orthostatic hypotension (dizziness or lightheadedness upon standing or changes of body position). Currently, the most effective alpha-blocking agent with the fewest undesirable side effects is phenoxybenzamine (Dibenzyline). Other sympatholytic or antiadrenergic agents that you may encounter include: methyldopa (Aldomet), guanethidine (Ismelin), prazosin (Minipress), tolazoline (Priscoline), phentolamine (Regitine), and reserpine (Serpasil).

Miscellaneous Drugs Used in Hand Conditions

Nifedipine (Adalat, Procardia) is a calcium channel blocker that commonly is employed in the treatment of hypertension and other cardiovascular diseases. Nifedipine works on the vascular smooth muscle to cause dilation of blood vessels and increases peripheral blood flow. It also may reverse the signs of vasomotor instability, and for these reasons may be useful in the treatment of Raynaud's syndrome and RSD. It also is sometimes used after microvascular surgery. Nifedipine has been shown to decrease vasospasm and may decrease the frequency and severity of attacks in patients with Raynaud's syndrome.

Amitriptyline (Elavil) is a tricyclic antidepressant used in the treatment of RSD, neuralgias, and other chronic pain disorders of the upper extremity. Amitriptyline is of benefit in RSD patients because many of them have some degree of clinical depression, but it also produces vasodilation and has analgesic action. Amitriptyline commonly causes drowsiness, orthostatic hypotension, and marked anticholinergic side effects, including dry mouth, blurred vision, tachycardia, urinary retention, and slowed gastric emptying. It can be very dangerous in overdoses, and this should be remembered in patients with severe depression or suicidal tendencies.

Capsaicin (Zostrix) is a topical ointment derived from the red capsicum pepper. It has shown promise in the local relief of hyperalgesia, hypersensitivity of the skin, and pain associated with various neuropathies as well as some arthritic conditions. Topical application of this medication may be helpful in some patients with RSD.

Gabapentin (Neurontin) is an anticonvulsant drug that is used to treat some forms of epilepsy. It also is used by some hand surgeons in the treatment of RSD and neuropathic pain or phantom pains after peripheral nerve injuries. Its mechanism of action in these conditions is unclear.

Drugs of Abuse and Their Negative Effects in Hand Rehabilitation

Nicotine

Nicotine, found in cigarettes, cigars, chewing tobacco, snuff, and pipe tobacco, causes peripheral vasoconstriction, increased heart rate, and elevated blood pressure. Nicotine has an adverse effect on wound healing in the hand therapy patient. Vasoconstriction decreases the blood supply to bone, muscle, and soft tissue, causing a delay in overall healing; this is especially true for those who have undergone microvascular procedures such as flap application or replants, after which smoking is definitely contraindicated. These effects often are more pronounced in the elderly or debilitated patient, who already may have conditions that adversely affect healing and circulation. Nicotine also can alter the activity of other concomitant prescription and over-the-counter medications. Remember that drugs used to help with smoking cessation typically contain nicotine and if patients smoke while taking these medications, the level of nicotine in the bloodstream increases dramatically and may be dangerous. Smoking cessation drugs include: Habitrol, Nicoderm CQ, Nicorette gum, Nicotrol, and ProStep.

Alcohol

Because alcohol is water soluble, it affects every living cell in the body. In contrast to nicotine, moderate doses of alcohol can cause vasodilation, especially in cutaneous vessels. Alcohol also is a central nervous system depressant that affects not only reasoning but also memory and coordination. Alcohol commonly has a profound effect on therapy because it may influence understanding of and compliance with wound care as well as clinical and home exercise programs. Chronic alcohol abuse may cause gastrointestinal distress and interfere with normal digestion and may be accompanied by poor nutrition, often leading to impaired wound healing. When alcohol is combined with other prescription or nonprescription drugs such as pain medications or sedatives, it may cause overdose, liver failure, or death.

Caffeine

Caffeine is a drug that few people consider when taking a medical history. Caffeine is found not only in coffee but in many beverages, foods, and medications. It may cause vasoconstriction in the hand therapy patient, resulting in numbness and pain in the extremities. Caffeine also may exacerbate previous medical problems such as hypertension, tachycardia, cardiac arrhythmias, and coronary artery disease. Many hand patients, because of their altered work and activity schedules, increase their intake of coffee and caffeine substantially. Common medications that contain caffeine include: Anacin (Aspirin), ergotamine (Cafergot), butalbital (Esgic, Fioricet, Fiorinal), Excedrin (Aspirin), orphenadrine (Norgesic), and ergotamine (Wigraine).

Bibliography

Drug Evaluations Annual 1992. Chicago, 1991, American Medical Association.

Gellman H, Nichols D: Reflex sympathetic dystrophy in the upper extremity, *J Am Acad Orthop Surg* 5:313, 1997.

Green DP, editor: *Operative hand surgery,* ed 3, New York, 1993, Churchill Livingstone.

Physician Assistants' Prescribing Reference, Winter 1997-1998, New York, 1997, Prescribing Reference, Inc.

Physicians' Desk Reference, ed 52, Montvale, NJ, 1998, Medical Economics Company, Inc.

List of Drugs Commonly Encountered in Hand Therapy*

Drug name	Indication/Drug category
Adalat (nifedipine)	hypertension, Raynaud's
Advil (ibuprofen)	NSAID
alcohol	CNS depressant
Aldomet (methyldopa)	hypertension/sympatholytic
Aleve (naproxen)	NSAID
amitriptyline (Elavil)	depression, neuropathic pain
amoxicillin/clavulanate (Augmentin)	antibiotic
ampicillin/sulbactam (Unasyn)	antibiotic
Anacin (aspirin)	NSAID, anticoagulant
Anaprox (naproxen sodium)	NSAID
Ancef (cefazolin IV)	antibiotic
Ansaid (flurbiprofen)	NSAID
ardeparin (Normiflo)	anticoagulant
Aristocort (triamcinolone)	corticosteroid
aspirin	NSAID, anticoagulant
Augmentin (amoxicillin/clavulanate)	antibiotic
azithromycin (Zithromax)	antibiotic
Bayer (aspirin)	NSAID, anticoagulant
betamethasone (Celestone)	corticosteroid
Biaxin (clarithromycin)	antibiotic
Bufferin (aspirin)	NSAID, anticoagulant
butalbital (Esgic, Fioricet, Fiorinal)	migraine headache/caffeine
butorphanol (Stadol)	narcotic analgesic
Cafergot (ergotamine)	migraine headache/caffeine
caffeine	stimulant
capsaicin (Zostrix)	neuropathic pain
Ceclor (cefaclor)	antibiotic
cefaclor (Ceclor)	antibiotic
cefadroxil (Duricef)	antibiotic
cefazolin (Kefzol, Ancef)	antibiotic
Cefotan (cefotetan)	antibiotic
cefotaxime (Claforan)	antibiotic
cefotetan (Cefotan)	antibiotic
cefprozil (Cefzil)	antibiotic
ceftazidime (Fortaz)	antibiotic
Ceftin (cefuroxime)	antibiotic
ceftriaxone (Rocephin)	antibiotic
cefuroxime (Ceftin)	antibiotic
Cefzil (cefprozil)	antibiotic
Celestone (betamethasone)	corticosteroid
cephalexin (Keflex)	antibiotic
Cipro (ciprofloxacin)	antibiotic
ciprofloxacin (Cipro)	antibiotic
Claforan (cefotaxime)	antibiotic
clarithromycin (Biaxin)	antibiotic
Cleocin (clindamycin)	antibiotic
clindamycin (Cleocin)	antibiotic
Clinoril (sulindac)	NSAID

*Note: Common trade names are capitalized; generic names are in lower case.

Appendix 1 Drugs Commonly Encountered in Hand Therapy

Drug name	Indication/Drug category
codeine	narcotic analgesic
cortisone	corticosteroid
Coumadin (warfarin)	anticoagulant
danaparoid (Orgaran)	anticoagulant
Darvocet-N (propoxyphene)	narcotic analgesic
Darvon (propoxyphene)	narcotic analgesic
Daypro (oxaprozin)	NSAID
Decadron (dexamethasone)	corticosteroid
Deltasone (prednisone)	corticosteroid
Demerol (meperidine)	narcotic analgesic
Depo-Medrol (methylprednisolone)	corticosteroid
dexamethasone (Decadron)	corticosteroid
Dibenzyline (phenoxybenzamine)	hypertension/sympatholytic
diclofenac (Voltaren)	NSAID
diflunisal (Dolobid)	NSAID
Dilaudid (hydromorphone)	narcotic analgesic
dipyridamole (Persantine)	anticoagulant
Dolobid (diflunisal)	NSAID
Dolophine (methadone)	narcotic analgesic
doxycycline (Vibramycin)	antibiotic
Duricef (cefadroxil)	antibiotic
E-mycin (erythromycin)	antibiotic
E.E.S. (erythromycin)	antibiotic
Ecotrin (aspirin)	NSAID, anticoagulant
Elavil (amitriptyline)	depression, neuropathic pain
enoxaparin (Lovenox)	anticoagulant
ergotamine (Cafergot, Wigraine)	migraine headache/caffeine
erythromycin (E-mycin, E.E.S.)	antibiotic
Esgic (butalbital)	migraine headache/caffeine
etodolac (Lodine)	NSAID
Excedrin (aspirin, caffeine)	NSAID, anticoagulant/caffeine
Feldene (piroxicam)	NSAID
fenoprofen (Nalfon)	NSAID
Fioricet (butalbital)	migraine headache/caffeine
Fiorinal (butalbital)	migraine headache/caffeine
Flagyl (metronidazole)	antibiotic
Floxin (ofloxacin)	antibiotic
flurbiprofen (Ansaid)	NSAID
Fortaz (ceftazidime)	antibiotic
gabapentin (Neurontin)	seizures, RSD/neuropathic pain
guanethidine (Ismelin)	hypertension/sympatholytic
Habitrol (nicotine)	smoking cessation
heparin	anticoagulant
hydrocodone (Lorcet, Lortab, Vicodin)	narcotic analgesic
hydromorphone (Dilaudid)	narcotic analgesic
ibuprofen (Advil, Motrin, Nuprin)	NSAID
Indocin (indomethacin)	NSAID
indomethacin (Indocin)	NSAID
Ismelin (guanethidine)	hypertension/sympatholytic
Keflex (cephalexin)	antibiotic
Kefzol (cefazolin)	antibiotic
Kenalog (triamcinolone)	corticosteroid
ketoprofen (Orudis)	NSAID

Appendix 1 Drugs Commonly Encountered in Hand Therapy

Drug name	Indication/Drug category
ketorolac (Toradol)	NSAID
Lodine (etodolac)	NSAID
Lorcet (hydrocodone)	narcotic analgesic
Lortab (hydrocodone)	narcotic analgesic
Lovenox (enoxaparin)	anticoagulant
Medrol (methylprednisolone)	corticosteroid
meperidine (Demerol)	narcotic analgesic
methadone (Dolophine)	narcotic analgesic
methyldopa (Aldomet)	hypertension/sympatholytic
methylprednisolone (Depo-Medrol, Medrol)	corticosteroid
metronidazole (Flagyl)	antibiotic
Minipress (prazosin)	hypertension/sympatholytic
morphine (MS Contin, Roxanol)	narcotic analgesic
Motrin (ibuprofen)	NSAID
MS Contin (morphine)	narcotic analgesic
nabumetone (Relafen)	NSAID
nafcillin (Unipen)	antibiotic
nalbuphine (Nubain)	narcotic analgesic
Nalfon (fenoprofen)	NSAID
Naprosyn (naproxen)	NSAID
naproxen (Aleve, Anaprox, Naprosyn)	NSAID
Neurontin (gabapentin)	seizures, RSD/neuropathic pain
Nicoderm CQ (nicotine)	smoking cessation
Nicorette gum (nicotine)	smoking cessation
nicotine	stimulant
Nicotrol	smoking cessation
nifedipine (Adalat, Procardia)	hypertension, Raynaud's
Norgesic (orphenadrine)	muscle relaxant/caffeine
Normiflo (ardeparin)	anticoagulant
Nubain (nalbuphine)	narcotic analgesic
Nuprin (ibuprofen)	NSAID
ofloxacin (Floxin)	antibiotic
Orgaran (danaparoid)	anticoagulant
orphenadrine (Norgesic)	muscle relaxant,caffeine
Orudis (ketoprofen)	NSAID
oxaprozin (Daypro)	NSAID
oxycodone (Percocet, Percodan, Tylox)	narcotic analgesic
Pen-Vee K (penicillin V)	antibiotic
penicillin V (Pen-Vee K)	antibiotic
pentazocine (Talwin)	narcotic analgesic
Percocet (oxycodone)	narcotic analgesic
Percodan (oxycodone)	narcotic analgesic
Persantine (dipyridamole)	anticoagulant
phenoxybenzamine (Dibenzyline)	hypertension/sympatholytic
phentolamine (Regitine)	hypertension/sympatholytic
piroxicam (Feldene)	NSAID
prazosin (Minipress)	hypertension/sympatholytic
prednisone (Deltasone)	corticosteroid
Priscoline (tolazoline)	hypertension/sympatholytic
Procardia (nifedipine)	hypertension, Raynaud's
propoxyphene (Darvocet-N, Darvon)	narcotic analgesic
Prostep (nicotine)	smoking cessation
Regitine (phentolamine)	hypertension/sympatholytic

Appendix 1 Drugs Commonly Encountered in Hand Therapy

Drug name	Indication/Drug category
Relafen (nabumetone)	NSAID
reserpine (Serpasil)	hypertension/sympatholytic
Rocephin (ceftriaxone IV)	antibiotic
Roxanol (morphine)	narcotic analgesic
Serpasil (reserpine)	hypertension/sympatholytic
Stadol (butorphanol)	narcotic analgesic
sulindac (Clinoril)	NSAID
Talwin (pentazocine)	narcotic analgesic
Ticlid (ticlopidine)	anticoagulant
ticlopidine (Ticlid)	anticoagulant
tolazoline (Priscoline)	hypertension/sympatholytic
Toradol (ketorolac)	NSAID
tramadol (Ultram)	non-narcotic analgesic
triamcinolone (Aristocort)	corticosteroid
triamcinolone (Kenalog)	corticosteroid
Tylox (oxycodone)	narcotic analgesic
Ultram (tramadol)	non-narcotic analgesic
Unasyn (ampicillin/sulbactam)	antibiotic
Unipen (nafcillin)	antibiotic
Vibramycin (doxycycline)	antibiotic
Vicodin (hydrocodone)	narcotic analgesic
Voltaren (diclofenac)	NSAID
warfarin (Coumadin)	anticoagulant
Wigraine (ergotamine)	migraine headache, caffeine
Zithromax (azithromycin)	antibiotic
Zostrix (capsaicin)	neuropathic pain

Appendix 2
Nutrition

Amy Mills, *OTR/L*

The following is a quick nutritional reference for therapists. This appendix will assist therapists in discussing optimal nutrition with their patients. While compiling information for this section, the contributor selected vitamins, minerals, and food supplements, as well as their benefits and cautions, with the hand therapy patient in mind. Further study is recommended for an in-depth evaluation of this subject. Vitamins, minerals, or supplements that contain extensive precautions or are controversial are omitted from this section.

Vitamins

Vitamin	Benefits*	Cautions†
Vitamin B1 (Thiamine)	Enhances circulation; assists blood formation; optimizes brain function	
Vitamin B2 (Riboflavin)	Assists red blood cell formation, antibody production, and cell respiration and growth; people with carpal tunnel syndrome may benefit from use of this vitamin in combination with B6	
Vitamin B3 (Niacin)	Assists nervous system function and circulation	A flush, usually harmless, may occur after ingestion of niacin supplements; those who are pregnant, diabetic, or have glaucoma, gout, liver disease, or peptic ulcers should use cautiously because amounts over 500 mg daily may cause liver damage if taken for prolonged periods
Vitamin B5 (Pantothenic acid)	Assists stress reduction and production of neurotransmitters	
Vitamin B6 (Pyridoxine)	Assists sodium and potassium balance; required by nervous system; assists immune system function; decreases water retention; thought to be helpful for treatment of carpal tunnel syndrome and other common peripheral nerve pathologies	
Vitamin B12 (Cyanocobalamin)	Helps prevent nerve damage; maintains fatty sheaths that cover and protect nerve endings	
Folic acid	Needed for red blood cell formation; aids in proper functioning of white blood cells, thereby strengthening immunity	Those with a hormone related cancer or convulsive disorder must not take high doses of folic acid for extended periods
Vitamin C (Ascorbic acid)	Assists tissue growth and repair; enhances immunity; guards against infection; promotes healing of wounds and burns	Pregnant women should not take more than 5000 mg daily because infants may become dependent on this supplement and develop scurvy when deprived of the accustomed megadoses after birth; if aspirin and vitamin C are taken together, stomach irritation may occur
Vitamin D	Especially important for normal growth and development of bones and teeth in children; benefits immune system; assists blood clotting	Should not be taken without calcium; toxicity may result from taking more than 65,000 international units over a period of years; excessive amounts may cause vomiting, diarrhea, weight loss, and kidney damage
Vitamin E	Improves circulation; necessary for tissue repair; assists blood clotting/healing; reduces scarring in some wounds; synergistic relationship with Vitamin C (effectiveness enhanced when taken together)	Those taking a blood thinner should not take more than 1200 international units of vitamin E daily; those with diabetes, rheumatic heart disease, or overactive thyroid, should not take more than the recommended dosage; if hypertensive, start with small amounts such as 200 mg daily and gradually increase dosage
Vitamin K	Necessary for blood clotting; aids in bone formation and repair	Large doses of synthetic vitamin K should not be taken during the last few weeks of pregnancy because it can be toxic for newborns; megadoses can cause flushing and sweating; excessive amounts of the synthetic vitamin may cause jaundice
Vitamin P (Bioflavonoids)	Used extensively in athletic injuries for relieving pain, bruises; has an antibacterial effect; promotes circulation	Very high doses may cause diarrhea

*The benefits listed in this table have been indicated to be effective according to the cited references.
†Blank spaces indicate no significant cautions associated with use according to the cited references.

Minerals

Minerals	Benefits*	Cautions†
Boron	Small amount needed for healthy bones and metabolism of calcium	No more than 3 mg should be taken daily
Calcium	Vital for strong bones; aids in transmission of nerve impulses	Calcium supplements should not be taken by those with history of kidney stones or kidney disease; may interfere with effects of verapamil (Calan, Isoptin, Verelan), a calcium channel blocker sometimes prescribed for hypertension or cardiac problems
Copper	Aids in formation of bone, hemoglobin, and red blood cells; works in balance with zinc and vitamin C to form elastin; necessary for healing; promotes healthy nerves and joints; essential for collagen formation	High doses may result in a rare metabolic condition (Wilson's disease)
Germanium	Improves cellular oxygenation; helps fight pain; keeps immune system functioning	
Iron	Oxygenates red blood cells; aids immune system function	Iron supplements should not be taken if active infection is present because extra iron can increase bacterial growth in the body; high doses can lead to cirrhosis of the liver
Magnesium	Helps prevent calcification of soft tissue; aids in bone formation; maintains body pH balance	Diarrhea may result if large doses are consumed
Manganese	Required for normal bone growth and reproduction and formation of cartilage and synovial fluid	
Phosphorus	Aids in bone formation; promotes normal cell function	
Potassium	Promotes healthy nervous system; helps control water retention with sodium	Excess can result in muscular weakness or death
Silicon	Aids in formation of collagen for bones and connective tissue; aids in calcium absorption in early stages of bone formation	Inhalation of small silicon particles into the lungs may lead to silicosis
Sodium	Helps maintain proper water balance; helps control blood pH	Large doses can cause high blood pressure
Sulfur	Necessary for collagen synthesis	
Vanadium	Needed for cellular metabolism; aids in production of bone	High doses may cause lung irritation
Zinc	Required for protein synthesis; aids in collagen formation; promotes healthy immune system function; assists in wound healing	More than 100 mg daily can depress the immune system; excess amounts may lead to vomiting, nausea, fever, and diarrhea

*The benefits listed in this table have been proven to be effective according to the cited references.
†Blank spaces indicate no significant cautions associated with use.

Natural Food Supplements

Natural Food Supplements	Benefits*	Cautions†
Alfalfa	Good for arthritis pain; contains chlorophyll, which aids in healing of infection and burns	May reactivate symptoms in people with quiescent systemic lupus
Aloe vera	Skin healer and moisturizer; good for treatment of burns and cuts	Should be used only topically for therapeutic purposes described here
Barley grass	Acts as an antiinflammatory	
Bovine cartilage	Accelerates wound healing; reduces inflammation; helpful in treatment of rheumatoid arthritis	
Cayenne	Relieves pain when applied topically	
Fish oil	Relieves arthritis	Not for diabetics because of the high fat content of this oil (but diabetics should consume fish for essential fatty acids)
Flaxseed oil or flaxseed	Decreases pain, inflammation, and edema associated with arthritis	
Garlic	Stimulates immune system; acts as a natural antibiotic	
Glucosamine	Involved in formation of tendons, skin, bones, and ligaments; can be helpful for tendonitis and bursitis	
Honey	Promotes healing; natural antiseptic; good salve for burns and wounds	Not to be taken by babies under one year of age, or those with diabetes or hypoglycemia
Kelp	Beneficial for sensory nerves and spinal cord	
Lactobacillus bifidus	Helps maintain healthy intestinal flora when antibiotics are taken	
Sea cucumber	Relieves arthritis	
Sea mussel	Helps relieve pain and stiffness associated with arthritis	
Shark cartilage	Relieves arthritis; promotes healthy immune system	Should not be taken by pregnant women, children, or those who have had recent heart attacks or surgery

*The benefits listed in this table have been proven to be effective according to the cited references.
†Blank spaces indicate no significant cautions associated with use.

References

Balch JF, Balch, PA: *Prescription for nutritional healing: A practical A-Z reference to drug-free remedies using vitamins, minerals, herbs, and food supplements*, ed 2, Garden City Park, New York, 1997, Avery Publishing Group.

Peterson MS: *Eat to compete: A guide to sports nutrition*, ed 2, St. Louis, 1996, Mosby.

Appendix 3

Resource List of Vendors

Amy Mills, *OTR/L*

This appendix provides a quick reference to many companies and the types of products they offer. The categories selected indicate each company's chief product line in reference to hand therapy. This is not an all-inclusive listing and is not intended to endorse any specific company or product.

Appendix 3 Resource List of Vendors

Companies	Splinting Products	CPM Products	Wound Care Products
Advanced Therapy Products PO Box 3420, Glen Allen, VA 23058 800-548-4550, 804-747-0676 (fax) www.richmond.infi.net/~atp	X		X
Alimed 297 High Street, Dedham, MA 02026 800-225-2610, 800-437-2966 (fax) www.alimed.com	X		X
Austin Medical Equipment 1900 South Mannheim Rd, Westchester, IL 60154 800-382-0300, 800-422-0515 (fax)			
Bailey Manufacturing Company PO Box 130, Lodi, OH 44254 800-321-8372, 800-224-5390 (fax)			
Baltimore Therapeutic Equipment 7455 L New Ridge Rd, Hanover, MD 21076 800-331-8845, 410-850-5244 (fax) www.bteco.com		X	
Bio-concepts, Inc. 2424 E. University, Phoenix, AZ 85034-6911 800-421-5647, 602-273-6931 (fax) www.bio-con.com			
Biodex Medical Systems Brookhaven R&D Plaza, 20 Ramsay Rd, Box 702 Shirley, NY 11967-0702 800-224-6339, 516-924-9338 (fax) www.biodex.com	X		
Bio Med Sciences 101 Technology Dr, Bethlehem, PA 18015 800-257-4566, 610-974-8831 (fax) www.silon.com	X		X
Bio Technologies 2160 N. Central Road, Suite 204 Fort Lee, NJ 07024 800-971-2468, 201-947-4495 (fax)	X		
DeRoyal/LMB 200 DeBusk Ln, Powell, NJ 37849 800-935-6197 www.deroyal.com	X		X
Dynasplint 770 Ritchie Hwy., Suite W 21 Severna Park, MD 21146-3937 800-638-6771	X		
Dynatronics Corporation 7030 Park Centre Dr, Salt Lake City, UT 84121 801-568-7000, 801-568-7711 (fax) www.dynatron.com			
Empi 599 Cardigan Rd, St. Paul, MN 55126-4099 800-328-2536 ext. 1773 www.empi.com	X		

Appendix 3 Resource List of Vendors   265

Burn/Scar Products	Exercise Products	Work Conditioning Software Products	ADL Products	Thermal Modality Products	Electrotherapy Products	Ergonomic Products
	X	X		X	X	X
X	X		X	X	X	X
	X		X	X	X	
	X	X				
	X	X				
X						
	X			X	X	
X						
			X	X		X
				X	X	
					X	

Appendix 3 Resource List of Vendors

Companies	Splinting Products	CPM Products	Wound Care Products
Ergodyne 1410 Energy Park Dr, Suite One St. Paul, MN 55108 800-225-8238, 651-642-1882 (fax) www.ergodyne.com			
Ergoscience, Inc. 4131 Cliff Rd, Birmingham, AL 35222 205-595-4536, 205-592-9528 (fax)			
Fiskars, Inc. 7811 West Stewart Ave Wausau, WI 54401 800-950-0203, 715-848-3657 (fax) www.Fiskars.Fi/f.1100.htm			
Greenleaf Medical 3145 Porter Dr, Bldg A202 Palo Alto, CA 94304 800-925-0925, 650-843-3645 (fax) www.greenleafmed.com			
Iomed 3385 W. 1820 South Salt Lake City, UT 84104 800-621-3347, 801-972-9072 (fax) www.iomed.com			
Jobst PO Box 653, Toledo, OH 43697-0653 800-537-1063, Ohio 800-228-2736 419-691-4511 (fax) HYPERLINK http://www.beirsdorf.com www.beirsdorf.com			X
Joint Active Systems 2600 S. Raney Street, Effingham, IL 62401 800-879-0117, 217-347-3384 (fax) www.bonuttiresearch.com	X		
Joint Jack Company 108 Britt Rd, East Hartford, CT 06118 860-568-7338, 860-568-9588 (fax)	X		
Jtech Medical Industries 357 West 910 South, Heber City, UT 84032 800-985-8324, 435-657-2700 (fax) www.Jtechmed.com			
Kinesis Corporation 22121 17th Ave. SE, Suite 112, Bothell, WA 98021 800-454-6374, 425-402-8181 (fax) www.kinesis-ergo.com			
Lafayette Instruments PO Box 5729, Lafayette, IN 47903 800-428-7545, 765-423-4111 (fax) www.licmef.com			
Mettler Electronics Corporation 1333 S. Claudina St, Anaheim, CA 92805 800-854-9305, 714-635-7539 (fax) www.mettlerelec.com			

Burn/Scar Products	Exercise Products	Work Conditioning Software Products	ADL Products	Thermal Modality Products	Electrotherapy Products	Ergonomic Products
		X				X
						X
						X
		X				
					X	
X						
		X				
						X
		X				
				X	X	

Appendix 3 Resource List of Vendors

Companies	Splinting Products	CPM Products	Wound Care Products
North Coast Medical, Inc. 187 Stauffer Blvd, San Jose, CA 95125-1042 800-821-9319, 408-283-1950 (fax) www.ncmedical.com	X		X
Sammons Preston 4 Sammons Ct, Bolingbrook, IL 60440 800-323-5547, 800-547-4333 (fax) www.sammonspreston.com	X		X
Silver Ring Splint Company PO Box 2586, Charlottesville, VA 22902 804-971-4052, 804-971-8828 (fax) www.silverringsplint.com	X		
Smith & Nephew PO Box 1005, Germantown, WI 53022 800-228-3693, 414-251-7758 (fax) www.easy-living.com	X		X
The Blankenship Group 3620 Eisenhower Pkwy, Macon, GA 31206 800-248-8846, 912-781-8566 (fax) www.blankenshipsystem.com			
Tetra Medical Supply Corporation 6364 West Gross Point Rd, Niles, IL 60714-3916 800-621-4041, 847-647-9034 (fax) www.tetramed.com	X		
The Healthy Back Store 8245 Backlick Rd, Springfield, VA 22079 800-4MY-BACK, 703-339-0671 (fax) www.healthyback.com/hbs/newstuff.qry			
Home Medical of America 10901 Roosevelt Boulevard, Suite D100 St. Petersburg, FL 33716 800-289-1938, 727-579-0259 (fax)	X	X	
Upper Extremity Net 401 N. Michigan Ave, Chicago, Il 60611-4267 312-321-6866, 312-321-5194			
U. E. Tech P.O. Box 2145, Edwards, CO 81632 800-736-1894, 970-926-8870 (fax)	X		
Valpar PO Box 5767, Tucson, AZ 85703-5767 800-528-7070, 520-292-9755 (fax) www.valparint.com			
OrthoLogic/Sutter Corporation 1275 W. Washington St, Tempe, AZ 85281 800-225-1814, 888 301 0080 (fax) www.orthologic.com	X	X	
Henley International 120 Industrial Blvd, Sugar Land, TX 77478 800-237-8749, 281-276-7176 (fax) www.henleyhealth.com			

Burn/Scar Products	Exercise Products	Work Conditioning Software Products	ADL Products	Thermal Modality Products	Electrotherapy Products	Ergonomic Products
X	X		X	X		X
X	X		X	X	X	X
X	X		X	X	X	X
		X				
				X		
						X
				X	X	
		X				
	X			X	X	
		X				
				X	X	
	X			X	X	

Appendix 4

Internet Websites

Amy Mills, *OTR/L*

Since the invention of the World Wide Web, therapists and other healthcare professionals have had limitless information available at their fingertips. This appendix provides a sampling of what is available on the Internet regarding therapy, surgery, professional organizations, health, and medicine related to the hand and upper extremity.

Amazon Books
www.amazon.com
Online bookstore that includes a varied selection of hand therapy books.

American Academy of Orthopaedic Surgeons
www.aaos.org
Online information source regarding the association and its research, products, patient education brochures, and legislative information.

American Academy of Wound Management
members.aol.com/woundnet
Information on wound care and board certification for clinicians and others involved in wound management.

American Association for Hand Surgery
www.handsurgery.org
Comprehensive website that includes membership information, related links, newsletter information, and important information on grant funds for research.

American College of Rheumatology
www.rheumatology.org
Includes patient information, a search index, related links, and research information.

American Medical Association
www.ama-assn.org
American medical news; online publication for coverage of current issues in medicine.

American Occupational Therapy Association
www.aota.org
Online information source for the occupational therapy profession.

American Physical Therapy Association
www.apta.org
Online information source for the physical therapy profession.

American Society of Hand Therapists
www.asht.org
Includes a directory and marketplace, as well as various member services.

American Society of Plastic and Reconstructive Surgeons
www.plasticsurgery.org
Provides background on a wide variety of cosmetic and reconstructive surgery procedures, as well as web links.

American Society for Surgery of the Hand
www.hand-surg.org
Online American society for surgery of the hand; informational and member service site.

Arthritis Foundation
www.arthritis.org
Online information related to arthritis and the foundation.

Appendix 4 Internet Websites

Bayscenes
www.bayscenes.com
Forum for exchange of ideas and knowledge in field of physical medicine and rehabilitation; serves as a resource for residents and other health care professionals.

B. C. Professional Firefighter's Burn Fund Home Page
www.vanserve.org/home.html
Provider information on burn treatment, therapeutic management, and links to other websites.

Belcher's Hand Surgery Site
www.pncl.co.uk/~belcher/home.htm
HJCR Belcher, MS, FRCS, Queen Victoria Hospital. Surgical information site for various hand procedures, as well as links to other resources on the web.

Buncke Clinic
www.summit.stanford.edu/bunke
World wide web journal of reconstructive plastic surgery.

Community Health Research Methods
isu.indstate.edu/gabanys/course341/341start.htm
An excellent research site designed by Steve G. Gabany at Indiana online research class.

CTD News Online
ctdnews.com
Practical information about cumulative trauma disorders. Includes standards, guidelines, conferences, and seminars.

Drug InfoNet
www.druginfonet.com
Comprehensive prescription information website that includes detailed descriptions of drugs as well as contraindications and warnings.

Eaton's Hand Surgery Links
www.eatonhand.com
By Charles Eaton, MD. Hand surgery information that includes anatomy, clip art images, slide show, and links to other helpful sources.

Ergoweb
www.ergoweb.com
Ergonomics website.

Hand Therapy Certification Commission
www.htcc.org
Includes news about certification, eligibility requirements, and recertification information.

Healing Touch International
www.healingtouch.net
Information about the use of healing touch as well as future course dates, locations, and membership in this organization.

Healthseek
www.healthseek.com
Offers a healthcare forum for sharing of ideas, questions, etc.

Health Answers
www.healthanswers.com
A site specifically for health care professionals; offers health news and its own search engine.

Indiana Hand Center
www.indianahandcenter.com
Devoted to information regarding the Indiana hand center, its history, physicians, hand conference, and educational information and resources.

International Food Information Council
www.ificinfo.health.org
Extensive nutrition website.

International Hand Library
www.handlibrary.org
Not-for-profit library and archives in Louisville, KY, with detailed collection of health information on hand and upper extremity.

Mosby
www.mosby.com
Provides access to books, articles, and periodicals published by Mosby.

National Board for Certification in Occupational Therapy
www.nbcot.org
Online information source for occupational therapy profession.

Occupational Health and Safety Administration (OSHA)
www.osha.gov
Online resource for information related to communicable diseases, regulations, standards, etc.

Occupational Therapy Internet World
www.mother.com/~ktherapy/ot
Comprehensive occupational therapy information source with other related links, as well as a directory and online newsletter.

Orthopaedic Web Links
www.bonehome.com/owl.html
Offers information on various orthopaedic surgery topics, including the hand.

Professional Examination Service
www.proexam.org
Information related to the organization and its testing.

PT Central
www.ptcentral.com
Offers thorough review of upper extremity muscles.

Wheeless' Textbook of Orthopaedics
www.medmedia.com/med.htm
Extremely comprehensive information source developed by C.R. Wheeless, MD.

Worldortho
www.worldortho.com
Complete interactive website maintained by the Department of Orthopaedic Surgery at Nepean Hospital, Sydney, Australia.

World Wide Wounds
www.smtl.co.uk/world-wide-wounds
Features wound care journal devoted to wound management, care, and dressings.

Appendix 5

Self Review

Following are 100 questions for you to answer as a self review of the material you have learned in this text. An answer key can be found at the end of this review. Detailed explanations of these answers have not been provided because the information can be found in the text. This appendix has been perforated so that you can tear it out, photocopy it, and test yourself repeatedly.

1. Which structure is responsible for metacarpophalangeal joint contractures in Dupuytren's disease?

   A. Pretendinous cord
   B. Spiral cord
   C. Lateral cord
   D. Retrovascular cord

2. Which of the following is the excursion distance for digital flexors?

   A. 2 to 3 cm
   B. 3 to 4 cm
   C. 4 to 5 cm
   D. 6 to 7 cm

3. In general, postoperative treatment for tendon transfers should include immobilization for:

   A. 1 week
   B. 3 to 4 weeks
   C. 6 weeks
   D. 12 weeks

4. Which tendon transfer for median nerve palsy uses the palmaris longus?

   A. Huber
   B. Stiles Bunnell
   C. Camitz
   D. Rolye-Thompson

5. Which is the most common primary bone tumor in the hand?

   A. Enchondroma
   B. Glomerulus tumor
   C. Volar wrist ganglion
   D. Lipoma

6. A patient presents to your clinic with complaints of persistent numbness in the index and long fingers. She reports that the numbness increases when she drives or does needlepoint. She also reports frequently waking up at night with pain in her hand. Which is the most likely diagnosis?

   A. Compression of the ulnar nerve at Guyon's canal
   B. Compression of the ulnar nerve at the cubital tunnel
   C. Compression of the median nerve at the wrist
   D. Compression of the radial nerve at the arcade of Frohse

7. You are treating a patient with a diagnosis of pronator syndrome. Which of the following is not a potential site of compression in pronator syndrome?

   A. The arcade of Struthers
   B. The lacertus fibrosus
   C. The pronator teres
   D. The arch of the flexor digitorum superficialis

275

8. You are treating a patient who complains of pain in the forearm, as well as weakness affecting the thumb and index fingers. Evaluation reveals minimal function of the flexor digitorum profundus to the index and long fingers, and decreased function of the flexor pollicis longus. Sensation is normal. Which syndrome might this patient have?

A. Carpal tunnel syndrome
B. Anterior interosseous nerve syndrome
C. Radial nerve palsy
D. Posterior interosseous nerve syndrome

9. Which of the following is not a site of compression in radial tunnel syndrome?

A. Fibrous bands anterior to radial head
B. Recurrent radial vessels
C. Tendinous margin of the extensor carpi radialis brevis
D. The arcade of Frohse
E. All of the above are sites of compression

10. You are treating a patient who complains of dorsal wrist pain with numbness affecting the thumb, index, and long fingers. The patient has severe shooting pain with thumb and wrist motion. Which diagnosis might be appropriate for this patient?

A. Radial tunnel syndrome
B. Carpal tunnel syndrome
C. Wartenberg's syndrome
D. Pronator syndrome

11. You are treating a patient who complains of intermittent pain along the medial proximal forearm and numbness in the small and ring fingers. He reports waking at night with numbness in the hand and pain in his arm. The patient also has a positive Tinel's sign at the medial epicondyle. Which diagnosis might be appropriate for this patient?

A. Carpal tunnel syndrome
B. Cubital tunnel syndrome
C. Pronator syndrome
D. Anterior interosseous nerve syndrome

12. Which of the following is not a compression site of the ulnar nerve in cubital tunnel syndrome?

A. Medial head of the triceps
B. Aponeurosis of the flexor carpi ulnaris
C. Ligament of Struthers
D. All of the above are compression sites for the ulnar nerve

13. Which of the following is a contraindication for replantation of digits?

A. Proximal phalanx level amputation of the thumb in a 40-year-old man
B. Multiple digit amputation in a 65-year-old woman
C. Distal fingertip amputation in a 35-year-old man
D. Distal tip amputation in a 7-year-old child

14. You are treating a patient after his replant. Venous outflow appears to be a problem. What should you do?

A. Lower the limb
B. Elevate the limb
C. Put the dressing on tighter
D. Make the limb colder

15. What is the maximal warm ischemic time that will not produce deleterious effects for digit replantation?

A. 2 hours
B. 6 hours
C. 12 hours
D. 24 hours

16. Pinch strength is achieved primarily by muscular innervation supplied by:

A. The deep branch of the ulnar nerve
B. The anterior interosseous nerve
C. The posterior interosseous nerve
D. The deep branch of the median nerve

17. Perception of touch in the fingertips is mediated by:

A. Nonmyelinated C fibers
B. Large, myelinated group A-beta fibers
C. Small, myelinated free nerve endings
D. Myelinated C fibers

18. The deep motor branch of the ulnar nerve enters the hand through the:

A. Carpal tunnel
B. Cubital tunnel
C. Guyon's canal
D. Hunter's canal

19. An advancing Tinel's sign along the course of a repaired nerve is:

A. Indicative of the number of regenerating axons progressing down the nerve
B. The only way to predict return of nerve function
C. An indication of the presence of both sensory and motor axons distal to the repair site
D. An indication of nerve regeneration, but not a predictive value

20. By week three, a sutured wound has which percentage of its tensile strength?

A. 15%
B. 35%
C. 50%
D. 75%

21. A pathologic process similar to Dupuytren's disease occurs in which of the following?

A. Albright's disease
B. Ledderhose's disease
C. Dercum's disease
D. Paschen's disease

22. A patient exhibits tenderness in the snuffbox. Which bone might be fractured?

A. Lunate
B. Triquetrum
C. Scaphoid
D. Trapezium

23. Sudden, forcible flexion of the distal phalanx avulsing the extensor tendon has been termed:

A. Boutonniere deformity
B. Boxer's fracture
C. Mallet finger
D. Jersey finger

24. Stenosing tenosynovitis involving the abductor pollicis longus and the extensor pollicis brevis is termed:

A. de Quervain's disease
B. Preiser's disease
C. Intersection syndrome
D. Wartenberg's syndrome

25. Which of the following muscles abducts the fingers?

A. Volar interossei
B. Dorsal interossei
C. Lumbricals
D. Flexor pollicis longus

26. As the median nerve courses through the carpal tunnel, it innervates which muscle first after crossing the wrist?

A. Pronator quadratus
B. Opponens pollicis
C. Abductor pollicis brevis
D. Flexor pollicis brevis

27. When manual muscle testing the supinator, which nerve are you evaluating?

A. Radial nerve
B. Musculocutaneous nerve
C. Ulnar nerve
D. Median nerve

28. The resisted middle finger test is used to evaluate irritation of which nerve?

A. Median
B. Radial
C. Ulnar
D. Musculocutaneous

29. The muscle found in extensor compartment five is the:

A. Extensor pollicis brevis
B. Extensor carpi ulnaris
C. Extensor digitorum communis
D. Extensor digiti minimi

30. Which dermatome provides sensory innervation to the middle finger?

A. C5
B. C6
C. C7
D. C8

31. A distal radius fracture presenting with volar displacement of the distal fragment is called a:

A. Colles' fracture
B. Essex-Lopresti fracture
C. Smith's fracture
D. Galeazzi fracture

32. Which of the following is not an intraarticular fracture?

A. Bennett's
B. Barton's
C. Monteggia
D. All of the above are intraarticular fractures

33. Ganglion cysts occur frequently and are most often present where?

A. At the dorsal scapholunate interval
B. At the volar scapholunate interval
C. At the volar lunotriquetral interval
D. At the dorsal lunotriquetral interval

34. Stress loading is a treatment used for reflex sympathetic dystrophy. Lois Carlson recommends how many minutes of scrubbing for the initial treatment?

A. 3 minutes
B. 6 minutes
C. 9 minutes
D. 15 minutes

35. Which of the following is *not* one of the four cardinal signs of reflex sympathetic dystrophy?

A. Pain
B. Swelling
C. Heat
D. Discoloration

36. Which of the following is the most common rheumatoid thumb deformity?

A. Swan-neck deformity
B. Lateral instability of the interphalangeal joint
C. Boutonniere deformity
D. None of the above

37. Which of the following thumb muscles is innervated by two nerves?

A. Opponens pollicis
B. Flexor pollicis longus
C. Abductor pollicis brevis
D. Flexor pollicis brevis

38. Which of the following muscles should be the first to be reinnervated after a laceration of the median nerve above the elbow?

A. Pronator teres
B. Supinator
C. Palmaris longus
D. Flexor carpi radialis

39. When should rehabilitation be initiated after a tenolysis?

A. On the same day
B. 4 to 5 days postoperatively
C. 7 to 10 days postoperatively
D. 14 days postoperatively

40. Which structure(s) centralize(s) the tendons of the extensor digitorum communis over the metacarpophalangeal joints?

A. Transverse fibers
B. Collateral ligaments
C. Sagittal bands
D. Oblique retinacular ligament

41. Which of the following is the anatomical term for the communications between the extensor tendons on the dorsum of the hand?

A. Sagittal bands
B. Lateral bands
C. Juncturae tendinea
D. Interosseous membrane

42. Which of the following are the primary receptors for tactile gnosis?

A. Merkel cells
B. Meissner cells
C. Pacinian corpuscles
D. Ruffini end-organ

43. Which is the first sensation to return after nerve repair?

A. Light touch
B. Pain and temperature
C. Deep pressure
D. Moving two-point discrimination

44. Which of the following is the classification for the least complicated nerve injury?

A. Neuronotmesis
B. Neuralgia
C. Neuropraxia
D. Neuroma

45. Which percentage of range of motion is lost with a radiocarpal fusion?

A. 12%
B. 27%
C. 55%
D. 80%

46. Which muscle is most commonly involved in a rotator cuff repair?

A. Subscapularis
B. Infraspinatus
C. Supraspinatus
D. Teres major

47. You are treating a patient with limited wrist extension. Which type of joint mobilization will help to increase wrist extension?

A. Volar glide
B. Dorsal glide
C. Radial glide
D. Ulnar glide

48. You are treating a burn patient who has blisters. The patient would be placed in which burn classification?

A. First-degree
B. Second-degree
C. Third-degree
D. Fourth-degree

49. You are treating a patient with ulnar nerve problems. You notice a positive Froment's sign. Which muscle is atrophied?

A. Abductor pollicis brevis
B. Adductor pollicis
C. Opponens pollicis
D. Flexor pollicis brevis

50. Which of the following carpal bones does not articulate with the lunate?

A. Trapezium
B. Triquetrum
C. Hamate
D. Capitate
E. Scaphoid

51. Which of the following tendons does not originate off of the ulna?

A. Extensor indicis proprius
B. Extensor pollicis longus
C. Flexor pollicis longus
D. Abductor pollicis longus

52. Gamekeeper's thumb refers to:

A. Radial collateral ligament injury of the thumb at the metacarpophalangeal joint
B. Fracture at the base of the thumb
C. Ulnar collateral ligament injury of the thumb at the metacarpophalangeal joint
D. Fracture at the radial styloid

53. A positive Terry Thomas sign on a radiograph is indicative of:

A. Scapholunate dissociation
B. Scaphoid fracture
C. Lunotriquetral tear
D. Triangular fibrocartilage complex tear

54. What is the name of the test that Dellon developed?

A. Two-point discrimination
B. Semmes-Weinstein
C. Moving two-point discrimination
D. Ninhydrin

55. A patient presents with hyperextension of the thumb metacarpophalangeal joint with lateral pinch after an ulnar nerve lesion. This hand posture can be termed:

A. Froment's sign
B. Duchenne's sign
C. Jeanne's sign
D. Wartenberg's sign

56. The patient described in the previous question presents with a flattened metacarpal arch. What is the name for this clinical presentation?

A. Froment's sign
B. Masse's sign
C. Duchenne's sign
D. Wartenberg's sign

57. Paraffin should be applied at which temperature?

A. 160° F to 170° F
B. 125° F to 135° F
C. 102° F to 104° F
D. 80° F to 90° F

58. Which of the following is an example of conductive-type heat?

A. Hot pack
B. Fluidotherapy
C. Whirlpool
D. All of the above are conductive types of heat

59. Which type of prosthesis is a Pillet prosthesis?

A. Myoelectric hand
B. Above-elbow prosthesis
C. Prosthesis for shoulder disarticulation
D. Aesthetic prosthesis

60. You are manual muscle testing a patient's biceps. The patient is able to achieve full range of motion against gravity. He is not able to tolerate any resistance. Which muscle grade is he?

A. Trace
B. Poor
C. Fair
D. Good
E. Normal

61. Which structures pass through the quadrangular space?

A. Median nerve and brachial artery
B. Ulnar nerve and brachial artery
C. Axillary nerve and posterior circumflex artery
D. Axillary nerve and anterior circumflex humeral artery

62. The rotator cuff comprises which muscles?

A. Supraspinatus, infraspinatus, subscapularis, and teres minor
B. Supraspinatus, subscapularis, teres major, and infraspinatus
C. Supraspinatus, infraspinatus, teres major, and latissimus dorsi
D. Teres minor, infraspinatus, subscapularis, and coracobrachialis

63. All of the following muscles insert into the greater tuberosity, except:

A. Supraspinatus
B. Infraspinatus
C. Teres minor
D. Subscapularis

64. The mobile wad of Henry is composed of all of the following muscles, except:

A. Brachioradialis
B. Extensor carpi radialis longus
C. Extensor digitorum communis
D. Extensor carpi radialis brevis

65. What is the normal "carrying angle" of the elbow in males?

A. 50 degrees valgus
B. 10 degrees valgus
C. 50 degrees varus
D. 10 degrees varus

66. You are treating a patient with a radial head fracture and a disruption of the distal radioulnar joint. What is this injury called?

A. Chauffeur's fracture
B. Monteggia's fracture
C. Bennett's fracture
D. Essex-Lopresti injury

67. What nerve is most commonly injured after elbow dislocation from valgus stress at the time of the dislocation?

A. Radial nerve
B. Median nerve
C. Ulnar nerve
D. None of the above

68. The tendon most frequently involved in lateral epicondylitis is the:

A. Extensor carpi radialis longus
B. Extensor carpi radialis brevis
C. Extensor digitorum communis
D. Extensor carpi ulnaris

69. A patient has sustained a severe injury to the elbow, and the surgeon has determined that fusion is the only option. In which position is the elbow usually fused to maximize function?

A. Flexed at 130°
B. Flexed at 90°
C. Flexed at 60°
D. Flexed at 30°

70. You are treating a patient who reports that he felt a "pop" in his shoulder while attempting to lift a bag of heavy groceries. You note a bulge in the anterior aspect of his right arm. What might have happened to this patient?

A. Rupture of the long head of the biceps
B. Rupture of the triceps
C. Distal humerus fracture
D. Proximal humerus fracture

71. You are treating a patient who displays winging of the scapula. Which nerve was injured?

A. Suprascapular
B. Subscapular
C. Long thoracic
D. Thoracodorsal

72. Which of the following is *not* a provocative test for thoracic outlet syndrome?

A. Adson's test
B. Allen's test
C. Wright's hyperabduction test
D. Costoclavicular maneuver

73. Which ligament(s) hold(s) the skin in place on the digit?

A. The oblique retinacular ligament
B. The transverse retinacular ligament
C. Cleland ligament
D. The collateral ligaments

74. When treating acute lateral epicondylitis, which of the following is recommended?

A. Wrist splint at 30° to 40° extension
B. Wrist splint with wrist at neutral
C. Wrist splint with wrist in slight flexion
D. No splint is indicated

75. In relation to sympathetic function, vasomotor refers to:

A. Skin color
B. Sweat
C. Gooseflesh response
D. Trophic nail changes

76. In reference to the Semmes-Weinstein monofilaments, monofilament number 3.22 correlates with:

A. Normal sensation
B. Diminished light touch
C. Diminished protective sensation
D. Loss of protective sensation

77. When fabricating a splint for a patient with ulnar nerve palsy, the therapist must take into consideration which of the following goals? The splint must:

A. Assist function of the thumb for tip prehension
B. Assist grasp by providing a stable wrist in extension
C. Prevent clawing and assist in grasp and release
D. Prevent overstretch of the wrist extensors

78. When performing manual muscle testing for the extensor digitorum communis, it is necessary to:

A. Position the forearm in pronation with wrist stabilized and ask the patient to extend the metacarpophalangeal joints with the interphalangeal joints flexed.
B. Have the forearm supinated and wrist stabilized and ask the patient to extend the metacarpophalangeal joints with the interphalangeal joints extended.
C. Have the forearm in neutral and the wrist stabilized and ask the patient to extend the metacarpophalangeal joints with the interphalangeal joints extended.
D. Have the forearm pronated and the wrist stabilized and ask the patient to extend the index finger while all other fingers are flexed.

79. According to the Clinical Assessment Committee of the American Society for Surgery of the Hand, when testing grip strength using the Jamar dynamometer, which handle position is recommended?

A. Position 1
B. Position 2
C. Position 3
D. Position 4
E. Position 5

80. In reference to extensor tendons, zone IV correlates with which anatomical structure of the hand?

A. Fingernail
B. Proximal phalanx
C. Sagittal band
D. Metacarpophalangeal joint

81. In reference to functional electrical stimulation, amplitude refers to:

A. Duration of treatment
B. Intensity
C. Duty cycle
D. Frequency

82. In relation to the muscle and nerve fibers in the strength duration curve, which of the following is true?:

A. Muscle fibers require low-intensity, short-duration current and nerve fibers require long-duration, high-intensity current before response.
B. Nerve fibers require low-intensity, short-duration current and muscle fibers require long-duration, high-intensity current before response.
C. Nerve fibers require long-duration, low-intensity current and muscle fibers require short-duration, high-intensity current before response.
D. Nerve and muscle tissues respond in an equal manner to elicit a response.

83. When treating a patient who has a proximal phalanx fracture with stable internal fixation, active and passive range-of-motion exercises should be initiated:

A. Between 1 and 3 days after surgery
B. 1 week after surgery
C. 3 to 4 weeks after surgery
D. 6 weeks after surgery

84. A 26-year-old male sustained a crush injury to the distal interphalangeal joint 3 months ago. The patient has difficulty performing prehension tasks primarily because of hypersensitivity. However, his occupation requires prehension tasks. The patient's insurance allows only one visit for hand rehabilitation. What should be done?

A. A Stax splint should be provided to protect the distal interphalangeal joint.
B. The patient should be instructed to wear latex gloves to decrease the irritation of the distal interphalangeal joint.
C. The patient should be given a transcutaneous electrical nerve stimulation unit.
D. The patient should be taught desensitization techniques.

85. In relation to ergonomic management, the recommended handle length for a hand-held tool is:

A. 4 cm
B. 9 cm
C. 11 cm
D. 15 cm

86. A complication that may occur after a distal radius fracture is:

A. Extensor pollicis longus rupture
B. Radial nerve compression
C. Median nerve compression
D. A and C are correct
E. B and C are correct

87. Which of the following are the two most important pulley structures in the finger?

A. A1 and A3
B. A3 and A5
C. A2 and A5
D. A2 and A4

88. What is the most common carpal coalition?

A. Scaphoid-triquetrum
B. Lunate-triquetrum
C. Hamate-triquetrum
D. Scaphoid-hamate

89. Which of the following does not serve as a border for the anatomic snuffbox?

A. Abductor pollicis longus
B. Extensor pollicis brevis
C. Extensor pollicis longus
D. Abductor pollicis brevis

90. Which of the following is not true about a myoelectric prosthesis?

A. It is considered a body-powered prosthesis.
B. It does not require a body harness.
C. It is powered by the amplified action potentials of underlying muscles.
D. It has no sensory feedback.

91. A patient presents to the clinic with a zone-IV flexor tendon laceration. Where is this zone?

A. Within the carpal tunnel
B. Proximal to the carpal tunnel
C. Within the fibro-osseous canal
D. At the level of palm

92. You are treating a patient in the clinic who has greater passive distal interphalangeal joint flexion with the proximal interphalangeal joint flexed than with it extended. Which structure is involved?

A. Sagittal band
B. Lateral band
C. Oblique retinacular ligament
D. Flexor digitorum profundus

93. Which of the following is considered the most severe form of nerve injury?

A. Neuropraxia
B. Neurotmesis
C. Axonotmesis
D. Wallerian degeneration

94. Which of the following is the most common ganglion to develop in the hand and the wrist?

A. Volar wrist ganglion
B. Mucus cyst
C. Dorsal wrist ganglion
D. Squamous-cell carcinoma

95. Which of the following is not true about the management of a patient with frostbite?

A. The frozen extremity should be allowed to rewarm at room temperature.
B. The patient's core body temperature should be restored with external warming and ingestion of warm fluids by mouth.
C. The frozen extremity should be rewarmed rapidly at 40° C to 44° C
D. All of the above are true statements

96. Which angle of pull is recommended when using dynamic splinting?

A. 30-degree angle
B. 60-degree angle
C. 90-degree angle
D. 120-degree angle

97. Where is Lister's tubercle located?

A. Distal ulna
B. Proximal ulna
C. Proximal radius
D. Distal radius

98. You are treating a patient with a proximal interphalangeal joint contracture of the middle finger. Which mobilization technique will help to increase extension?

A. Volar glide
B. Dorsal glide
C. Radial glide
D. Ulnar glide

99. Which grade of movement is used when performing a small amplitude of movement at the beginning of the range of motion to treat a painful joint?

A. Grade I
B. Grade II
C. Grade III
D. Grade IV

100. According to Gelberman, which amount of tendon glide is needed to stimulate intrinsic healing at the repair site without creating significant gap formation?

A. 1 to 2 mm
B. 3 to 4 mm
C. 4 to 6 mm
D. 8 to 10 mm

Answer Key

1. A, 2. D, 3. B, 4. C, 5. A, 6. C, 7. A, 8. B, 9. E, 10. C, 11. B, 12. C,
13. C, 14. B, 15. C, 16. A, 17. B, 18. C, 19. D, 20. A, 21. B, 22. C, 23. C,
24. A, 25. B, 26. C, 27. A, 28. B, 29. D, 30. C, 31. C, 32. C, 33. A, 34. A,
35. C, 36. C, 37. D, 38. A, 39. A, 40. C, 41. C, 42. A, 43. B, 44. C, 45. C,
46. C, 47. A, 48. B, 49. B, 50. A, 51. C, 52. C, 53. A, 54. C, 55. C, 56. B,
57. B, 58. A, 59. D, 60. C, 61. C, 62. A, 63. D, 64. C, 65. B, 66. D, 67. C,
68. B, 69. B, 70. A, 71. C, 72. B, 73. C, 74. A, 75. A, 76. B, 77. C, 78. A,
79. B, 80. B, 81. B, 82. B, 83. A, 84. D, 85. B, 86. D, 87. D, 88. B, 89. D,
90. A, 91. A, 92. C, 93. B, 94. C, 95. A, 96. C, 97. D, 98. B, 99. A, 100. B

References

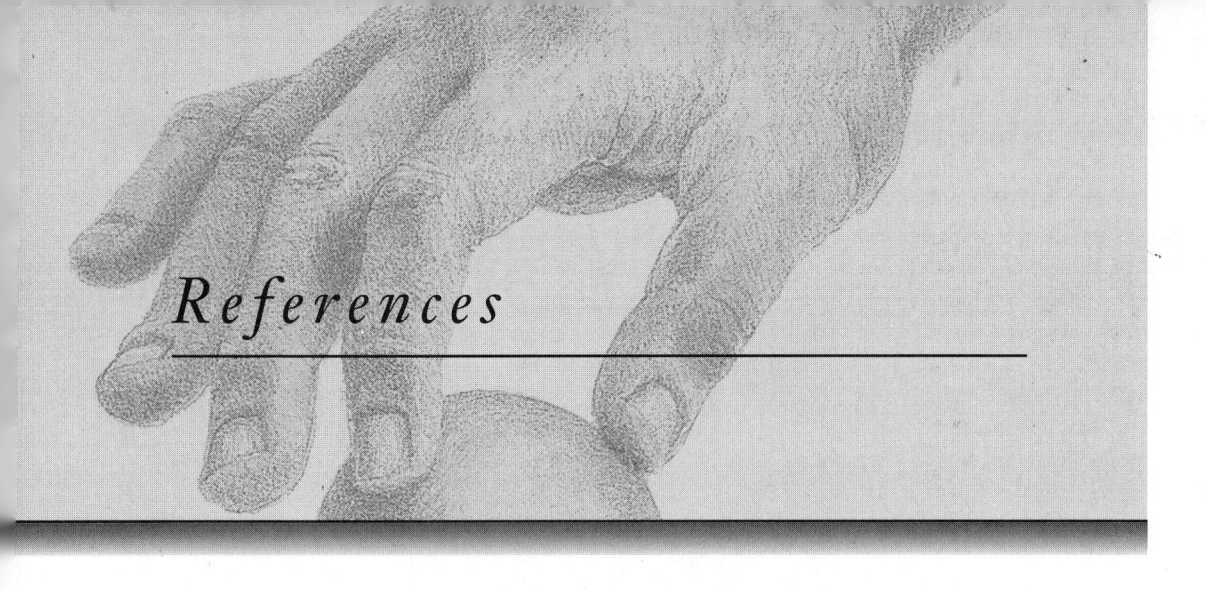

Ablove RH, Howell RM: The physiology and technique of skin grafting, *Hand Clin* 13:2, 1997.

Akelman E: Tumors of the hand and forearm, *Hand Clin* 11:2, 1995.

Almquist EE: Kienbock's disease, *Hand Clin* 3:1, 1987.

Alverez O, Rozint J, Wiseman D: Moist environment for healing: Matching the dressing to the wound, *Wound* 1:35, 1989.

American Medical Association: *Drug evaluation annual 1992*, Chicago, 1992.

American Society for Surgery of the Hand: *Hand surgery update*, Rosemont, Ill, 1996, American Academy of Orthopaedic Surgeons.

Anderson JE: *Grant's atlas of anatomy*, ed 8, Baltimore, 1983, Williams & Wilkins.

Arnheim D, Prentice W: *Principles of athletic training*, ed 8, St. Louis, 1993, Mosby.

Atkins DJ, Meier RH: *Comprehensive management of the upper-limb amputee*, New York, 1989, Springer-Verlag.

Aulicino P: Neurovascular injuries in the hands of athletes, *Hand Clin* 6:455, 1990.

Backhouse KM, Catton WT: An experimental study of the functions of the lumbrical muscles in the human hand, *J Anat* 88:133, 1954.

Balch Jr. JF, Balch P: *Prescription for nutritional healing*, ed 2, Garden City Park, NY, 1997, Avery Publishing Group.

Baratz ME, Divelbiss B: Skeletal fixation in the upper extremity, *Hand Clin* 13:4, 1997.

Barnes J: *Myofascial release* I, Presented Clearwater, Fla, January, 1996.

Basti J et al: Management of proximal humeral fractures, *J Hand Ther* 7:2, 1994.

Beasley RW: General considerations in managing upper-limb amputations, *Orthop Clin North Am* 12:743, 1981.

Bednar J, Osterman L: Carpal instability: evaluation and treatment, *J Am Acad Orthopedic Surg*, 1993.

Bell-Krotoski J: A study of peripheral nerve involvement underlying physical disability of the hand in Hansen's disease, *J Hand Ther* 5:3, 1992.

Berger R: The anatomy and basic biomechanics of the wrist joint, *J Hand Ther* 9:2, 1996.

Blair WF: *Techniques in hand surgery*, Baltimore, 1996, Williams & Wilkins.

Blank JE, Cassidy C: The distal radioulnar joint in rheumatoid arthritis, *Hand Clin* 12:93, 1996.

Bonutti PM et al: *Static progressive stretch to reestablish elbow range of motion, clinical ortopaedics, and related research*, Philadelphia, 1994, JB Lippincott.

Bowker JH, Michael JW: *Atlas of limb prosthetics: Surgical, prosthetic, and rehabilitation principles*, St. Louis, 1992, Mosby.

Brand PW, Hollister A: *Clinical mechanics of the hand*, ed 2, St. Louis, 1993, Mosby.

Brandt KD: *Diagnosis and nonsurgical management of osteoarthritis*, 1996, Professional Communications, Inc.

Brecker L: Jenny McConnell offers new techniques for problem shoulders, *Advance for Physical Therapists* December, 1993.

Brennwald J: Bone healing in the hand, *Clin Orthop* 2:4, 1987.

Brotzman SB: *Clinical orthopaedic rehabilitation*, St. Louis, 1996, Mosby.

Browner BD et al: *Skeletal trauma*, Philadelphia, 1992, WB Saunders.

Burton R, Pellegrini V: Surgical management of basal joint arthritis of the thumb. Part two: ligament reconstruction with a tendon interposition arthroplasty, *J Hand Surg*, 11A:3, 1986.

Butler DS: *Mobilization of the nervous system*, New York, 1991, Churchill Livingstone.

Calliet R: *Shoulder pain*, ed 3, Philadelphia, 1991, F.A. Davis Company.

Carlson L, Watson K: Treatment of reflex sympathetic dystrophy using the stress-loading program, *J Hand Ther*, 1988.

Carroll R: Acute calcium deposits in the hand, *JAMA*, 157:422, 1995.

Casanova JS, editor: *Clinical assessment recommendations*, ed 2, Chicago, 1992, American Society of Hand Therapists.

Centers for Disease Control (CDC), Atlanta, Ga.

Clark GC et al, editors: *Hand rehabilitation*, ed 2, New York, 1996, Churchill Livingstone.

Clayton T: *Taber's cyclopedic medical dictionary*, ed 17, Philadelphia, 1993, F.A. Davis Company.

Coe M, Trumble T: Biomechanical comparison of methods used to treat Kienbock's disease, *Hand Clin* 9:3, 1993.

Cohen M: Fractures of the carpal bones, skeletal fixation in the upper extremity, *Hand Clin* 13:4, 1997.

Conrad III EU, Enneking WF: *Clinical symposia: common soft tissue tumors*, 42, #1, Ciba-Geigy, New York, 1990.

Cooney WP, Linscheid RL, Dobyns JH: *The wrist: diagnosis and operative treatment*, St. Louis, 1998, Mosby.

Coppard BM, Lohman H: *Introduction to splinting: a critical thinking and problem-solving approach*, St. Louis, 1996, Mosby.

Crossland M: *Overview of chronic wound healing problems*, presented at 17th annual meeting ASHT, September, 1994, Washington, DC.

Cyriax J: Diagnosis of soft tissue lesions, *Textbook of orthopedic medicine*, ed 8, London, 1982, Bailliere Tindall.

Day HJB: *The ISO/ISPO classification of congenital limb deficiency*. In Bowker JH, Michael JW, editors: *Atlas of limb prosthetics: surgical, prosthetic, and rehabilitation principles*, St. Louis, 1992, Mosby.

DeLee J, Drey D: *Orthopaedic sports medicine*, Philadelphia, 1994, WB Saunders.

Dellon AL: *Evaluation of sensibility and re-education of sensation in the hand*, Baltimore, 1981, Williams & Wilkins.

Dellon AL: *Somatosensory testing and rehabilitation*, Bethesda, Md, 1997, American Occupational Therapy Association, Inc.

Diao E: Skeletal fixation in the upper extremity: Metacarpal fixation, *Hand Clin* 13:4, 1997.

Dictionary of titles, ed 4, revised 1991, U.S. Government Printing Office.

Donatelli R: Clinics in physical therapy: *Physical therapy of the shoulder*, ed 2, NY, 1991, Churchill Livingstone.

Dorland's medical dictionary, ed 24, Philadelphia, 1965, WB Saunders.

Duda-Huys S: *Joint mobilization: Hand therapy course review-study guide*, Atlanta, 1990.

Dumitru D: Reflex sympathetic dystrophy, *Physical Medicine and Rehab State-of-the-Arts Review* 5:1, 1991.

Eaton R, Malerich M: The volar plate arthoplasty in the proximal phalangeal joint: a review of ten years' experience, *J Hand Surg* 5:60, 1980.

Ejeskar A: Finger flexion force and hand grip strength after tendon repair, *J Hand Surg* 9:4, 1982.

Engkvist O, Lundburg G: Rupture of the extensor pollicis longus tendon after fracture of the lower end of the radius: a clinical and microangiographic study, *Hand Clin* 11:76, 1979.

Esquenazi A, Meier RH: Rehabilitation in limb deficiency: 4-limb amputation, *Arch Phys Med Rehabil* 77:3, 1996.

Evans R: Natalie Barr lecture, *J Hand Ther* 10:1, 1997.

Evans R, Thompson DE: The application of force to healing tendons, *J Hand Ther*, 6:4, 1993.

Falkenberg S, Schultz D: Ergonomics for the upper extremity: Occupational diseases of the hand, *Hand Clin* 9:2, 1993.

Federal Register, Department of Labor, Part II, Occupational Safety and Health Administration, December, 1991.

Fess E, Philips CA: *Hand splinting: principles and methods*, ed 2, St. Louis, 1987, Mosby.

Flatow EL, editor: *Orthop Clin North Am* 28:2, 1997.

Florida Administrative Code Biomedical Waste, Chapter 64, June, 1997.

Floyd W, Troom J: Tumors of the hand and forearm, *Hand Clin* 11:2, 1995.

Freeland A, Jabaley ME, Hughes JL: *Stable fixation of the hand and wrist*, New York, 1986, Springer-Verlag.

Frymoyer KW: Orthopedic Knowledge Update 4, 1993.

Giannakopoulos PN et al: Tumors of the hand and forearm, *Hand Clin* 11:2, 1995.

Gilberman KH: *Operative nerve repair and reconstruction*, Philadelphia, 1991, JB Lippincott.

Giurintano DJ: Basic biomechanics, *J Hand Ther* 8:2, 1995.

Green DP: *Operative hand surgery*, ed 3, New York, 1993, Churchill Livingstone.

Greenfield B, Syen D: *Brachial plexus lesions: physical therapy of the shoulder*. In *Clinics in physical therapy*, ed 2, NY, 1991, Churchill Livingstone.

Grothe G: The impact of compliance on rehabilitation of patients with mallet finger, *J Hand Ther* 7:1, 1994.

Hardy SGP, Hardy MA: Reflex sympathetic dystrophy: the clinician's perspective, *J Hand Ther* 10:2, 1997.

Hareau J: What makes treatment for reflex sympathetic dystrophy successful? *J Hand Ther* 9:4, 1996.

Hastings H, Ernest J: Dynamic external fixation for fractures of the proximal interphalangeal joint, *Hand Clin* 9:4, 1993.

Hastings II H, Graham JJ: The classification and treatment of heterotopic ossification about the elbow and forearm, *Hand Clin*, 10:3, 1994.

Hawkins R, Bell R, Lippitt S: *Atlas of shoulder surgery*, St. Louis, 1996, Mosby.

Hayes K: *Manual for physical agents*, ed 4, Stanford, Conn, 1993, Appleton & Lange.

Hecox B, Mehreteab TA, Weisberg J: *Physical agents: a comprehensive text for physical therapists*, Stanford, Conn, 1994, Appleton & Lange.

Herndon DN: *Total burn care*, Philadelphia, 1996, WB Saunders.

Hodges PL: *Surgical flaps*. In *Selected readings in plastic surgery*, Waco, Tex, 1992, Baylor University Medical Center.

Holderman V: Principles of splinting. Presented for Hand Therapy Review Course, Chicago, 1992.

Hopkins H, Smith H, editors: *Willard and Spackman's occupational therapy*, ed 7, Philadelphia, 1988, JB Lippincott.

Hoppenfeld S: *Physical examination of the spine and extremities*, Norwalk, Conn, 1976, Appleton-Century-Crofts.

Hoppenfeld S, de Boer P: *Surgical exposures in orthopedics: the anatomic approach*, Philadelphia, 1994, JB Lippincott.

Howard FM: Compression neuropathies in the anterior forearm, *Hand Clin* 2:4, 1986.

Hunter J, Mackin E, Callahan A: *Rehabilitation of the hand: surgery and therapy*, ed 4, St. Louis, 1995, Mosby.

Hunter JM, Schneider LH, Mackin EJ: *Tendon and nerve surgery in the hand: a third decade*, St. Louis, 1997, Mosby.

Idler R: General principles of patient evaluation in nonoperative management of cubital syndrome, *Hand Clin* 12:2, 1996.

Jacobson MD et al: Architectural design of the intrinsic hand, *J Hand Surg* 17:804, 1992.

Jaffe R, Chidgery L, LaStayo P: The distal radioulnar joint: anatomy and management of disorders, *J Hand Ther* 9:2, 1996.

Jain S: Rehabilitation in limb deficiency. 2: The pediatric amputee, *Arch Phys Med Rehabil* 77:3, 1996.

Johnson S: Ergonomic hand tool design, *Hand Clin* 9:—, 1993.

Jones B, Stern P: *Hand Clin*ics: Interphalangeal joint arthrodesis, *Hand Clin* 10:2, 1994.

Kandel ER, Schwartz JH: *Principles of neuroscience*, ed 2, New York, 1985, Elsevier.

Kasdan ML: *Occupational hand injuries*. In *Occupational medicine: state-of-the-art reviews*, Philadelphia, 1989, Hanley & Belfus.

Kimura J: Principles and pitfalls of nerve conduction studies, *Ann Neurol* 16:418, 1984.

King II T: The effect of water temperature on hand volume during volumetric measurement using the water displacement method, *J Hand Ther* 6:202, 1993.

Kisner C, Colby L: *Therapeutic exercise: Peripheral joint mobilization*, Philadelphia, 1985, F.A. Davis Company.

Kleiman WB: American society for surgery of the hand, 17:3, 1989.

Kleinert H: Flexor tendon injuries, *Surg Clin North Am* 61:2, 1981.

Knapp, Rebecca Grant: *Basic statistics for nurses*, ed 2, New York, 1985, John Wiley & Sons.

Laseter GE, Carter PR: Management of distal radius fractures, *J Hand Ther* 9:2, 1996.

Lee S: The use of modalities within the framework of occupational therapy. Presented March, 1995, Ft. Lauderdale, Fla.

Leibozic SJ: Internal fixation for small joint arthrodesis in the hand and the interphalangeal joints, *Hand Clin* 13:2, 1997.

Lennard T et al: *Physiatric procedures in clinical practice*, Philadelphia, 1995, Hanley & Belfus.

Lichtman DM: The distal radial ulnar joint. In *The wrist and its disorders*, Philadelphia, 1988, WB Saunders.

Light T, Bednar M: Management of intraarticular fractures of the metacarpophalangeal joint, *Hand Clin* 10:2, 1994.

Lister G: *The hand: diagnosis and indication*, London, New York, 1984, Churchill Livingstone.

Loth T, Wadsworth C: *Orthopaedic review for physical therapists*, St. Louis, 1998, Mosby.

Ludlow KS, Cox JA, Hurst L: Pillar pain as a postoperative complication of carpal tunnel release: A review of the literature, *J Hand Ther* 10:4, 1997.

van der Laan L, Goris RJA: Reflex sympathetic dystrophy: an exaggerated regional inflammatory response, *Hand Clin* 13:3, 1997.

Maddy L, Meyerdierks E: Dynamic extension assist splints of acute central slip lacerations, *J Hand Ther* 10:3, 1997.

Magee D: *Orthopedic physical assessment*, ed 2, Philadelphia, 1992, WB Saunders.

Malick MH, Kasch M: *Manual of management of specific hand problems*, Pittsburgh, 1984, AREN Publishing.

Malick MH: *Manual on static splinting*, ed 3, Pittsburgh, 1985, AREN Publishing.

Malone JM, Fleming LL, Robertson J: Immediate, early, and late postsurgical management of upper-limb amputation, *J Rehabil Res* 21:1, 1984.

Malone TR, McPoil TG, Nitz AJ: *Orthopaedics and sports physical therapy*, ed 3, Philadelphia, 1997, Mosby.

Markinson R: Tendinitis and related inflammatory conditions seen in musicians, *J Hand Ther* 5:2, 1992.

Marks P, Warner J, Irrgang J: rotator cuff disorders of the shoulder, *J Hand Ther* 7:2, 1994.

McCollister EC: *Surgery of the musculoskeletal system*, ed 2, New York, 1990, Churchill Livingstone.

McCulloch JM, Kloth L, Feedar J: *Wound healing alternatives in management*, ed 2, Philadelphia, 1995, F.A. Davis Company.

McFarlane R: Dupuytren's disease, invitational lecture, ASHT 19th annual meeting, *J Hand Ther* 10:1, 1997.

Meredith JM: Comparison of three myoelectrically controlled prehensors and the voluntary-opening split hook, *Am J Occup Ther* 48:10, 1994.

Meyer T: *Review book for physical therapy licensing exam*, vol 1 & 2, 1997, Midwest Hi-Tech Publishers.

Meyerdierks E, Werner F: Limited wrist arthrodesis: a laboratory study article, *J Hand Surg* 12:4, 1987.

Michlovitz SL: *Thermal agents in rehabilitation*, ed 3, Philadelphia, 1996, F.A. Davis Company.

Miles W: Soft tissue trauma, *Hand Clin* 2:1, 1986.

Milford L: *Tumors and tumorous conditions of the hand*. In *The hand*, St. Louis, 1988, Mosby.

Millender LH, Louis DS, Simmons BP: *Occupational disorders of the upper extremity*, New York, 1992, Churchill Livingstone.

Moberg E: Nerve repair in hand surgery: an analysis, *Surg Clin North Am* 48:985, 1968.

Mosby's medical nursing and allied health dictionary, ed 4, St. Louis, 1994, Mosby.

Murphy LD: Joint Mobilization, ASHT - A Comprehensive Review of Hand Therapy, June, 1995.

Nalebuff E: Surgery of psoriatic arthritis of the hand, *Hand Clin* 12:3, 1996.

Nelson C, Sawmiller S, Phalen G: Ganglions of the wrist and hand, *J Bone Joint Surg Am* 54:A, 1972.

Netter FH: *Anatomy, physiology, and metabolic disorders.* In *The Ciba collection of medical illustration*, vol 8, Musculoskeletal System, West Caldwell, NJ, 1987-1991, Ciba-Geigy Corp.

Norkin C, White DJ: *Measurement of joint motion: a guide to goniometry*, Philadelphia, 1995, F.A. Davis Company.

Norris C: *Sports injuries: diagnosis and management for physiotherapists*, Oxford, 1993, Butterworth-Heineman Ltd.

Oates SD, Daley RA: Thoracic outlet syndrome, *Hand Clin* 12:4, 1996.

Orenstein HH: Hand I: fingernails and soft tissue trauma: infections, tumors and reconstruction. In *Selected reading in plastic surgery*, vol 6, Waco, Tex, 1992, Baylor University Medical Center.

Palmer AK: Triangular fibrocartilage disorders: injury patterns and treatment *Arthroscopy* 6:125, 1990.

Pascarelli E, Quilter D: *Repetitive strain injury: a computer user's guide*, New York, 1994, John Wiley & Sons.

Pedretti LW: *Occupational therapy practice skills for physical dysfunction*, ed 4, St. Louis, 1996, Mosby.

Peimer CA, editor: *Surgery of the hand and upper extremity*, New York, 1996, McGraw-Hill.

Peterson MS: *Eat to complete: A guide to sport nutrition*, ed 2, St. Louis, 1996, Mosby.

Pettrone FA: *Athletic injuries of the shoulder*, New York, 1995, McGraw-Hill.

Physician assistants' prescribing reference, New York, 1997, New York Prescribing Reference, Inc.

Physicians' desk reference, ed 52, Montvale, NJ, 1998, Medical Economics Company, Inc.

Plancher KD: Carpal and cubital tunnel surgery, *Hand Clin* 12:2, 1996.

Portney LG, Watkins MP: *Foundations of clinical research: applications to practice*, Stanford, Conn, 1993, Appleton & Lange.

Prasartritha T, Liupolvanish P, Rojanakit A: A study of the posterior interosseous nerve and the radial tunnel in thirty Thai cadavers, *J Hand Surg* 18:1, 1993.

Pratt N: Anatomy and biomechanics of the shoulder, *J Hand Ther*, 7:2, 1994.

Prosser R, Conolly WB: Complication following surgical treatment for Dupuytren's contracture, *J Hand Ther* 9:4, 1996.

Prosser R, Herbert T: The management of carpal fractures and dislocations, *J Hand Ther* 9:2, 1996.

Putz-Anderson V: *Cumulative trauma disorders: a manual for musculoskeletal disease of the upper extremity*, New York, 1988, Taylor & Francis.

Ranney D: *Chronic musculoskeletal injuries in the workplace*, Philadelphia, 1977, WB Saunders.

Raemon JP: Étude pathogénique de la maladie de Kienböck, *Ann Chir Main* 1:240, 1982.

Rayhack JM: The history and evolution of percutaneous pinning of displaced distal radius fractures. *Orthop Clin North Am* 24:2, 1993.

Reagan DS, Linscheid RL, Dobyns JH: Lunotriquetral sprains *J Hand Surg* 9A:502, 1984.

Reiner M, Lohman W: *Medical management program for cumulative trauma disorders of the upper-extremity*, St. Paul, 1992, Hand Rehab, Inc.

Richards R, Staley M: *Burn care and rehabilitation principles and practice*, Philadelphia, 1994, F.A. Davis Company.

Rockwood Jr CA, Green DP: *Fractures in adults*, ed 2, Philadelphia, 1984, JB Lippincott.

Rockwood C, Matsen F: *The shoulder*, vols 1 and 2, Philadelphia, 1990, WB Saunders.

Ryu J et al (Mayo Clinic Group): Functional ranges of motion of the wrist joint, *J Hand Surg* 16:3, 1991.

Sailer SM: The role of splints in rehabilitation in the treatment of carpal and cubital syndrome, *Hand Clin* 12:2, 1996.

Saunders HD: *Evaluation, treatment and prevention of musculoskeletal disorders*, 1985, Viking Press.

Schenck R: Intraarticular fractures of the phalanges, *Hand Clin* 10:2, 1994.

Schneider LH: Fractures of the distal interphalangeal joint, *Hand Clin* 10:2, 1994.

Schreuders TAR, Stam HJ: Strength measurements of lumbrical muscles, *J Hand Ther* 9:4, 1996.

Sears HH: Approaches to prescription of bodypowered and myoelectric prosthesis, *Phys Med Rehabil Clin North Am* 2:2, 1991.

Sieg K, Adams SP: *Illustrated essentials of musculoskeletal anatomy*, ed 2, Gainsville, Fla, 1985, Megabooks.

Silver Ring Splint Company Catalog, Charlottesville, Va, 1994.

Simmons BP, Mckenzie: Symptomatic carpal coalition, *J Hand Surg* 10:1A, 1985.

Skirven T: Therapy post wrist arthroscopy, American Society of Hand Therapists, A Comprehensive Approach to Challenging Wrist Problems, Chicago, April, 1995.

Smith JW, Aston SJ: *Grabb and Smith's plastic surgery*, ed 4, Boston, 1991, Little, Brown and Company.

Sneider S (guest editor), Karzel R: Evaluation and treatment of the rotator cuff, *Orthop Clin North Am* 24:1, 1993.

Spiegel SR: *Adult myoelectric upper-limb prosthetic training.* In Atkins DJ, Meier RH, editors: *Comprehensive management of the upper-limb amputee*, New York, 1989, Springer-Verlag.

Spinner M: *Kaplan's functional and surgical anatomy of the hand*, ed 3, Philadelphia, 1984, JB Lippincott.

Stanley B, Tribuzi S: *Concepts in hand rehabilitation*, Philadelphia, 1992, F.A. Davis Company.

Stirrat CR: Rheumatoid arthritis of the hand and wrist: Metacarpophalangeal joint and rheumatoid arthritis of the hand, *Hand Clin*, 12:3, 1996.

Strickland J: Biologic rationale, clinical application, and results of early motion following flexor tendon repair, *J Hand Ther*, 1989.

Strickland J: Flexor tendon injuries: a scientific rationale for management. Presented at Hand Care '96, Indianapolis, Ind, 1996.

Swanson AB: Congenital limb defects classification & treatment, Clinical Symposia, 33:3, CIBA, 1981.

Taleisnik J: *The wrist*, New York, 1985, Churchill Livingstone.

Thomas D, Moutet F, Guinard D: Postoperative management of extensor tendon repairs in zone V, VI, & VII, *J Hand Ther* 4:9, 1996.

Thomes L, Thomes B: Early mobilization method of surgically repaired Zone III extensor tendons, *J Hand Ther* 8:3, 1995.

Thorson EP, Szabo R: *Tendonitis of the wrist and elbow in occupational hand injuries*. In Kosdan M, editor: *Occupational medicine*, vol 4, Philadelphia, 1989, Hanley & Belfus.

Travell JG, Simons DG: *Myofascial pain and dysfunction: the trigger point manual*, Baltimore, 1983, Williams & Wilkins.

Trombly CA: *Occupational therapy for physical dysfunction*, ed 4, Baltimore, 1995, Williams & Wilkins.

Tubiana R, Thomine JM, Mackin E: *Examination of the hand and wrist*, London, 1996, Martin Dunitz, Ltd.

Vasudevan SV, Melvin JL: Upper-extremity edema control: rationale of the techniques, *Am J Occup Ther* 33:8, 1979.

Walsh M: Therapist management of thoracic outlet syndrome, *J Hand Ther* 7:2, 1994.

Walters KJ: Understanding intrinsic and extrinsic tendon tightness and how to correct the problem. Presented at Indiana Hand Care, Indianapolis, Indiana, 1996.

Warner JJP: *J Am Acad Orthopedic Surgeons* 5:3, 1997.

Warwick L, Seradge H: Early versus later range of motion following cubital tunnel surgery, *J Hand Ther*, 8:245, 1995.

Watson H, Goodman M, Johnson T: Limited wrist arthrodesis, part two: intercarpal and radiocarpal combinations, *J Hand Surg*, 1981.

Wehbe MA: Tendon gliding exercise, *Am J Occup Ther* 41:3, 1987.

Werner F, An K: Biomechanics of the elbow and forearm difficulty: Disorders of the elbow and forearm, *Hand Clin* 10:3, 1994.

Westra V: OSHA and the proposed ergonomic standard. Presented at the Applied Ergonomics Professional Residency Program, Orlando, Fla, 1994.

Wiedrich T: A Comprehensive Approach to Challenging Wrist Problems, ASHT Continuing Education, Chicago, April, 1995.

Wilder RT et al: Reflex sympathetic dystrophy in children: clinical characteristics and follow-up of 70 patients, *J Bone Joint Surg* 74:6, 1992.

Wong GY, Wilson PR: Classification of complex and regional pain syndrome: new concepts, *Hand Clin* 3:3, 1997.

Wright T, Michlovitz S: Management of carpal instabilities, *J Hand Ther* 9:2, 1996.

Wyalett-Rendall J: Sensibility evaluation and rehabilitation *Orthop Clin North Am* 19:43, 1988.

Yaremchuk MJ: Plastic surgery inservice exam: Hand and extremities.